AF352191

RN TO
MOOR
ES LIB

LATES

FUNCTIONAL ASPECTS OF THE NORMAL, HYPERTROPHIED, AND FAILING HEART

DEVELOPMENTS IN CARDIOVASCULAR MEDICINE

Lancée, C.T., ed.: Echocardiology, 1979. ISBN 90–247–2209–8.
Baan, J., Arntzenius, A.C., Yellin, E.L., eds.: Cardiac dynamics. 1980. ISBN 90–247–2212–8.
Thalen, H.J.T., Meere, C.C., eds.: Fundamentals of cardiac pacing. 1970. ISBN 90–247–2245–4.
Kulbertus, H.E., Wellens, H.J.J., eds.: Sudden death. 1980. ISBN 90–247–2290–X.
Dreifus, L.S., Brest, A.N., eds.: Clinical applications of cardiovascular drugs. 1980. ISBN 90–247–2295–0.
Spencer, M.P., Reid, J.M., eds.: Cerebrovascular evaluation with Doppler ultrasound. 1981. ISBN 90–247–2348–1.
Zipes, D.P., Bailey, J.C., Elharrar, V., eds.: The slow inward current and cardiac arrhythmias. 1980. ISBN 90–247–2380–9.
Kesteloot, H., Joossens, J.V., eds.: Epidemiology of arterial blood pressure. 1980. ISBN 90–247–2386–8.
Wackers, F.J.T., ed.: Thallium-201 and technetium-99m-pyrophosphate myocardial imaging in the coronary care unit. 1980. ISBN 90–247–2396–5.
Maseri, A., Marchesi, C., Chierchia, S., Trivella, M.G., eds.: Coronary care units. 1981. ISBN 90–247–2456–2.
Morganroth, J., Moore, E.N., Dreifus, L.S., Michelson, E.L., eds.: The evaluation of new antiarrhythmic drugs. 1981. ISBN 90–247–2474–0.
Alboni, P.: Intraventricular conduction disturbances. 1981. ISBN 90–247–2483–X.
Rijsterborgh, H., ed.: Echocardiology. 1981. ISBN 90–247–2491–0.
Wagner, G.S., ed.: Myocardial infarction. Measurement and intervention. 1982. ISBN 90–247–2513–5.
Meltzer, R.S., Roelandt, J., eds.: Contrast echocardiography. 1982. ISBN 90–247–2531–3.
Amery, A., Fagard, R., Lijnen, R., Staessen, J., eds.: Hypertensive cardiovascular disease; pathophysiology and treatment. 1982. ISBN 90–247–2534–8.
Bouman, L.N., Jongsma, H.J., eds.: Cardiac rate and rhythm. 1982. ISBN 90–247–2626–3.
Morganroth, J., Moore, E.M., eds.: The evaluation of beta blocker and calcium antagonist drugs. 1982. ISBN 90–247–2642–5.
Rosenbaum, M.B., ed.: Frontiers of cardiac electrophysiology. 1982. ISBN 90–247–2663–8.
Roelandt, J., Hugenholtz, P.G., eds.: Long-term ambulatory electrocardiography. 1982. ISBN 90–247–2664–8.
Adgey, A.J., ed.: Acute phase of ischemic heart disease and myocardial infarction. 1982. ISBN 90–247–2675–1.
Hanrath, P., Bleifeld, W., Souquet, eds.: Cardiovascular diagnosis by ultrasound. Transesophageal, computerized, contrast, Doppler echocardiography. 1982. ISBN 90–247–2692–1.
Roelandt, J., ed.: The practice of M-mode and two-dimensional echocardiography. 1983. ISBN 90–247–2745–6.
Meyer, J., Schweizer, P., Erbel, R., eds.: Advances in noninvasive cardiology. 1983. ISBN 0–89838–576–8.
Morganroth, Joel, Moore, E.N., eds.: Sudden cardiac death and congestive heart failure: Diagnosis and treatment. 1983. ISBN 0–89838–580–6.
Perry, H.M., ed.: Lifelong management of hypertension. ISBN 0–89838–582–2.
Jaffe, E.A., ed.: Biology of endothelial cells. ISBN 0–89838–587–3.
Surawicz, B., Reddy, C.P., Prystowsky, E.N., eds.: Tachycardiac. 1984. ISBN 0–89838–588–1.
Spencer, M.P., ed.: Cardiac Doppler diagnosis. ISBN 0–89838–591–1.
Villareal, H.V., Sambhi, M.P., eds.: Topics in pathophysiology of hypertension. ISBN 0–89838–595–4.
Messerli, F.H., ed.: Cardiovascular disease in the elderly. 1984. ISBN 0–89838–596–2.
Simoons, M.L., Reiber, J.H.C., eds.: Nuclear imaging in clinical cardiology. ISBN 0–89838–599–7.
Ter Keurs, H.E.D.J., Schipperheym, J.J., eds.: Cardiac left ventricular hypertrophy. ISBN 0–89838–612–8.
Sperelakis, N., ed.: Physiology and pathophysiology of the heart. ISBN 0–89838–615–2.
Messerli, F.H., ed.: Kidney in essential hypertension. 1983. ISBN 0–89838–616–0.
Sambhi, M.P., ed.: Fundamental fault in hypertension. ISBN 0–89838–638–1.
Marchesi, D., ed.: Ambulatory monitoring: Cardiovascular system and allied applications. ISBN 0–89838–642–X.
Kupper, W., Macalpin, R.N., Bleifeld, W., eds.: Coronary tone in ischemic heart disease. ISBN 0–89838–646–2.
Sperelakis, N., Caulfield, J.B., eds.: Calcium antagonists: Mechanisms of action on cardiac muscle and vascular smooth muscle. ISBN 0–89838–655–1.
Godfraind, T., Herman, A.S., Wellens, D., eds.: Entry blockers in cardiovascular and cerebral dysfunctions. ISBN 0–89838–658–6.
Morganroth, J., Moore, E.N., eds.: Interventions in the acute phase of myocardial infarction. ISBN 0–89838–659–4.

FUNCTIONAL ASPECTS OF THE NORMAL, HYPERTROPHIED, AND FAILING HEART

edited by

FRANCIS L. ABEL, M.D., Ph.D.
Professor and Chairman
Department of Physiology
University of South Carolina
  School of Medicine
Columbia, South Carolina

and

WALTER H. NEWMAN, Ph.D.
Professor of Pharmacology
Medical University of South Carolina
Charleston, South Carolina

Martinus Nijhoff Publishing
A member of the Kluwer Academic Publishers Group
Boston/The Hague/Dordrecht/Lancaster

Distributors for North America:
Kluwer Academic Publishers
190 Old Derby Street
Hingham, MA 02043

for all other countries
Kluwer Academic Publishers Group
Distribution Centre
P.O. Box 322
3300 AH Dordrecht
The Netherlands

QP
111
.2
.F86
1983

Library of Congress Cataloging in Publication Data

International Society for Heart Research. American
   Section. Meeting (5th : 1983 : Hilton Head, S.C.)
   Functional aspects of the normal, hypertrophied, and
failing heart.

   (Developments in cardiovascular medicine)
   Includes bibliographical references.
   1. Heart--Congresses. 2. Coronary arteries--Congres-
ses. 3. Heart--Hypertrophy--Congresses. 4. Heart
failure--Congresses. I. Abel, Francis L., 1931-   .
II. Newman, Walter H. III. Title. IV. Series.
[DNLM: 1. Coronary Circulation--congresses. 2. Heart--
physiology--congresses. 3. Heart Enlargement--
physiopathology--congresses. 4. Heart Failure, Conges-
tive--physiopathology--congresses. 5. Muscle, Smooth,
Vascular--physiology--congresses. W1 DE997VME /
WG 200 16135 1983f]
QP111.2.I58 1983   616.1'29   84-10137
ISBN 0-89838-665-9

Copyright 1984 © by Martinus Nijhoff Publishing, Boston

All rights reserved. No part of this publication may be reproduced, stored in a retrieval system, or transmitted in any form or by any means, mechanical, photocopying, recording, or otherwise, without written permission of the publisher, Martinus Nijhoff Publishing, 190 Old Derby Street, Hingham, Massachusetts 02043.

CONTENTS

CONTRIBUTORS

F.L. ABEL, M.D., Ph.D.

Department of Physiology
University of South Carolina
    School of Medicine
Columbia, South Carolina 29208

J.C. ALLEN, Ph.D.

Cardiovascular Science Section
Department of Medicine
Baylor College of Medicine
1200 Moursund Avenue
Houston, Texas 77030

N.R. ALPERT, Ph.D.

Department of Physiology and Biophysics
University of Vermont College of Medicine
Burlington, Vermont 05405

S.P. BISHOP, D.V.M., Ph.D.

University of Alabama
Birmingham, Alabama 35294

M. BOND, Ph.D.

Pennsylvania Muscle Institute
University of Pennsylvania
    School of Medicine
B42 Anatomy-Chemistry Building G3
Philadelphia, Pennsylvania 19104

R.D. BUKOSKI, Ph.D.

Department of Physiology
Giltner Hall
Michigan State University
East Lansing, Michigan 48824

J.M. CANTY, JR., M.D.

Department of Medicine
State University of New York at Buffalo
School of Medicine
Clinical Center, Room CC169
462 Grider Street
Buffalo, New York 14215

J.B. CAULFIELD, M.D.

Department of Pathology
University of South Carolina
    School of Medicine
Columbia, South Carolina 29208

D. CHARLEMAGNE, Ph.D.

Institut National de la Sante
  et de la Recherche Medicale
Batiment I.N.S.E.R.M.
Hopital Lariboisiere
41, Boulevard de la Chapelle
75010 Paris, France

K.S. DHALLA

Experimental Cardiology Section
Department of Physiology
Faculty of Medicine
University of Manitoba
Winnipeg, Canada R3E 0W3

N.S. DHALLA, Ph.D.

Experimental Cardiology Section
Department of Physiology
Faculty of Medicine
University of Manitoba
Winnipeg, Canada R3E 0W3

H.F. DOWNEY, Ph.D.

Department of Physiology
University of Texas Health Science Center
    at Dallas
PO Box 225999
Dallas, Texas 75235

M.B. FRANKIS

Department of Pharmacology
Medical University of South Carolina
171 Ashley Avenue
Charleston, South Carolina 29425

R.A. GOLDSTEIN, M.D.

Department of Medicine
University of Texas Medical Science Center
Houston, Texas 77030

R. GOULETTE

Department of Physiology and Biophysics
University of Vermont College of Medicine
Burlington, Vermont 05405

D.M. GRIGGS, JR., M.D.

Department of Physiology
University of Missouri School of Medicine
Columbia, Missouri 65212

N. HAUGAARD, Ph.D.

Department of Pharmacology G3
University of Pennsylvania
   School of Medicine
Philadelphia, Pennsylvania 19104

M.E. HESS, Ph.D.

Department of Pharmacology G3
University of Pennsylvania
   School of Medicine
Philadelphia, Pennsylvania 19104

J.C. KHATTER, Ph.D.

Experimental Cardiology Section
Department of Physiology
Faculty of Medicine
University of Manitoba
Winnipeg, Canada R3E 0W3

T. KITAZAWA, Ph.D.

Department of Pharmacology
School of Medicine
Juntendo University
2-1-1, Hongo, Bunkyo-ku
Tokyo 113, Japan

F.J. KLOCKE, M.D.

Department of Medicine
State University of New York at Buffalo
   School of Medicine
Clinical Center, Room CC169
462 Grider Street
Buffalo, New York 14125

E.G. LAKATTA, M.D.

Cardiovascular Section
National Institute on Aging
Gerontology Research Center
4940 Eastern Avenue
Baltimore, Maryland 21224

L. LELIEVRE, Ph.D.

Institut National de la Sante
    et de la Recherche Medicale
Batiment I.N.S.E.R.M.
Hopital Lariboisiere
41, Boulevard de la Chapelle
75010 Paris, France

C.J. LIMAS, M.D.

Department of Medicine
Cardiovascular Section
University of Minnesota School of Medicine
Minneapolis, Minnesota 55455

R.Z. LITTEN, Ph.D.

Department of Physiology and Biophysics
University of Vermont College of Medicine
Burlington, Vermont 05405

J.H. McNEILL, Ph.D.

Faculty of Pharmacy Science
University of British Columbia
2146 East Mall
Vancover, British Columbia
Canada V6T 1W5

R.E. MATES, PH.D.

Mechanical Engineering
State University of New York at Buffalo
Clinical Center, Room CC172
462 Brider Street
Buffalo, New York 14215

J.J. MERCADIER, Ph.D.

Institut National de la Sante
    et de la Recherche Medicale
Batiment I.N.S.E.R.M.
Hopital Lariboisiere
41, Boulevard de la Chapelle
75010 Paris, France

D.F. MICHIEL, M.S.

Experimental Cardiology Section
Department of Physiology
Faculty of Medicine
University of Manitoba
Winnipeg, Canada R3E OW3

J.R. MILLER, Ph.D.

Department of Pharmacology
School of Medicine
Vanderbilt University
Nashville, Tennessee 37232

M.P. MOFFAT, Ph.D.

Experimental Cardiology Section
Department of Physiology
Faculty of Medicine
University of Manitoba
Winnipeg, Canada R3E OW3

L.A. MULIERI, Ph.D.

Department of Physiology and Biophysics
University of Vermont College of Medicine
Burlington, Vermont 05405

S.S. NAVRAN, Ph.D.

Department of Medicine
Baylor College of Medicine
1200 Moursund Avenue
Houston, Texas 77030

W.H. NEWMAN, Ph.D.

Department of Pharmacology
Medical University of South Carolina
171 Ashley Avenue
Charleston, South Carolina 29425

V. PANAGIA, M.D., Ph.D.

Experimental Cardiology Section
Department of Physiology
Faculty of Medicine
University of Manitoba
Winnipeg, Canada R3E OW3

J.M. PFEFFER, Ph.D.

Department of Medicine
Harvard Medical School
Brigham and Women's Hospital
75 Francis Street
Boston, Massachusetts 03115

M.A. PFEFFER, M.D., Ph.D.

Department of Medicine
Harvard Medical School
Brigham and Women's Hospital
75 Francis Street
Boston, Massachusetts 03115

G.N. PIERCE, Ph.D.

Experimental Cardiology Section
Department of Physiology
Faculty of Medicine
University of Manitoba
Winnipeg, Canada R3E 0W3

L. RAPPAPORT, Ph.D.

Institut National de la Sante
    et de la Recherche Medicale
Batiment I.N.S.E.R.M.
Hopital Lariboisiere
41, Boulevard de la Chapelle
75010 Paris, France

J.L. SAMUEL, Ph.D.

Institut National de la Sante
    et de la Recherche Medicale
Batiment I.N.S.E.R.M.
Hopital Lariboisiere
41, Boulevard de la Chapelle
75010 Paris, France

L. SCHINE, M.S.

Department of Physiology and Biophysics
University of Vermont College of Medicine
Burlington, Vermont 05405

K. SCHWARTZ, Ph.D.

Institut National de la Sante
    et de la Recherche Medicale
Batiment I.N.S.E.R.M.
Hopital Lariboisiere
41, Boulevard de la Chapelle
75010 Paris, France

C.L. SEIDEL, Ph.D.

Department of Medicine
Baylor College of Medicine
1200 Moursund Avenue
Houston, Texas   77030

H. SHUMAN, Ph.D.

Pennsylvania Muscle Institute
University of Pennsylvania
    School of Medicine
B42 Anatomy-Chemistry Building G3
Philadelphia, Pennsylvania   19104

P.J. SILVER, Ph.D.

Experimental Therapeutics
Wyeth Laboratories, Inc.
P.O. Box 8299
Philadelphia, Pennsylvania   19101

P.K. SINGAL, Ph.D.

Experimental Cardiology Section
Department of Physiology
Faculty of Medicine
University of Manitoba
Winnipeg, Canada R3E OW3

M.J. SOLE, M.D.

Division of Cardiology
Toronto General Hospital
101 College Street
Toronto, Ontario M5G 1L7
Canada

A.P. SOMLYO, M.D.

Pennsylvania Muscle Institute
University of Pennsylvania
    School of Medicine
B42 Anatomy-Chemistry Building G3
Philadelphia, Pennsylvania   19104

A.V. SOMLYO, Ph.D.

Pennsylvania Muscle Institute
University of Pennsylvania
    School of Medicine
B42 Anatomy-Chemistry Building G3
Philadelphia, Pennsylvania   19104

L.A. SORDAHL, Ph.D.

Division of Biochemistry
University of Texas Medical Branch
Galveston, Texas   77550

H.L. STONE, Ph.D.

Department of Physiology and Biophysics
University of Oklahoma Health Science Center
P.O. Box 26901
Oklahoma City, Oklahoma   73190

J.T. STULL, Ph.D.

Department of Pharmacology
University of Texas Health Science Center
   at Dallas
5323 Harry Hines Boulevard
Dallas, Texas   75235

B. SWYNGHEDAUW, M.D.

Institut National de la Sante
   et de la Recherche Medicale
Batiment I.N.S.E.R.M.
Hopital Lariboisiere
41, Boulevard de la Chapelle
75010 Paris, France

S.B. TAO, M.D.

Electron Microscopic Laboratory
Shanxi Medical College
Peoples Republic of China
TAIYUAN, Shanxi

B.S. TUANA, Ph.D.

Experimental Cardiology Section
Department of Physiology
Faculty of Medicine
University of Manitoba
Winnipeg, Canada R3E OW3

P.M. VANHOUTTE, M.D., Ph.D.

Department of Physiology and Pharmacology
Mayo Clinic 921-C
The Guggenheim Building
Rochester, Minnesota   55905

A.J. WASSERMAN, Ph.D.

Pennsylvania Muscle Institute
University of Pennsylvania
    School of Medicine
B42 Anatomy-Chemistry Building G3
Philadelphia, Pennsylvania   19104

J.G. WEBB, Ph.D.

Department of Pharmacology
Medical University of South Carolina
171 Ashley Avenue
Charleston, South Carolina   29425

PREFACE

These Proceedings are from the Fifth Annual Meeting of the American Section of the International Society for Heart Research held at Hilton Head Island, South Carolina, September 21-24, 1983. The program and abstracts were published in the Journal of Molecular and Cellular Cardiology, Vol. 15, Supplement 4, September 1983, Academic Press.

This Symposium Proceedings consists of three sections. Section I deals with the mechanical factors and their influence on coronary blood flow in the normal and failing heart. Section II is developed around the area of vascular smooth muscle and the factors that may control it which ultimately play such an important role in the regulation of coronary blood flow. Section III is primarily devoted to the mechanical aspects of the function of the heart in both hypertrophy and failure including the molecular changes in the myocyte, alterations in neural control, and in inotropic responsiveness of the hypertrophied and failing heart. The editors hope that these three areas encompass a significant body of new and ongoing information that will be helpful to those who work in these areas as well as those who treat patients with varying degrees of myocardial failure or with compromised coronary circulations.

The editors express their appreciation to all the contributors and to Ms. Jeri B. McClain for assisting in the organization and compiling of this volume.

Francis L. Abel, M.D., Ph.D.
Professor and Chairman
Department of Physiology
University of South Carolina
School of Medicine
Columbia, South Carolina

Walter H. Newman, Ph.D.
Professor of Pharmacology
Department of Pharmacology
Medical University of South
   Carolina
Charleston, South Carolina

<u>ACKNOWLEDGEMENTS</u>

Members of the Organizing Committee for the 1983 meeting of the International Society for Heart Research, American Section, gratefully acknowledge the support of the National Institutes of Health, Grant Number HL-30581. Contributions from the following organizations were instrumental to the Committee in conducting the meeting:

Abbott Laboratories
American Cyanamid Company
American Heart Association - South Carolina
    Affiliate
Beckman Company
Burroughs Wellcome Company
Culpepper Foundation
Drug Science Foundation, Medical University of
    South Carolina
Fujisawa Smith-Kline Company
International Society for Heart Research,
    American Section
Merck and Company, Inc.
Searle Pharmaceuticals, Inc.
Sigma Xi, University of South Carolina Chapter
Smith Kline - Beckman
University of South Carolina
University of South Carolina School of Medicine
Upjohn Company

I
ROLE OF MECHANICAL FACTORS IN THE REGULATION OF CORONARY BLOOD
FLOW IN NORMAL AND FAILING HEARTS

Section I of this volume deals with the role of
mechanical factors in the regulation of coronary blood flow
in the normal and the failing heart. Some metabolic aspects
are necessarily included because of the inseparable
interaction between metabolic and mechanical factors in
almost any type of experimental study on the coronary
system. This section begins with a microscopic study of the
relationship between the coronary capillary system and the
surrounding myocytes, demonstrating the presence of collagen
fibers, and relating possible effects of the collagen matrix
to the changes in diameter of the coronary vessels and the
disappearance of collagen to a possible effect on the no
reflow phenomena.

The first paper deals with the overall structural to
capillary relationship and does not attempt to further
define these changes at the various myocardial levels. It
is followed by a discussion of the relationship of some
mechanical factors to filling of the coronary vessels in the
heart-lung preparation. This paper deals strictly with
inflow into the coronary vessels and alteration of the
inflow pattern with heart rate and arterial pressure and
with removal of aortic ejection by using a reservoir system
and forcing the heart to eject through a separate cannula.

The next paper shows more of the flow relationships
occurring in the intramyocardial portions of the coronary
bed by looking at pressure and flow relationships obtained
from long diastoles in paced animals. The possible roles of
collateral flows on coronary flow and capacitance are
discussed in this paper. The author particularly stresses
the relationship of varying capacitance during the cardiac
cycle and the problem with estimating coronary resistance
from end diastolic pressure and flow relationships.

The following paper relates flow through the wall of the myocardium, as estimated by microsphere studies in normal and maximally dilated coronary vessels, with the dilation produced by hypoxia and by coronary occlusion. An interesting aspect of this paper is that hypoxia may actually produce a greater hyperemic response than does coronary occlusion alone. There is also a distinctly different time course of the hyperemic response in the subepicardial versus subendocardial layers. The authors indicate that hypoxia may play a role in the effects on coronary blood flow during strenuous exercise. Obviously the difference between the flow seen with occlusion and hypoxic perfusion also has a number of clinical implications.

The last paper in the section deals with the distribution of transmural flow when autoregulation is eliminated by reducing the perfusing pressure below the autoregulatory level; comparison studies are made of coronaries perfused at 85 mm mercury versus 45 mm mercury with distinctly different results. Not only does the distribution across the myocardial wall vary, thereby changing the endo-epicardial ratio, but the distribution of creatine phosphate, inorganic phosphate, and lactate also varied across the wall. The variation with perfusion pressure occurred whether or not the end diastolic pressure was increasing or if the ventricle was failing due to the low perfusion pressure. This study again argues for the lack of appropriate mechanisms to perfuse the endocardium during conditions of not only failure but also reduction of arterial driving pressure and must be related to fundamental concepts relative to how endocardial flow is normally maintained at high levels despite the subjection of the endocardial vessels to much higher extravascular pressures during systole. These concepts may relate to some of the thoughts in the first paper relative to structural effects, i.e., the relationship of the collagen fibers to the capillary vessels.

In summary, this series of articles addresses and summarizes some of the major problems in understanding the mechanisms whereby blood flow into, through, and out of the coronary circulation is regulated in the normal and failing heart. While it provides few definitive answers it indicates the areas to which much of the current coronary research is addressed and some of the major problems still to be solved. In a symposium of this type the authors are encouraged to put forth new theories which may or may not be subsequently justified and need not be as rigorously defended as in an original article in a scientific journal. The authors have by and large done this and it is hoped the reader will examine these theories in the spirit in which they are offered as proposing some new ways of looking at the coronary system, thoughts regarding some novel approaches to current problems in the field, and hypotheses which should be considered but which are not yet scientifically well validated.

1

CAPILLARY MYOCYTE RELATIONSHIPS IN THE VENTRICULAR WALL

JAMES B. CAULFIELD AND SUN BEN TAO

Blood flow through the myocardium is markedly affected by phasic contractions which result in pressure changes across the myocardium. These pressures range from ventricular cavity pressure (120-150 mmHg) at the endocardium to near intrathoracic pressure at the epicardium during systole. Wall pressures during diastole are far lower. Consideration of these phenomena has led to two somewhat dissimilar ideas of myocardial flow: a) the systolic forces are simply compressive and impede circulation to the ventricular wall during contraction and b) that systole is an essential component of coronary blood flow, having a massaging effect that increases outflow during systole permitting greater diastolic flow subsequently (1,2). More recently each of these views has been refined and extended to include the idea of a "waterfall" phenomenon in the heart and the suggestion that during systole there is a positive "intramyocardial pump" action (3,4).

Our recent data indicated that the myocytes are tightly coupled to the capillaries and that not only must compressive effects be considered, but also geometric rearrangements of the heart since the capillaries at least are so tightly coupled to the myocytes that their length as well as radius will be affected during systole and diastole.

MATERIALS AND METHODS

Morphologic Data

Most tissues and especially muscles contract when exposed to fixatives used for microscopy, both light and electron. If structural parameters are to be evaluated as in the heart during systole and diastole it is necessary in some way to counteract the displacement that occurs when tissue is exposed to fixatives. This has been accomplished using both isolated papillary muscle and intact ventricles (5). The data to be presented is based on a variety of methods for obtaining heart muscle at either diastolic or systolic lengths. The methods used provided essentially identical information regarding the extracellular matrix of the heart. The length of the muscle i.e. diastolic or systolic was the determining factor for collagen strut distribution, not the fixative used (6).

Hearts from 18 dogs were fixed by various techniques including instillation of 5% buffered glutaraldehyde into the left and right main coronary arteries or the heart was sliced perpendicular to the long axis and small pieces fixed by immersion in 5% buffered glutaraldehyde. Fourteen of the dogs had a double ligature placed on the left anterior descending coronary artery prior to fixation. In this situation portions of myocardium from the outflow region of the ligated vessel and the posterior free wall were obtained and fixed at $\frac{1}{2}$, 1, 2, 3, 24 hours and 7 and 14 days after ligation.

Initial fixation was obtained using a buffered glutaraldehyde with a total tonicity of 590 mOsmol. The osmolarity of the vehicle, 290, seems to be the most important factor (7). Using this fixative and subsequent appropriate fixation and dehydration techniques, minimal evidence of cell damage was noted by either transmission or scanning electron microscopy (7).

Two papillary muscles were removed from 12 rabbits and placed in 30 ml of Krebs bicarbonate buffer gassed with 95% O_2 and 5% CO_2 (8). After 30 min of equilibration, muscle prepartions were adjusted to maximal contraction length or rest length and stimulated 12 times per minute using 4msec duration impluses. The muscles were allowed to equilibrate under these conditions for 15 minutes. With 12 of the preparations, the bathing medium was replaced with 5% buffered glutaraldehyde, resulting in fixation at rest length or maximal contraction length. With 12 papillary muscles equilibrated at rest or maximal contraction length, the bathing medium was replaced with one containing ethylenediaminete- traacetic acid (EDTA), and stimulations continued for 20 min past the last recorded contraction. At this time, the EDTA-containing bathing medium was replaced with 5% buffered glutaraldehyde. One-half (six) of the muscles were fixed at rest length, and one-half at maximal contraction length as determined previously.

RESULTS

Left ventricular myocardium from various laboratory animals as well as humans was examined by light microscopy, scanning electron microscopy and occassionally transmission electron microscopy (6). The collagen matrix of the ventricle was qualitatively similar in all species examined although quantitative differences could be appreciated (9). The extracellular collagen matrix of the heart is reasonably analagous to that seen in skeletal muscle (10). There is a weave of collagen fibrils that surrounds groups of myocytes separating the myocardium into discrete units as described by Spotnitz et al (11). Extending from one weave pattern to the next are long thick bundles of collagen in a tendon like configuration. The weave itself is connected to the subjacent myocytes by short collagen struts. Each myocyte within a group is connected to all contiguous myocytes by short straight collagen struts that insert nearly perpendicular to the basal laminae of each cell (Fig. 1). There are many longitudinally arranged collagen struts that originate and insert into the basal lamina of a given myocyte. These may extend for less than a sarcomere, or cross over 3-4 Z lines. These are sufficient in number and distribution to prevent excessive stretch of the myocytes.

The capillaries lie between myocytes and run parallel to the long axis of the myocytes. An occasional capillary crosses a myocyte perpendicular to the long axis and joins the next capillary. The distribution seen by scanning electron microscopy is essentially the same as that previously described by others (12,13). Each capillary is connected to all contiguous myocytes by collagen struts. In many cases these struts insert nearly perpendicular to the basal lamina of the capillary and extend for some distance around the myocyte to insert tangentially into the basal lamina (14) (Fig. 2). The number and distribution of these struts would ensure that the capillary moves consonant with the myocyte throughout the cardiac cycle. Thus, all of the capillaries and myocytes enclosed by a weave of collagen are tightly interconnected and would function as a unit. The myocytes enclosed by a weave are only loosely connected to adjacent groups and displacement of one group relative to adjacent groups is much more likely.

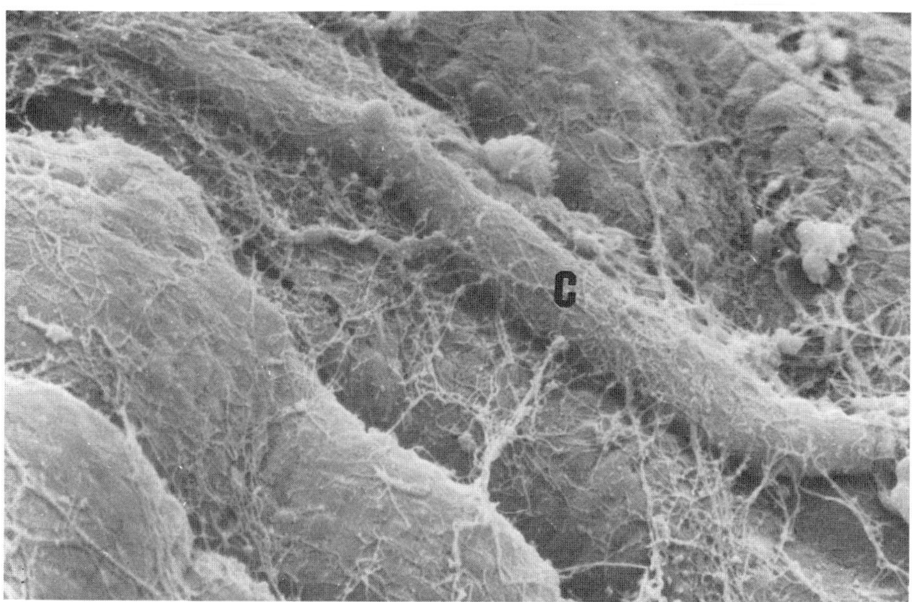

Fig. 1   Canine posterior left ventricle showing normal profusion of collagen struts that interconnect the myocytes (M).   3000x

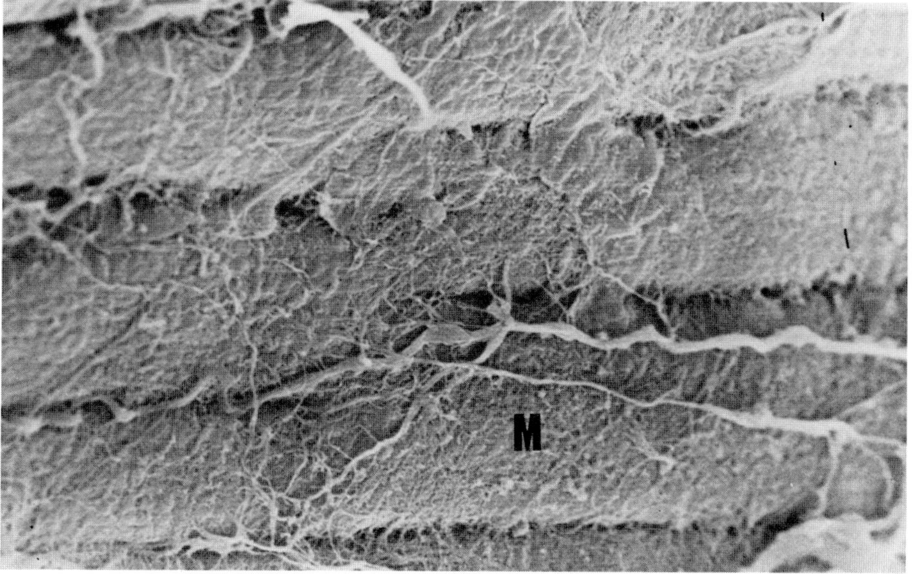

Fig. 2   Canine posterior left ventricle showing normal complex array of capillary (C) and myocyte collagen strut interconnections.   3000x

Examination of myocardial tissue in the region of the outflow of the ligated anterior descending artery at 1 hr post occlusion presents an essentially normal appearance of the collagen matrix. The control tissue from the posterior aspect of the free wall was normal at all time periods. At two hours a radical change occurs in the ischemic area in that very little of the collagen matrix is visible (Fig. 3). The basal laminae of the myocytes is visible and in many regions has holes in it. These rents may be quite large and mitochondria are visible suggesting complete breakdown of the sarcolemma/basement membrane complex and necrosis of the cell (15). At the lateral regions of ischemia there is loss of most of the collagen matrix with preservation of the basement membrane (Fig. 4). In this region the longitudinally oriented collagen struts are visible (16). Somewhat further removed from the central necrotic region there is evidence of some loss of the collagen struts with what appears to be retraction or contraction of some of the collagen matrix elements (Fig. 5). The basement membrane is intact showing ruffling with attachment in the Z band region indicating contraction of the cells. Thus, the loss of collagen struts extends beyond the area of definite necrosis for 2–5 mm. At 24 hours breakdown of the plasma membrane/sarcolemma complex is far more complete and cellular necrosis far easier to define. At this time loss of the collagen matrix at the lateral borders of the infarct extends for about 5 mm. At the endocardial surface of the infarct at 2 hrs. and subsequently Purkinjie fibers are present and appear to be viable. Loss of the collagen struts tethering these cells to their neighbors has occurred at 2 hrs. The loss of collagen struts is easily documented by scanning electron microscopy. Whether this loss is due to enzymatic degradation to amino acids and small peptides or is simply a depolymerization cannot be answered by scanning electron microscopy.

After two hours of LAD occlusion the myocyte to capillary struts are lost (Fig. 6). In this figure the capillary measures from 1.6 to 2.3 micra in diameter, a considerable reduction from that seen in Figure 2, a normal area which measures 6.6 micra in diameter. Though measurements are not highly accurate with a scanning electron microscope, the rather consistent reduction of capillary diameter to

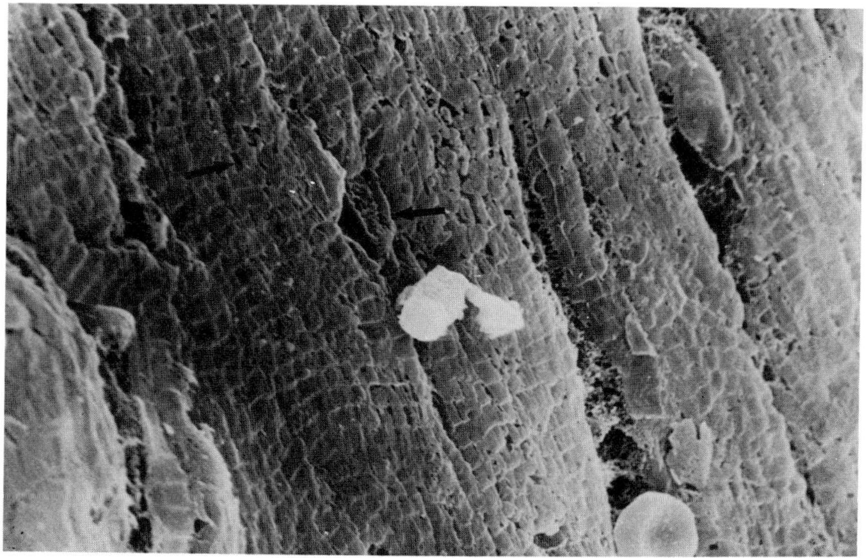

Fig. 3   Area in outflow region 2 hours after ligation of the anterior
descending artery.   There is extensive loss of collagen struts and
breakdown of the basal lamina/plasma membrane complex (arrows)
suggesting cell death. 3000x

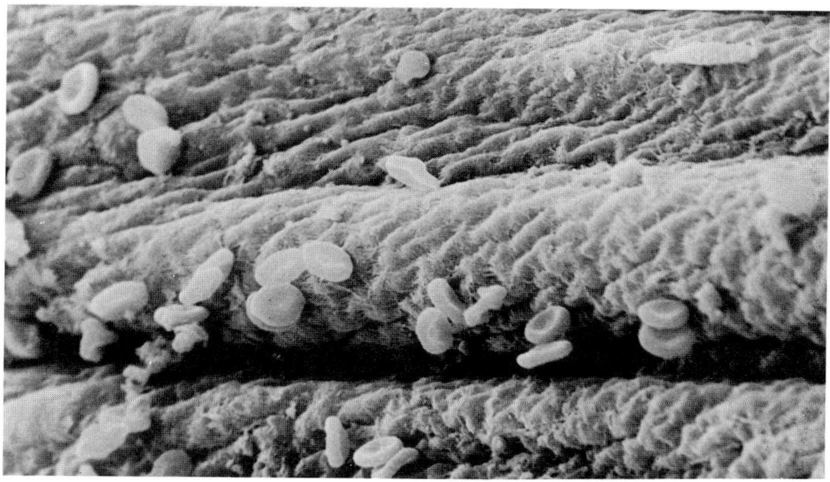

Fig. 4   Area lateral to area of necrosis 2 hours after coronary artery
ligation. Erythrocytes are visible as well as virtually total loss of
the struts that interconnect the myocytes. Many of the longitudinally
arranged struts are still visible. The basal lamina/plasma membrane
complex is intact and is ruffled suggesting that these cells are not
necrotic. 1500x

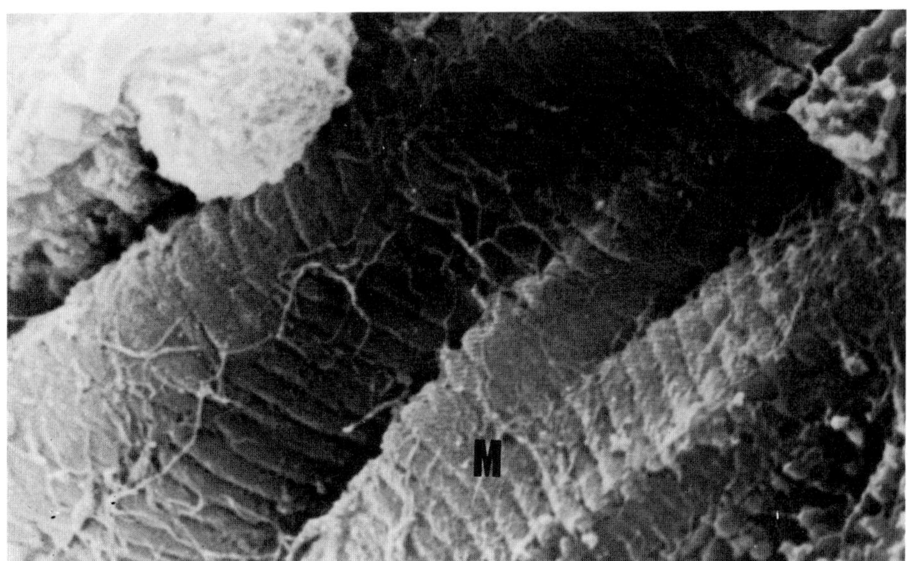

Fig. 5   Myocytes near the necrotic area with intact basal laminae, partial loss of the collagen matrix and suggestions of contraction. 4500x

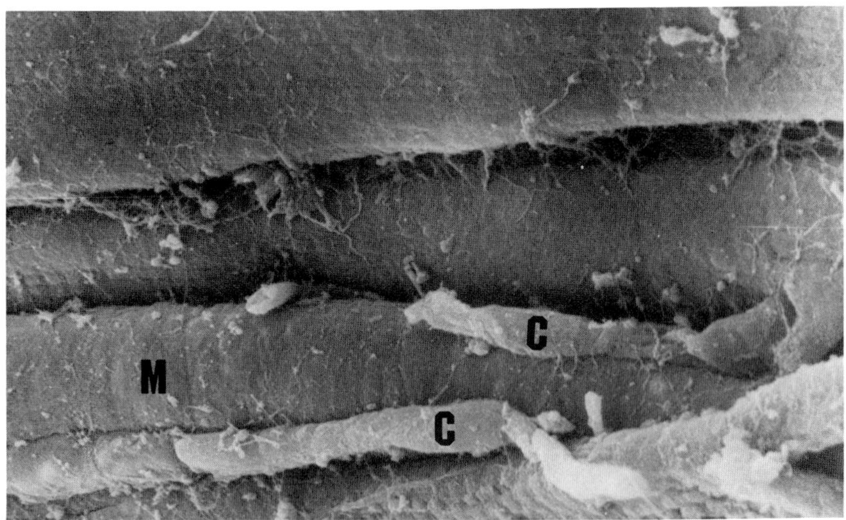

Fig. 6   Area near necrotic cells. These cells appear not to have contracted but have an intact basal lamina. Much of the collagen matrix has disappeared and the capillaries (C) range from about 1.6-2.2 micra in diameter. 3000x

one-third of that seen in normal areas processed similarly is probably reliable and strongly suggests a marked alteration in capillary length.

An important aspect of this work involves measurement of coronary artery flow during diastole, isovolumetric contraction and systole. Details of the methods and results of this work appear in the next chapter (17). The pertinent observation is the marked increase in flow occurring during isovolumetric contraction. This can account for as much as 20-50% of systolic flow (5). Since systolic flow accounts for 25-30% of total coronary flow this brief but substantial flow during isovolumetric contraction may be important to overall myocardial metabolism.

DISCUSSION

Systolic flow has been shown to occur by a number of investigators (18,19,20). The distribution of flow across the myocardium during systole is apparently sensitive to compressive forces being higher in the epicardial region than the endocardial region (18). However, during most of systole not only are compressive effects occurring, but also a rather marked rearrangement of the ventricular wall associated with ejection which may have an effect on blood flow.

Dividing coronary artery flow into an isovolumetric phase and ejection phase permits some separation of compressive effects from geometric changes. During isovolumetric contraction an increase in coronary flow velocity has been demonstrated (5,17). This flow can account for 20-50% of total systolic which is 25-30% of total coronary flow. The isovolumetric flow correlates with wall tension but not work parameters. This observation can be coupled with the known geometric changes occurring during isovolumetric contraction, a marked lengthening of the long axis of the heart with little or no change in the short axis which would result in rearrangement of the myocytes to accomodate this increase and a concommitant increase in the length of the capillaries providing a larger volume for blood to enter (21). This increase in length may more than offset the increase in wall pressure occurring during isovolumetric contraction and permit the large flow measured during isovolumetric contraction. During ejection with marked and rapid decrease in sarcomere length, the capillaries tethered to the myocytes would shorten. This rearrangement in distribution associated with the increase in wall pressure would account for the increased velocity of red cells in capillaries and venules during ejection that has been photographed on the epicardial surface (22,23).

The arrangement of the capillaries in parallel with the myocytes and closely coupled to them by collagen struts would be an explanation of the massaging effect proposed by Wiggers or its extension the intramyocardial pump of Spann et al (2,4). The arteries and veins are not in parallel with the myocytes and the precise effect of wall pressure or geometric rearrangement of the ventricular wall on these structures is not clear. They do have a complex collagen net surrounding and attached to them, which may alter simple compressive effects.

In many portions of the ischemic region the collagen matrix disappears within 2 hrs. following ligation of a coronary artery. This is associated with marked stretching of sarcomeres to 3.5 micra (24). Presumably the stress that causes sarcomere lengthening can also result in stretching of the capillaries. The loss of collagen is also associated with realignment of the slippage of the muscle bundles (25,26). The loss of the collagen matrix with its attendent distortion of the ventricular wall occurs at the time of the "no reflow" phenomenon i.e. with ligation of a coronary artery for 1 hr. and then release there is blood flow throughout the ischemic area whereas at 1½-2 hrs. post ligation with removal of the ligature no flow occurs into the ischemic area (27). This lack of flow is associated with a change in the point of maximum vascular resistance from the arteriole to the capillary (28). This is easily explicable on the basis of the marked alterations in the organization of ventricular wall associated with loss of the collagen supporting structures, and with the continued stress of systole. That the lack of reflow involves more than capillary endothelial alteration is attested to by the very different reaction of skeletal muscle when made ischemic. Intervals of ischemia to the hind legs of dogs for intervals of 18 hrs are not associated with a "no-reflow" phenomenon, but rather very good flow through muscle with release of the ligature (29). One must conclude that structural alterations are important in the heart or that the metabolism of vascular endothelial cells in the hind limb and the heart are totally dissimilar. The latter seems unlikely in view of the 9 fold time increase in ischemia to skeletal muscle over the heart that still permits good reflow.

<u>CONCLUSIONS</u>

There is a complex array of collagen struts in the heart that tightly couples the myocytes to the capillaries. This arrangement would ensure that the capillaries move concordant with the myocytes throughout the cardiac cycle. The tethering effect would lengthen the capillaries during isovolumetric contraction as the long axis of the heart increases and would help explain increased coronary artery flow during this period. Loss of the collagen strut matrix as occurs within 2 hrs. after coronary artery ligation in the ischemic area would explain the structural rearrangements that occur as well as the no reflow phenomenon. The tight tethering of the myocytes to the capillaries would help explain the massaging effect of systole proposed by Wiggers as well as the intramyocardial pumping action of Spann <u>et</u> <u>al</u>.

REFERENCES

1. Sabiston DC, Gregg DE: Effect of cardiac contraction on coronary blood flow. Circulation (15):14-20, 1957.
2. Wiggers CJ: The interplay of coronary vascular resistance and myocardial compression in regulating coronary flow. Circ Res (2): 271-279, 1954.
3. Downey JB, Kirk ES: Inhibition of coronary blood flow by a vascular waterfall mechanism. Circ Res (36):753-760, 1975.
4. Spann JAE, Breuls NPW, Laird JD: Diastolic-systolic coronary flow differences are caused by intramyocardial pump action in the anesthetized dog. Circ Res (49):584-593, 1981.
5. Caulfield JB, Borg TK, Abel FL: The effects of systole on left ventricular blood flow. In: Chazov E, Saks V, Rona G (eds) Advances in myocardiology. Plenum Pub Corp, 1983, pp 379-393.
6. Caulfield JB, Borg TK: The collagen network of the heart. Lab Invest (40):364-372, 1979.
7. Arborgh B, Bell P, Brunk V, Collins VP: The osmotic effect of glutaraldehyde during fixation: A transmission electron microscopy, scanning electron microscopy and cytochemical study. J Ultrast Res (56):339-350, 1976.
8. Ingebretsen WR, Becker E, Friedman WF, Mayer SE: Contractile response of cardiac and skeletal muscle to isoproteronal covalently linked to glass beads. Circ Res (40):474-484, 1977.
9. Borg TK, Ranson WF, Moslehy FA, Caulfield JB: Structural basis of ventricular stiffness. Lab Invest (44):49-54, 1981.
10. Adams RD: In: Diseases of muscle. A study in pathology, 3rd edition, Harper and Row, Hagerstown, Maryland, 1975, pp 46-48.
11. Spotnitz HM, Sonnenblick EH: Structural conditions in the hypertrophied and failing heart. Am J Cardiol (32):398-410, 1973.
12. Bassingthwaighte JB, Yipintsoi T, Harvey RB: Microvasculature of the dog left ventricular myocardium. Microvasc Res (7):229-249, 1974.
13. Coulson RL, Grayson J, Irvine M: Observations on coronary collateral communications and the control of flow in the circulation in the dog. J Physiol (208):563-581, 1970.
14. Borg TK, Caulfield JB: Collagen in the heart. Fed Proc (40):2037-2041, 1981.
15. Caulfield JB, Klionsky B: Myocardial ischemia and early infarction. An electron microscopic study. Am Jour Path (35):489-523, 1959.
16. Robinson TF, Cohen-Gould L, Factor S: Skeletal framework of mammalian heart muscle. Lab Invest (49):482-498, 1983.
17. Abel FL: Role of mechanical factors in coronary inflow. In: Abel FL and Newman WH (eds) Functional aspects of the normal, hypertrophied and failing heart. Martinus Hijhoff, Mass, 1984.
18. Hess DS, Bache RJ: Transmural distribution of myocardial blood flow during systole in the awake dog. Circ Res (38):5-15, 1976.
19. Kreuzer H, Schoeppe W: Das verhalten des bruckes in der herzewand. Pfluegers Arch (278):181-198, 1963.
20. Kreuzer H, Schoeppe W: Fur entstehung der differenz zwischen systolischem myokard und ventrikeldruck. Pfluefers Arch (278): 199-208, 1963.

21. Olsen CO, Rankin JS, Arentzen CE, Ring WS, McHale, PA, Anderson RW: The deformational characteristics of the left ventricle in the conscious dog. Circ Res (49):843-855, 1981.
22. Tillmans H, Ikeda S, Hansen H, Sarma JS, Fauvel JM, Bing RJ: Microcirculation in the ventricle of the dog and turtle. Circ Res (34): 561-569, 1974.
23. Tillmans H, Leinberger H, Thederon H, Steinhausen M, Kubler W: Pressure-velocity-diameter relations in the microvessels of the heart. In: Gaehtgens P (ed) Abstract of XI european conference for microcirculation, bibliotheca anatomica no. 20. S. Karger Basel, 1981, pp 484-489.
24. Crozatier B, Ashof M, Franklin D, Ross J: Sarcomere length in experimental myocardial infarction: evidence for sarcomere overstretch in dyskinetic ventricular regions. J Mol Cell Cardiol (9):785-797, 1977.
25. Weiseman HF, Udvarhelyi S, Bush DE, Bulkley BH: Cardiac remodeling in infarct expansion: differential distortion of the inner wall. Circ (68):part II, 1983, pp III-195 (abst).
26. Weisman HF, Bush DE, Kallman CH, Weisfeldt ML, Bulkley BH: Cellular mechanisms of infarct expansion: stretch vs. slippage. Circ (68):part II, 1983, pp III-253 (abst).
27. Kloner RA, Ganote CE, Jennings RB: The "no-flow" phenomenon after temporary coronary occlusion in the dog. Jour Clin Invest (54): 1496-1508, 1974.
28. Grayson J, Davidson JW, Fitzgerald-Finch A, Scott C: The functional morphology of the coronary microcirculation in the dog. Microvasc Res (8):20-43, 1974.
29. Miller HH, Wlech CS: Quantitative studies on the time factors in arterial injuries. Ann Surg (130):428-438, 1949.

Supported by NIH Grant 5 R01 HL27533

2

ROLE OF MECHANICAL FACTORS IN CORONARY INFLOW

FRANCIS L. ABEL

The coronary vessels pass through the walls of the myocardium in such a way that ventricular contraction may compress the coronary vessels sufficiently to decrease systolic blood flow. While numerous studies demonstrate that systolic flow is smaller than diastolic flow in individual vessels (17, 21, 23), few, if any, studies have been made of the components of <u>total</u> coronary blood flow during the cardiac cycle. During exercise the systolic flow component may increase along with the diastolic flow (25). The increase in systolic flow apparently occurs despite a decrease in systolic time, an increase in myocardial tension, and considerable evidence that systole does indeed compromise flow as shown by an increase in flow in fibrillating and asystolic hearts (26, 13). This led Wiggers (32) to propose a revised massaging theory, emphasizing the importance of systolic compression for effective venous emptying and subsequent arterial inflow. It is likely that mechanisms exist to prevent complete stoppage of systolic flow even during the most vigorous myocardial contractions; for the most part these have not been described or have been looked at from the viewpoint of flow in individual coronary vessels rather than for the total coronary system.

Recently we have been using an isolated heart-lung preparation to measure total coronary blood flow during the injection of pharmacological agents (1, 2). As systolic arterial pressure (afterload) was increased in that preparation, along with peak ventricular pressure and intramyocardial tension, coronary flow also markedly increased. This might be because of an accompanying increase in cardiac work and oxygen consumption. However, since these preparations were well supplied with oxygen ($P_0{}^2$ > 150 mmHg), with venous oxygen saturations of 80-90%, and were doing relatively small amounts of work, metabolic factors would not be expected to play such a large role in causing the responses. We thus chose to experimentally alter arterial pressure and heart rate while measuring total coronary flow, along with systolic and diastolic coronary inflow, to evaluate how these mechanical factors may alter total coronary flow and the systolic/diastolic flow ratio for filling the first part of the coronary vessels.

MATERIALS AND METHODS

The experiments were performed in twelve adult male mongrel dogs following anesthetization with sodium pentobarbital (30 mg/kg). Following insertion of a cuffed endotracheal tube and attachment to a ventilator to maintain respiration at 16/min with a tidal volume of about 10 ml/kg, a left thoracotomy in the fourth interspace was performed. The vena cava, azygos vein, aorta, pulmonary, brachiocephalic and left subclavian arteries were identified. A glass cannula was inserted into the left subclavian artery and connected to an open reservoir chamber which could be raised or lowered to control arterial pressure (Fig. 1). A T-tube connected the ventricular reservoir to a pump and heat exchanger. The output of the pump, after warming and debubbling the blood, was returned to the heart through a Bardic catheter inserted into the anterior aspect of the right ventricle. A polyethylene catheter inserted into the right atrium permitted continuous sampling of the right atrial inflow for oxygen saturation using a Waters oximeter or, in most experiments, content, using an A-V oxygen difference meter (and left atrial catheter for arterial sampling). A second catheter in the right atrium was also connected to a Statham pressure transducer for right atrial pressure measurement. A side arm from the subclavian cannula was connected to a Statham transducer to monitor the coronary reservoir pressure. A catheter-tipped high frequency transducer (Millar) was inserted into the left ventricle through a pulmonary vein for recording left ventricular pressure.

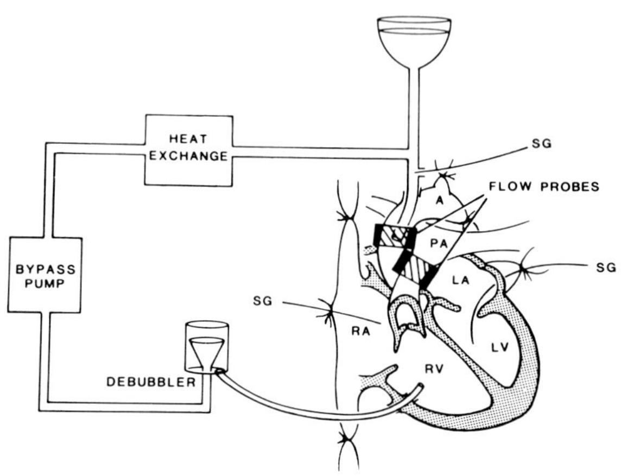

FIGURE 1. Diagram of heart-lung preparation. S.G. = strain gauge; heart = heat exchanger. See text for details.

The superior and inferior vena cava, azygos vein, aorta, and the brachiocephalic arteries were ligated in a sequence to prevent damage to the left ventricle from increased afterload. This consisted of bleeding the animal into the coronary reservoir then gradually occluding the aorta followed by ligating the veins. The resultant heart-lung preparation was thus totally isolated from the remainder of the animal as evidenced by the maintenance of a constant reservoir volume. Shortly after occluding the aorta and brachiocephalic arteries, brain death occurred, and neural outflow was assumed to cease. No additional adrenal secretions could enter the system, and no further anesthesia was given. The blood volume obtained was usually sufficient to fill the system, thereby eliminating the need for using a cross-matched animal or colloid solutions. The heat exchanger maintained temperature constant at 37°C.

Pulmonary artery flow was measured by a cannulating type electromagnetic flow probe inserted into the lumen of the pulmonary artery and connected to a pulsed electromagnetic flowmeter (5). Coronary flow was obtained by subtracting the bypass pump flow from the pulmonary artery flow. (The pulmonary artery flow is the sum of total coronary flow, except for Thebesian drainage into the left ventricle (estimated at less than 10% of left coronary flow (18)), and the known bypass pump flow. The bypass pump was previously calibrated and set at about 200 ml/min. If, for example, pulmonary artery flow, obtained by digital integration of the pulsatile flow signal were 400 ml/min, total mean coronary flow would be 200 ml/min.

The aorta was transected, and a second cannulating type flow probe was inserted into the ascending aorta just above (about 1 cm) the coronary ostia. This flow probe was connected by large (3/8" I.D.) silastic tubing to the reservoir chamber; the temporary subclavian cannula was then clamped off and removed. Flow in the aortic flow probe was forward during ejection and backward into the aortic root and coronary ostia during diastole. This flow was divided into true diastolic flow and flow during isovolumetric contraction. The isovolumetric contraction phase was calculated from the time of the beginning of the rise in ventricular pressure until the aortic flowmeter registered a forward flow. Diastolic timing was likewise taken from the left ventricular pressure waveform, using a computer program to evaluate maximal negative dp/dt (6) and the beginning of the rise of ventricular pressure.

Systolic flow was obtained by subtracting diastolic flow from total coronary flow. Note that this was not a pulsatile measurement of coronary inflow and could vary transiently with changes in ventricular or pulmonary compliance. Measurements were, therefore, made only during steady state conditions. Diastolic and isovolumetric inflow were phasically measured, systolic inflow was obtained by subtracting diastolic flow from the corresponding mean coronary flow value. Phasic non-isovolumetric systolic flow occurred into the coronary vessels between the aortic valves and the location of the aortic flow probe.

The Millar transducer was pre-calibrated with a known forcing. Prior to insertion, it was balanced and zeroed in a water bath at 37 °C. The zero pressure value was rechecked at the end of the experiment. The flowmeter probes were calibrated by pumping blood of equivalent hematocrit through them. The recording system filters were set at 3 db down at 20 Hz (minimum, often higher) for flow, arterial and venous pressures, and 3 db down at 120 Hz for ventricular pressure. The data were collected using an analog-to-digital converter sampling at a rate of 200 samples/sec/channel and processed on-line by a minicomputer (Nova 1200). The variables of interest were calculated and stored for later analysis on a floppy disk. The primary variables consisted of aortic pressure, right atrial pressure, left ventricular pressure, pulmonary flow, and aortic flow. From these were obtained the coronary flows described above, mean aortic pressure, aortic systolic and diastolic pressure, systolic time, diastolic time, maximal dp/dt, time to peak ventricular pressure (PVP time) (4), end diastolic pressure, heart rate, stroke volume, ventricular stroke work (from ventricular pressure and pulmonary flow), the integral of ventricular pressure during systole, cardiac output, cardiac work, and tension-time index. Most of the computer programs used to obtain these variables have been previously published (3).

Arterial and venous blood gases and pH were monitored at about 30-min intervals throughout the experiment. In early experiments, Van Slyke determinations of oxygen content were done to estimate oxygen consumption from the oximeter oxygen saturations, but in most of the experiments, oxygen content was determined using a Lex-O_2-Con (Lexington Instruments, Inc., Waltham, MA) and rapid changes assessed with an A-V oxygen difference meter (A-Vox Systems, Inc., San Antonio, TX). A-V difference was multiplied by mean coronary flow to obtain oxygen consumption. At the end of the experiment, the heart was removed and weighed.

The experimental procedures consisted of altering heart rate or aortic pressure. Heart rate was altered by blocking the AV node by electrocautery and electrically pacing the ventricles. The blocking procedure consisted of inserting a specially prepared electrode through a small incision in the right atrium and restraining it with a purse-string suture. The electrode consisted of a 2 mm diameter rod, connected to the electrocautery at one end and coated with insulation except for the bare tip. The external coronary sinus dimple was located, and the electrode was placed in the estimated location of the AV node. A short burst of electrocautery current usually produced a satisfactory block. A similar procedure has been published (27). Heart rate was altered over a range of approximately 60-240 beats/min, in increments of 20-40 beats/min, with a minimum of 1-2 min of data obtained at each setting (5-10 cardiac cycles processed by the computer program). During this procedure, aortic pressure was held constant at about 80 mmHg. Similarly with heart rate at about 130/min (since the heart was neurologically isolated, rate did not change with aortic pressure even without an AV block), aortic pressure was varied from 40-120 mmHg, in about 20 mmHg increments, by raising and lowering the aortic reservoir chamber. Sufficient time was allowed at each pressure or heart rate setting to avoid transient data. Thus, momentary changes in right heart volume or pulmonary vascular volume, which might alter pulmonary artery flow, were allowed to stabilize at each new pressure or rate before data were collected. Steady state was also observable by the constancy of the reservoir volume and the aortic pressure.

Statistical Data

Each animal was analyzed for his contribution to a given procedure by taking the mean of all cardiac cycles obtained at a given experimental condition (e.g., arterial pressure). All animals were then grouped to give the means and standard errors within a given arterial pressure or heart rate range, with each animal contributing only 1 point for each experimental procedure. Statistical significance was taken as $P \leq .05$ using a two-tailed paired t test (29) (also checked with a non-parametric Wilcoxon test [28]). For the correlation matrix, a non-parametric Spearman correlation coefficient (28) was calculated using the data as previously grouped by the variables heart rate and arterial pressure. Thus the experimental procedures, e.g. varying heart rate, resulted in several groups of data all of which were included in the final correlation matrix. In so far as one animal appears in several of these groups, he also appears that many times in the correlations. The Spearman matrix was also checked for errors by computing the Pearson product moment r; nearly identical results were obtained.

RESULTS

Table 1 (A and B) summarizes the overall data, obtained by varying mean aortic pressure or heart rate. Fig. 2 shows the percentage alterations in cardiac work, total coronary flow, and percent of flow as diastolic flow, as heart rate or mean aortic pressure (MAP) was varied. The 100% group was taken, for the aortic pressure experiment, as 80-100 mmHg and, for the heart rate experiments, as 100-140 beats/min. The figure shows that coronary flow increased when either heart rate or aortic pressure was increased. These increases were small, amounting to a mean of 1.8 ml/min/100 g Hg at the two pressure extremes and 0.4 ml/min/100 g/heart rate at the two extremes of rate. The percentage of total flow occurring in diastole, however, decreased, especially when heart rate was increased. Cardiac work increased when arterial pressure was increased, but the changes with heart rate were not significant. Oxygen consumption and tension-time index (Table 1) increased with both heart rate and arterial pressure, along with maximal dt/dt.

Table 2 gives the Spearman correlation coefficients for the two types of experiments. Spearman coefficients were also obtained for the two groups combined. Total coronary flow was significantly correlated ($P \leq .05$) with aortic pressure and heart rate only in the corresponding experimental group, i.e., correlated with aortic pressure only when aortic pressure was varied. Aortic pressure and heart rate were not correlated, demonstrating that they were

Table 1A.   Data Grouped by Arterial Pressure[+]

	Arterial Pressure (mmHg)			
	40-60	60-80	80-100	100-200
Mean Aortic Pressure	53.0 ± 1.0*	72.0 ± 1.0*	87.0 ± 1.0	105.0 ± 1.0*
End Diastolic Pressure	9.9 ± 0.8*	10.6 ± 1.0*	12.4 ± 1.4	14.2 ± 2.1
Peak Ventricular Pressure	82.0 ± 5.0*	106.0 ± 4.0*	122.0 ± 5.0	141.0 ± 7.0*
Maximal dp/dt	1.15± 0.10*	1.42± 0.15*	1.52± 0.15	1.60± 0.16
PVP Time[++]	133.0 ± 4.0	141.0 ± 5.0	132.0 ±10.0	143.0 ± 3.0
Systolic Time	205.0 ± 7.0*	216.0 ± 8.0	218.0 ± 8.0	231.0 ±10.0
Diastolic Time	258.0 ±15.0*	242.0 ±15.0	234.0 ±16.0	246.0 ±23.0
Heart rate	131.0 ± 4.0	133.0 ± 5.0	135.0 ± 5.0	129.0 ± 8.0
Cardiac Output	255.0 ±29.0*	299.0 ±28.0	322.0 ±33.0	342.0 ±46.0*
Cardiac Work	159.0 ±22.0*	248.0 ±28.0*	304.0 ±32.0	380.0 ±50.0*
Tension-Time Index	1422.0 ±96.0*	1948.0±116.0*	2345.0±159.0	2814.0±265.0
O_2 Consumption	4.6 ± 1.1*	5.6 ± 1.1	7.9 ± 2.0	4.7 ± 0.8
Total Coronary Flow	151.0 ±23.0*	197.0 ±25.0	225.0 ±29.0	245.0 ±41.0*
Systolic Flow	113.0 ±18.0*	152.0 ±20.0*	189.0 ±25.0	194.0 ±33.0
Diastolic Flow	49.0 ± 9.0*	55.0 ± 7.0	49.0 ± 9.0	51.0 ± 8.0
Isovolumetric Flow	41.0 ±24.0	38.0 ±22.0	56.0 ±33.0	41.0 ±15.0
% Systolic Flow	69.8 ± 3.4	73.0 ± 3.3	76.3 ± 2.3	78.9 ± 1.8
% Isovolumetric Flow	19.4 ±10.8	20.6 ±10.7	20.9 ±10.1	18.5 ± 8.0
N	10	11	10	6

* P ≤ .05 from 80-100 "control" group; 2-tailed paired t test.

[+] Mean ± SE. Pressures are in mmHg, flow in ml/min/100 g heart weight, times in millisec. Maximal dp/dt x 10^{-3}, cardiac work x 10^{-2}, tension-time index is mmHg·sec/min, oxygen consumption is ml/100 g/min.

[++] N for this variable is 3 less than Group N due to error in data acquisition.

N Number of animals.

Table 1B. Data Grouped by Heart Rate

	Heart Rate (Beats/Min)				
	60-100	100-140	140-180	180-220	220-260
Mean Aortic Pressure	71.0 ± 5.0	75.0 ± 5.0	76.0 ± 5.0	77.0 ± 4.0	80.0 ± 2.
End Diastolic Pressure	14.3 ± 2.5*	12.2 ± 1.7	11.5 ± 1.7	10.7 ± 1.0	15.3 ± 0.
Peak Ventricular Pressure	126.0 ± 8.0*	115.0 ± 5.0	113.0 ± 5.0	105.0 ± 4.0*	97.0 ± 4.
Maximal dp/dt	1.52± 0.16	1.42± 0.15	1.60± 0.15*	1.67± 0.11*	1.72± 0.
PVP Time[++]	136.0 ± 9.0*	126.0 ± 7.0	118.0 ± 6.0*	113.0 ± 1.0*	103.0 ± 4.
Systolic Time	227.0 ±11.0	220.0 ±13.0	201.0 ±10.0*	183.0 ± 8.0*	169.0 ± 8.
Diastolic Time	511.0 ±21.0*	310.0 ±11.0	185.0 ±13.0*	122.0 ±13.0*	79.0 ± 8.
Heart Rate	83.0 ± 3.0*	116.0 ± 2.0	158.0 ± 2.0*	199.0 ± 4.0*	243.0 ± 6.
Cardiac Output	279.0 ±33.0*	289.0 ±32.0	306.0 ±26.0*	318.0 ±20.0	330.0 ±22.
Cardiac Work	258.0 ±38.0	247.0 ±26.0	258.0 ±21.0	267.0 ±17.0	272.0 ±18.
Tension-Time Index	1508.0 ±50.0	1863.0±166.0	2283.0±222.0*	2414.0±215.0*	2610.0±261.
O_2 Consumption	3.3 ± 0.4*	4.9 ± 0.3	7.4 ± 0.6*	9.2 ± 1.1*	10.8 ± 1.
Total Coronary Flow	176.0 ±24.0*	189.0 ±26.0	206.0 ±21.0*	213.0 ±13.0	235.0 ±17.
Systolic Flow	123.0 ±19.0*	140.0 ±23.0	164.0 ±23.0*	200.0 ±15.0*	225.0 ±18.
Diastolic Flow	54.0 ±10.0	49.0 ±10.0	41.0 ±13.0	13.0 ± 8.0*	10.0 ± 5.
Isovolumetric Flow	31.0 ± 8.0	22.0 ±11.0	43.0 ± 6.0*	41.0 ± 9.0*	46.0 ±11.
% Systolic Flow	68.8 ± 4.9	72.3 ± 5.4	78.8 ± 6.5	93.7 ± 3.8*	95.8 ± 1.
% Isovolumetric Flow	19.4 ± 5.8	13.2 ± 5.6	22.7 ± 4.5	20.1 ± 4.7*	20.2 ± 5.
N	6	7	7	6	5

* $P \leq$ .05 from 100-140 group; 2 tailed paired t test; see Table 1A for other symbols.

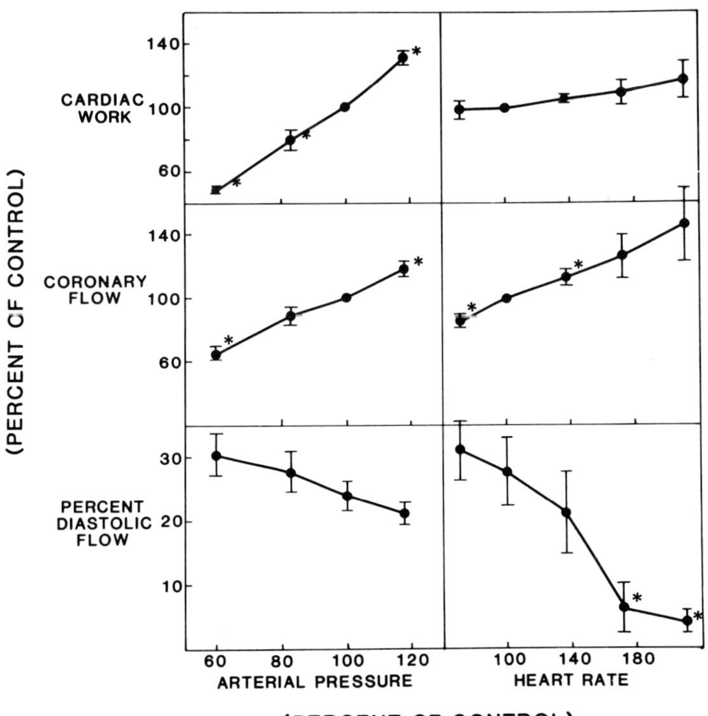

FIGURE 2. Percent changes in cardiac work, coronary flow, and percentage of flow in diastole versus arterial (aortic) pressure and heart rate. *$\underline{P} \leq$ .05 by two-tailed t test versus control (100%) group.

independently varied parameters. Systolic flow was also correlated with the varied parameters and highly correlated with total flow (combined coefficient = .853). In each group, total flow and systolic flow were also correlated with cardiac work, but not consistently with dt/dt, tension-time index, or oxygen consumption. Correlation with oxygen consumption and dt/dt occurred in the aortic pressure but not in the heart rate experiments, despite a greater

Table 2.   Spearman Correlation Coefficient

	A. Arterial Pressure Experiments				B. Heart Rate Experiments			
	Total Flow	Systolic Flow	Diastolic Flow	Isovolu-metric Flow	Total Flow	Systolic Flow	Diastolic Flow	Isovolu-metric Flow
Mean Aortic Pressure	.328*	.362*	.034	.127	-.116	.148	-.540*	-.207
Heart Rate	.087	.126	.135	.705*	.330*	.591*	-.635*	.368*
Peak Ventricular Pressure	.373*	.299*	.309*	.209	-.442*	-.664*	.565*	.041
Maximal dp/dt	.599*	.369*	.213	.221	-.077	-.142	.186	.480*
Systolic Time	-.157	-.009	-.171	-.112	-.327*	-.355*	.153	-.401*
Diastolic Time	-.090	-.180	.063	-.550	-.282	-.570*	.668*	-.323*
Cardiac Work	.888*	.719*	.320*	.004	.792*	.566*	.230	-.109
Tension-Time Index	.237	.246	.055	.322*	.088	.390*	-.651*	.222
O_2 Consumption	.295*	.477*	.644*	.702*	-.016	.257	-.523*	.487
Systolic Flow	.835*	1	.436*	.322*	.869*	1	-.496*	-.007
Diastolic Flow	.357*	.436*	1	.413*	-.051	-.496*	1	.094
Isovolumetric Flow	.032	.322*	.413*	1	.030	-.007	.094	1

* P $\leq$ .05, 2 tailed-test.

increase in oxygen consumption with changes in heart rate
(Table 1B) than with changes in aortic pressure (Table 1A).

Diastolic flow was positively correlated with oxygen
consumption and cardiac work only in the pressure
experiments; it was negatively correlated with heart rate,
tension-time index, and oxygen consumption in the rate
experiments. Isovolumetric flow was strongly correlated with
oxygen consumption in both groups (combined coefficient was
.503); it was also correlated with heart rate and dt/dt in
the heart rate experiments but not with cardiac work.
Overall correlation to dt/dt was .448. Interestingly, this
variable was never correlated with cardiac work, versus
systolic and diastolic flow, and also was not correlated
with total flow (combined coefficient = .148, not
significant). Thus, a different set of factors appeared to
be separately influencing this variable. We have previously
reported on its strong correlation with isovolumetric
pressure (9).

Summarizing the results, coronary flow was modestly
increased by both procedures. Changing heart rate increased
oxygen consumption but had less influence on cardiac work.
Tension time index, dt/dt and PVP time were also changed by
both procedures. Both procedures tended to increase the
percentage of coronary inflow occurring in systole, although
the only significant changes occurred with heart rate.
Total flow and systolic flow were correlated with the varied
parameters and with cardiac work. The correlation of total
and systolic flow with oxygen consumption varied with the
experimental procedure; they were correlated during the
aortic pressure experiments, even though oxygen consumption
increased in only one group, but not during the heart rate
experiments. Diastolic inflow was similar to total flow in
the aortic pressure group but not in the heart rate group;
it decreased as heart rate and oxygen consumption increased.
Isovolumetric flow correlated well with oxygen consumption
in both groups, but was not correlated with total flow or
cardiac work.

DISCUSSION

Considering the discrepancy between the results obtained for total coronary inflow versus flow in individual vessels (17, 21), several questions arise. The most obvious one is, could the results be in error because of phase lag either in the transducer placement or in the recording system? In order to prevent lag due to the transducer location, the aorta was opened between the branching of the brachiocephalic artery and the aortic valve, and a cannulating type of flow probe was inserted. Thus all but a small section, no more than 1-2 cm in length, of the aorta was replaced by the rigid flow probe and above that by the semi-rigid pump tubing. The phase lag in the recording system for the aortic flow probe was similar to that for the left ventricular pressure transducer used for systolic timing. Low-pass, one-stage RC filters were incorporated usually with 3 db points of 20-30 Hz but often opened up to 120 Hz where noise levels permitted. These considerations could not account for any serious phase lag in the pulsatile tracings. However, filling of the portion of aortic segment involved must be included as a part of the coronary inflow system being described.

The percentage of total coronary flow occurring during systole in this preparation was consistently high (Table 1), 69-96% of the total coronary flow (the overall mean $\pm$ SE was 77.5% $\pm$ 1.7%). This is much higher than usually reported. Flow during isovolumetric contraction was also significant ranging from 13 - 23% of total flow (overall mean 19.4% $\pm$ 2.5%). Fig. 3 illustrates the typical waveforms obtained and shows the small amount of diastolic flow and the phasic increase in flow occurring at the onset of left ventricular isovolumetric contraction.

It should be emphasized that the phasic tracings of coronary inflow are valid only for isovolumetric flow, before the aortic valve opens, and diastolic flow. The value for non-isovolumetric systolic flow is correct in magnitude, but since it does not enter the flow probe, it cannot be obtained as a phasic tracing. It is tempting to postulate that the variations from a smooth parabola in the

aortic ejection waveform (Fig. 3) represents some systolic
coronary inflow, but we have no way to quantitate this.

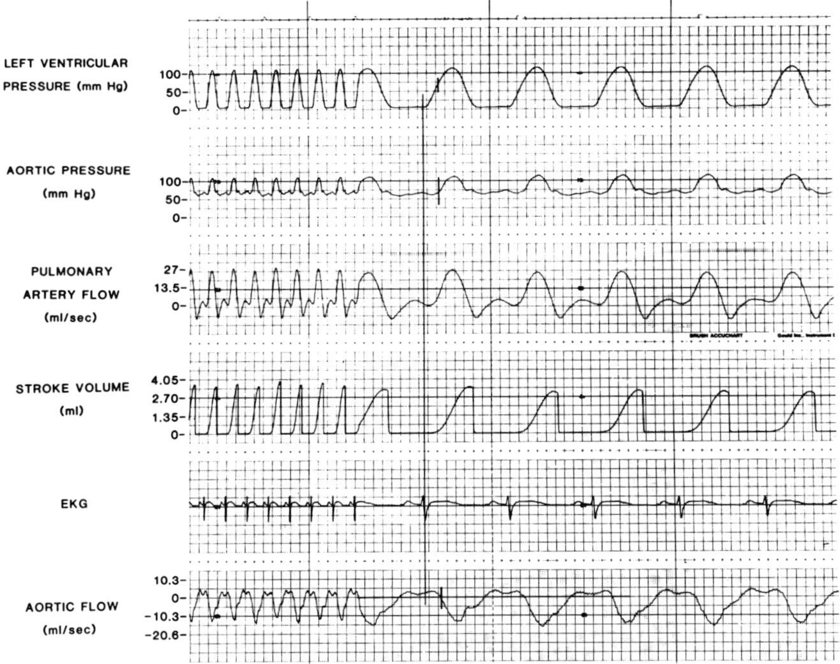

FIGURE 3. Typical flow patterns obtained from this preparation.
Stroke volume shown was from analog computer integration of
pulmonary artery flow. Lead II EKG. Time marks in seconds.
Aortic flow polarity is a positive deflection for flow downward through the probe into the coronary vessels. Negative
flow is ejection into the reservoir system.

We have recently demonstrated that this
sytolic/diastolic inflow ratio is also related to compliance
of the ascending aorta (7). In these experiments, the same
tubing arrangement was used, hence these data represent the
effects of heart rate and aortic pressure at a constant
aortic compliance.

The contribution of isovolumetric flow to systolic flow has previously been ignored. This flow may easily have been incorporated into diastolic flow, particularly when an on-line electronic integration was not used to compute the phasic flow areas (17). If one adds the isovolumetric flow to diastolic flow and subtracts it from systolic flow, systolic flow would be 55% of total flow. In addition, a portion of the total coronary flow, estimated at 15% (16), supplies the right ventricle, which should have a greater percentage of its flow occurring during systole.

If one considers that during ejection there is a rapidly moving forward volume of blood with associated swelling of the aortic root, and perhaps associated enlargement of the coronary ostia, it is reasonable to expect systolic filling of the coronary vessels in the same manner as systolic flow occurs into peripheral vessels arranged perpendicular to a large artery. The inertia of the forward moving blood would seem to inhibit diastolic filling. In fact, in most aortic flow probe tracings following the backflow during valve closure, little if any, coronary flow can be seen during diastole. This has always been explained as due to the relatively small (circa 5%) of cardiac output involved, but even when high-gain tracings are obtained with low noise content, very little diastolic coronary flow can be seen (unpublished observation).

As a test of this inertia hypothesis, we studied coronary flow when left ventricular ejection was forced to occur through a one-way valve from the ventricular apex. A second reservoir regulated ventricular afterload and a servo-operated pump maintained the level constant in a reservoir attached to the aorta. Aortic ejection was prevented by maintaining the aortic pressure reservoir at a higher level than the ventricular reservoir. Little or no aortic ejection could therefore occur, and coronary flow was measured from the aortic reservoir. In this preparation in 7 animals, total coronary flow averaged 338 ml/min with 29% of the flow occurring in systole and 71% in diastole (9). Fig. 4 shows the diastolic flow pattern from the aortic (coronary) flow probe and the typical pattern from a second flow probe around the left circumflex artery.

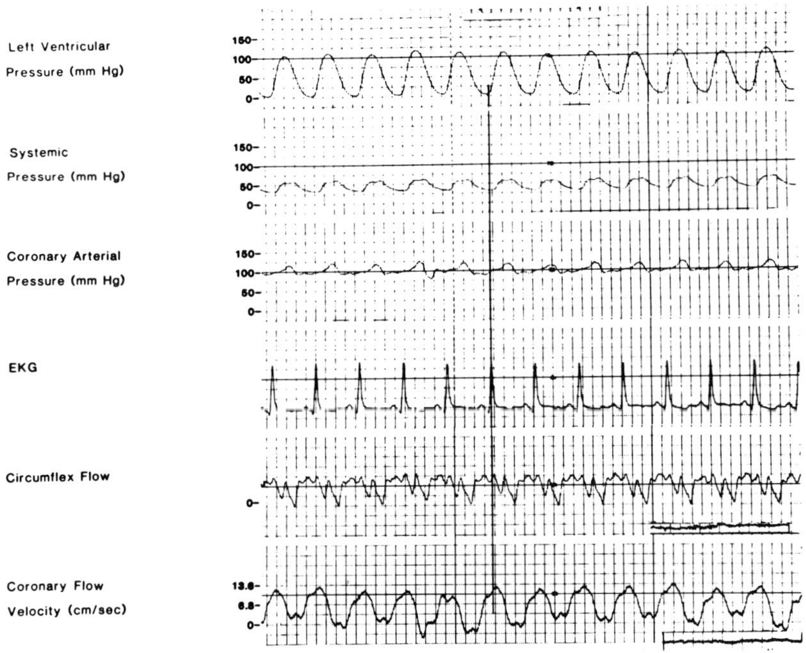

FIGURE 4.   Similar preparation as in Figure 1, but left
ventricle ejecting into a cannula inserted into the ventricular apex.   Low systemic pressure is an error caused by
artificial valve resistance, i.e., ventricular pressure
represents afterload seen by left ventricle.   Separate
reservoir for coronary flow.   Circumflex coronary flow
(uncalibrated) and "magnet off" tracings (inserts) to
illustrate vessel patterns and lack of EKG artifact.   See
text for details.   (From Abel FL: Modified starling heart-
lung preparation for measuring coronary vascular resistance,
Circ Shock 12:3, 1984.   Reprinted by permission of Alan R.
Liss, Inc.)

The predominance of diastolic flow is evident.   Systolic
flow represents primarily that flow occurring during
isovolumetric contraction and, to a lesser extent, that
during the ventricular pressure drop in midsystole.   The

inertial concept is also supported by our recent report on the dependence of systolic flow on aortic compliance (7). The more compliant the aorta, the more coronary inflow shifted to a diastolic pattern.

Could the increased systolic flow simply be related to vasodilation in the isolated heart-lung preparation? Although this possibility cannot be completely rejected, the preparation just discussed was also an isolated one. Moreover, this is not a completely dilated bed in that there is not a linear relationship between pressure with a zero-flow intercept pressure (20). Ten mg doses of papaverine given at the end of each experiment consistently produced a large (about 50%) increase in coronary flow. The preparation also showed reactive hyperemia to coronary occlusion. The coronary flow values presented (201 ml/min/100 gms) are about double the microsphere values of 109 ml/min/100 gms reported in awake animals (19).

The values for oxygen consumption are low. Cardiac output in this preparation is determined by the coronary flow and bypass pump flow--about 200 ml/min. Hence, cardiac work is also low, and oxygen consumption reflects the decreased work level. Likewise, maximal dp/dt reflect the low operating level and the low peak ventricular pressures produced by the reservoir system. To the extent that left ventricular tension is lower than normal, this may contribute to a decrease in compression of the coronary vessels during systole and a corresponding increase in systolic flow, although most of the flow probably pertains only to inflow into the first part of the coronary vessels.

Ideally, these measurements should be repeated in a normal unanesthetized animal, but no direct measurement technique is apparent. The systolic flow component here may appear as a distortion in the forward aortic flow curve, but there is no way to quantitate this in the intact animal. Most of the distortion appears to occur in late systole (Fig. 3), thus suggesting that this is also the timing of most of the systolic flow other than that occurring during isovolumetric contraction.

Thus it appears that in this preparation the majority of flow _into_ the coronary vessels is occurring in systole.

The runoff from the individual arteries presumably is occurring in diastole. Spaan et al. (31) have recently presented evidence for a to-and-fro phenomenon in the intramyocardial coronary vessels. This study indicates a large inflow into the epicardial vessels during systole. Even if systolic backflow also occurs up to the coronary ostia, it could not be seen due to the measurement site. Chilian and Marcus (11) have recently demonstrated a marked phasic difference in intramyocardial flow, as represented by septal artery flow, and epicardial flow. These effects were exacerbated by vasodilator drugs. Their data support the views that the epicardial vessels have an important capacitative function, even when the myocardial vessels are vasodilated. Although they obtained no quantitative measurement of volume flow, the systolic components of flow increased markedly with vasodilation. In view of previous estimates of the capacitance of the epicardial vessels, these results are somewhat high (11, 12). For a systolic coronary flow of 378 ml in a 200 gm heart (Table 1A), at a heart rate of 135, 2.8 ml/beat would need to be moved into the coronary vessels and attached aortic segment. While the latter segment cannot be quantitated in these studies, it was constant in a given animal. (In some instances the aortic flow cannula was within 3 mm of the coronary ostia.) Thus, systolic flow as seen here must extend some distance into the coronary system but, of course, involves both coronary vessels. Again, an important portion of this is isovolumetric flow, clearly greatly increased in the vasodilated state (11) and easily confused with diastolic flow.

The decrease in diastolic flow with heart rate has previously been described (23), with the increase in systolic flow ascribed to an active vasodilation process. These results concur with those findings but emphasize the importance of systolic flow at all levels of cardiac work and the importance of an early, seemingly mechanically related systolic flow component. This component may also be the factor that produces the increase in flow just after the "cove" in diastolic flow reported by Gregg et al. (17). Fig. 4 also shows this phenomenon in the circumflex vessel.

The association of coronary inflow primarily with systole and correlated with the metabolic state may have important implications for therapy in coronary disease particularly when associated with a decrease in myocardial contractile vigor. However, any associated increased rigidity of the coronary vessels, or for that matter, of the aorta, might change these relationships.

The mechanism whereby flow increases at a time when myocardial tension is also increasing is not clear. Rankin et al. (24) have described alterations in mechanical shape during contraction. Others have described collagen bundles extending from the capillaries to the supporting myocytes (10) and postulated that these may pull the capillaries open during contraction.

The resultant data may be considered relative to the concept of a critical closing pressure (15). The mean data points (Fig. 5) were matched using a geometric regression technique (29), i.e., an equation of the form $y = A \cdot x^\beta$ where A and B are constants. Fig. 5 shows the resultant sketched curves (dotted lines) for total and systolic flows (the standard error of the estimate was < .07 and the coefficient of correlation was > .97 for all curves). A linear model for aortic pressure versus diastolic flow was assumed. The first part of the diastolic flow versus heart rate was also assumed to be linear. Considering only the arterial pressure curve, one can ask which begins first as pressure is increased, systolic or diastolic flow? One is tempted to say that diastolic flow begins first in the beating heart, with systolic flow only occurring after aortic pressure has overcome some myocardial compression. Could the crossing points (dotted lines) of 11 mmHg (where diastolic flow is equal to total flow) and 20 mmHg (where diastolic flow is equal to systolic flow) represent these values? If so, the curves should be redrawn so that zero for total flow curves and the diastolic flow is at 11 mmHg and at 20 mmHg (solid lines) for systolic flow. The first part of the curve is usually assumed to be linear up to the point where autoregulation becomes manifest.

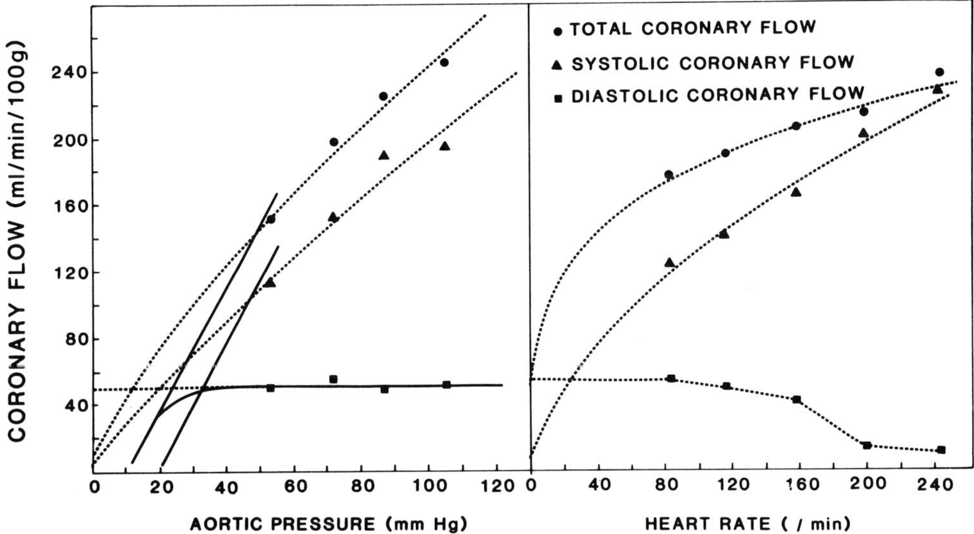

FIGURE 5. Total, systolic, and diastolic flow versus aortic pressure and heart rate. Total and systolic curves matched by geometric regression on mean values. See text for discussion.

The resultant postulated curves are shown by the solid lines in Fig. 5. Since we obtained no data at pressures less than 40 mmHg, they are estimates only. Besides the assumption that the model match produces curves crossing at the right points, it is assumed that: (1) diastolic flow is linear at low pressures and insensitive to overall pressure levels (see negative correlation coefficients [Table 2]); (2) systolic flow is sensitive to driving pressure and metabolic events (Table 2). The resultant conclusion is that flow is all diastolic at lower pressure levels. Most of the flow is also diastolic at very low heart rates.

These data then support the concept of a critical closing pressure which is increased during contraction. Whether or not this is also a part of a distant waterfall effect (14, 19) is not clear since these measurements were at the inflow. In regard to the substantial amount of systolic flow occurring during isovolumetric contraction, an active intramyocardial pump would appear to be involved (30).

The availability of data dependent on two different independent variables (i.e., aortic pressure and heart rate) also makes it possible to do a multiple regression analysis (29). Using a linear match, a family of curves was generated as shown in Fig. 6 (Total Flow = 24.2 + .26 HR + 1.83 AP; coefficient of correlation = .99, standard error of estimate = 5.0). These are similar to those of Laird et al.

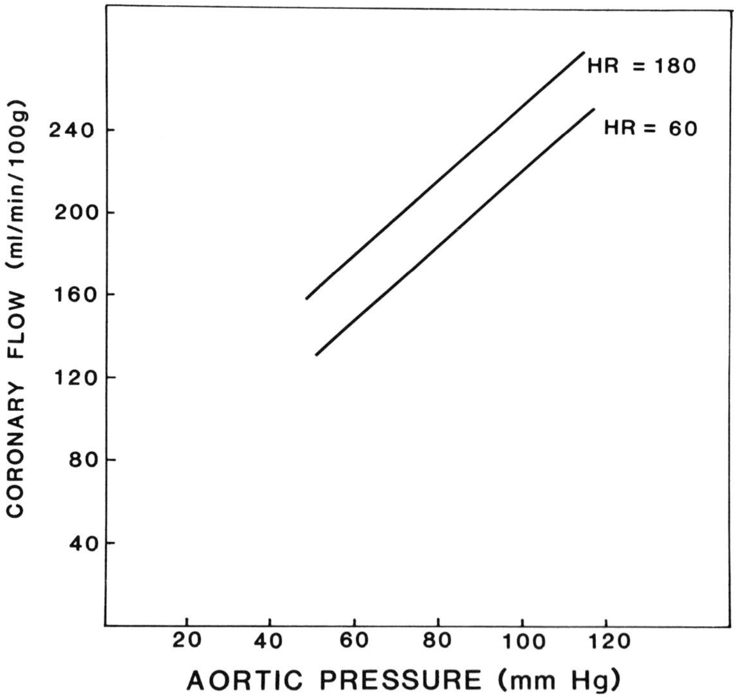

FIGURE 6. Predicted effects of heart rate and aortic pressure on coronary flow from multiple linear regression analysis of mean data. Actual curves are probably curvilinear.

(22) and show a much greater dependence on arterial pressure than on heart rate. This model has been discussed relative to the hypothesis of a single vasodilator substance (22). Again the generated data fails to show a proper low pressure intercept.

In summary, this study emphasizes the importance of mechanical factors in altering total coronary flow, and of systolic flow as the major inflow into epicardial vessels. Inflow can change dynamically to meet the metabolic needs of the myocardium during increases in pressure work or heart rate. No information was obtained, however, relative to how systolic flow might change to diastolic timing during passage through the coronary bed. Nineteen percent of total cardiac flow, about one fourth of systolic flow, occurred during isovolumetric contraction and was directly related to oxygen consumption. Total and systolic coronary flow were correlated with mean aortic pressure and with heart rate, when pressure and rate were independently varied. Diastolic flow did not increase as aortic pressure was increased and decreased markedly as heart rate was increased. When heart rate was increased systolic flow increased more than enough to keep total flow constant.

ACKNOWLEDGEMENTS

This work was partially supported by funds from the American Heart Association, South Carolina Affiliate: Public Health Service grants S08-RR-09093 and HL23700 from the National Institutes of Health: and by funds provided by Hoffman-LaRoche, Inc. The author acknowledges the capable technical assistance of Dr. E. Merrill Adams, Nancy Underwood, and Jay Castriotta.

REFERENCES

1.   Abel FL: Direct effects of ethanol on myocardial performance and coronary resistance. J Pharmacol Exp Ther (212):28-33, 1980.
2.   Abel FL: The effects of acetylstrophanthidin and glucocorticoids on canine left ventricular performance and coronary hemodynamics. Circ Shock (7):265-276, 1980.
3.   Abel FL, McCutcheon EP: Cardiovascular Function: Principles and Applications. Little, Brown, Boston, 1979, 424 pp.

4. Abel FL: Comparative evaluation of pressure and time factors in estimating left ventricular performance. J Appl Physiol (40):196-205, 1976.
5. Abel FL, Steinhoff F: Multiple-channel pulsed-field magnet driver. J Appl Physiol (23):121-124, 1967.
6. Abel FL: Maximal negative dp/dt as an indicator of end of systole. Am J Physiol (240):H676-H679, 1981.
7. Abel FL: Effects of aortic compliance on coronary blood flow. Fed Proc (42):1092, 1983.
8. Arts T, Kruger RTI, Garven WV, Lambregton GAC, Reneman RS: Propagation velocity and reflection of pressure wave in the canine coronary artery. Am J Physiol (237):H469-H474, 1979.
9. Caulfield JB, Borg TK, Abel FL: The effects of systole on left ventricular blood flow. **In**: Chazov E, Saks V, Rona G (eds) Advances in myocardiology 4. Plenum, New York, 1983, pp 379-393.
10. Caulfield JB, Borg TK: The collagen network of the heart. Lab Invest (40):364-372, 1979.
11. Chilian WM, Marcus ML: Phasic coronary blood flow velocity in intramural and epicardial coronary arteries. Circ Res (50):775-781, 1982.
12. Douglas JE, Greenfield JC, Jr: Epicardial coronary artery compliance in the dog. Circ Res (22):921-929, 1970.
13. Downey JM, Chagrasulis RW, Hemphill V: Quantitative study of intramyocardial compression in the fibrillating heart. Am J Physiol (237):H191-H196, 1979.
14. Downey JM, Kirk ES: Inhibition of coronary blood flow by a vascular waterfall mechanism. Circ Res (36):753-760, 1975.
15. Eng C, Jentzer JH, Kirk ES: Coronary capacitive effects on the high estimates of coronary critical closing pressure. Circulation (62):255, 1980.
16. Gregg DE, Fisher LC: Blood supply to the heart. **In**: Hamilton WF, Dorn P (eds) Handbook of physiology, Section 2, Circulation. American Physiological Society, Washington, 1963, vol. 2.
17. Gregg DE, Khouri EM, Rayford, CR: Systemic and coronary energetics in the resting unanesthetized dog. Circ Res (16):102-113, 1964.
18. Hammond GL, Austen WG: Drainage patterns of coronary arterial flow as determined from the isolated heart. Am J Physiol (212):1435-1440, 1967.
19. Hess DS, Bache RJ: Transmural right ventricular myocardial blood flow during systole in the awake dog. Circ Res (45):88-94, 1979.
20. Hoffman JIE, Buckberg GD: Transmural variations in myocardial perfusion. Prog Cardiol (5):37-89, 1976.
21. Khouri EM, Gregg DE, Lowensohn HS: Flow in the major branches of the coronary artery during experimental coronary insufficiency in the unanesthetized dog. Circ Res (23):99-109, 1968.

22. Laird JD, Breuls PN, Van Der Meer P, Spann JAE:
     Can a single vasodilator be responsible for both
     coronary autoregulation and metabolic vasodilation?
     Basic Res Cardiol (76):354-358, 1981.
23. Pitt B, Gregg DE: Coronary hemodynamic effects of
     increasing ventricular rate in the unanesthetized dog.
     Circ Res (22): 753-761, 1968.
24. Rankin JS, McHale PA, Arentzen CE, Ling D,
     Greenfield JC, Jr., Anderson RW: Three dimensional
     dynamic geometry of the left ventricle in the conscious
     dog. Circ Res (39):304-313, 1976.
25. Rayford CR, Huvos A, Khouri EM, Gregg DE: Some
     determinants of coronary flow in intact dogs.
     Physiologist (4):92, 1961.
26. Sabiston DC, Gregg DE: Effect of cardiac contraction
     on coronary blood flow. Circulation (15):14-20, 1957.
27. Shiang HH, Kupersmith J, Wiemann GF, Rhee CY,
     Litwak RS: Creating permanent complete heart block by
     indirect cauterization without atriotomy. Am J Physiol
     (233):H723-H726, 1977.
28. Siegel S: Nonparametric Statistics for the Behavioral
     Sciences. McGraw-Hill, New York, 1956, 312 pp.
29. Snedecor GW, Cochran WG: Statistical Methods 6th ed.
     Iowa State Press, Iowa, 1967.
30. Spann JAE, Breuls NPW, Laird JD: Diastolic-systolic
     coronary flow differences are caused by intramyocardial
     pump action in the anesthetized dog. Circ Res
     (49):584-553, 1981.
31. Spann JAE, Breuls NPW, Laird JD: Forward coronary
     flow normally seen in systole is the result of both
     forward and concealed back flow. Basic Res Cardiol
     (76):582-586, 1981.
32. Wiggers CJ: The interplay of coronary vascular
     resistance and myocardial compression in regulating
     coronary flow. Circ Res (2):271-279, 1954.

3

EVOLVING CONCEPTS OF CORONARY PRESSURE-FLOW RELATIONSHIPS

Francis J. Klocke, John M. Canty, Jr. and Robert E. Mates

Following Bellamy's 1978 report concerning diastolic coronary pressure-flow relationships (1), several laboratories have reinvestigated the relative roles of changes in driving pressure and resistance in physiological adjustments of coronary flow. Although most investigations have supported the position that coronary flow is influenced by a back pressure which exceeds coronary venous and/or left ventricular diastolic pressure, there has been concern that this

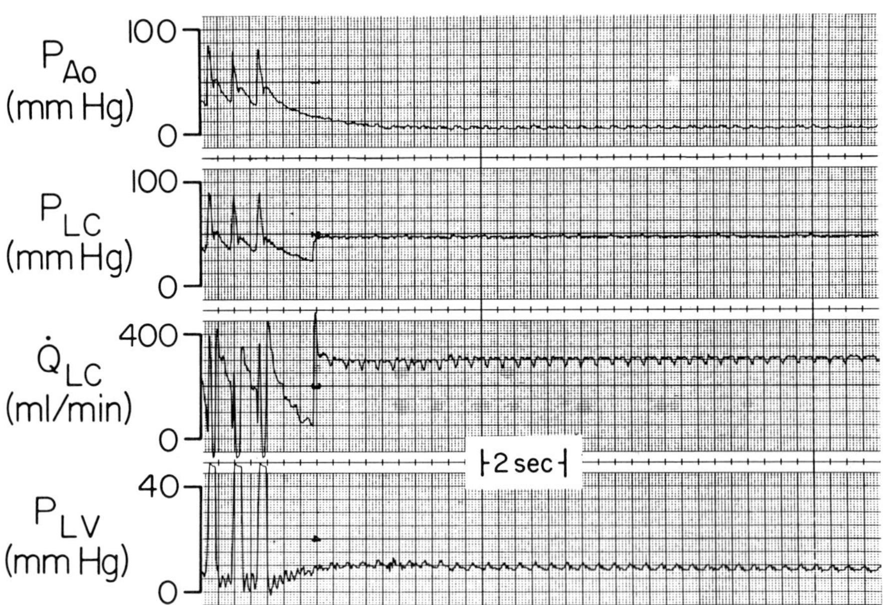

FIGURE 1.   Coronary inflow ($\dot{Q}_{LC}$) at constant inflow pressure (P_{LC}) during a long diastole in a bed vasodilated with adenosine. P_{Ao}, LV = aortic, left ventricular pressures. (Reprinted with permission, Am. J. Physiol. (243) [Heart Circ. Physiol. (12)]:H796-H802, 1982.)

finding is somehow a methodological peculiarity of the experimental approaches used to study it.

CHANGES IN BACK PRESSURE AND/OR CONDUCTANCE DURING LONG DIASTOLES

One concern has been that conductance and/or back pressure [which is commonly referred to as "zero-flow pressure" ($P_{f=\emptyset}$)] do not remain constant during a long diastole. Figure 1 examines this issue in the vasodilated bed of an open-chest heart blocked dog, showing aortic pressure, left circumflex pressure, circumflex inflow and left ventricular diastolic pressure. The circumflex artery has been cannulated and connected to a servovalve which allows the coronary bed to be perfused with any desired pressure waveform (2). During a long diastole following cessation of pacing, perfusion is switched from the usual aortic pressure waveform to a constant pressure level of 45 mm Hg. There is initially a transient overshoot in flow when constant pressure perfusion is initiated. This overshoot is no doubt capacitive in origin; a few hundred msec are required for flow to become steady even with the nearly "square wave" change in inflow pressure. For the subsequent 1$\emptyset$ seconds, flow remains constant with the usual atrial cove effects seen in heart-blocked preparations but no other evidence of a changing conductance or $P_{f=\emptyset}$, or of a more slowly discharging capacitance. This constancy of flow in the vasodilated bed is a regular finding as long as left ventricular pressure and coronary venous pressure remain constant.

Changes in $P_{f=\emptyset}$ and/or conductance are difficult problems during long diastoles in which autoregulation is operative. Figure 2 shows another analog record in which coronary perfusion pressure is raised to a new constant level shortly after the onset of a long diastole. After the initial transient, flow decreases continuously over the next several seconds, falling from 12$\emptyset$ to 7$\emptyset$ ml/min. This reduction in flow is thought to reflect the normal autoregulatory process, resulting in this case from an increase in perfusion pressure and the decrease in cardiac demand associated with cessation of pacing. While the magnitude of the autoregulatory response during a long diastole can be minimized in several ways, we find the response always to be present to some degree in beds which are not maximally vasodilated.

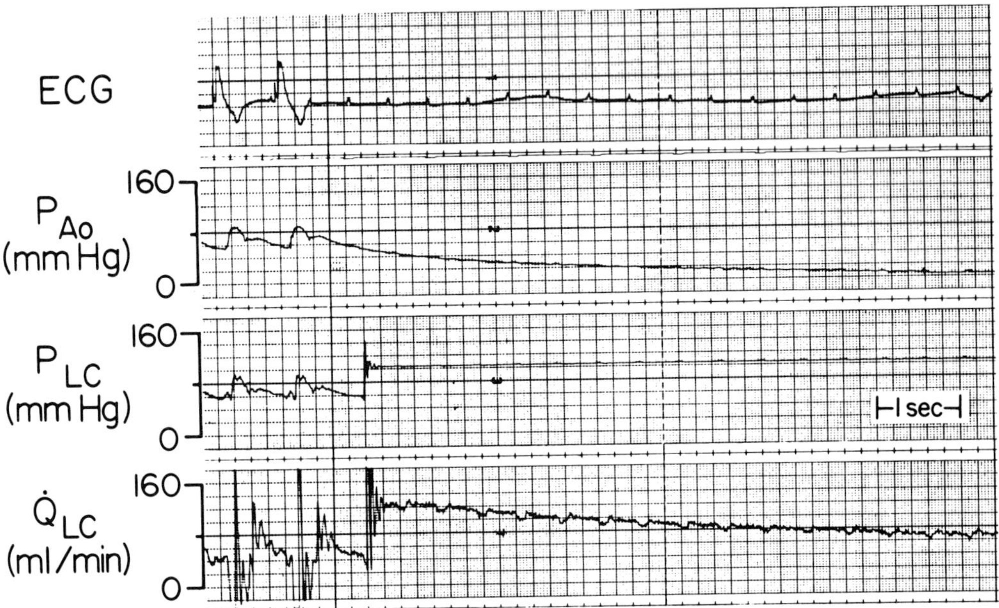

FIGURE 2.   Coronary inflow ($\dot{Q}_{LC}$) at constant inflow pressure (P_{LC}) during a long diastole in a bed with vasomotor tone intact. P_{Ao} = aortic pressure.

EFFECTS OF CAPACITANCE DURING LONG DIASTOLES

Reactive elements of impedance, i.e., inertia and capacitance, also require consideration. Current information suggests that inertial effects are small during long diastoles and these will not be considered further here. However, as originally pointed out by Eng, Jentzer and Kirk (3), effects of capacitive flow are an important issue.

Inflow measured in a proximal coronary artery necessarily underestimates flow in more distal portions of the bed as coronary inflow pressure falls. Conversely, measured inflow exceeds more distal flow when inflow pressure is increasing. The important question is the magnitude of this capacitive flow and its effects on the intercept and shape of experimentally determined pressure-flow relationships.

Although capacitance is distributed throughout the coronary bed, the major portion presumably lies on the venous side of the circulation. Two considerations suggest that the more distally located components of capacitance may affect diastolic pressure-inflow relationships less than proximal ones. As blood encounters increasing resistance upstream of the capillaries, variations in local intra-arterial pressure — and therefore variations in local intravascular volume — are damped progressively. In addition, if a vascular "waterfall" is present, capacitance located downstream to the waterfall point need not be involved in inflow regulation. For this latter reason, persistence of coronary venous outflow beyond the point of inflow cessation during a long diastole [as reported by some (4) but not all (5) workers] does not exclude a waterfall.

Efforts to elucidate effects of capacitive flow have led to new information about diastolic coronary input impedance. Experimental studies based on in vivo perturbations of inflow pressure with a sine wave or "ramp" function (6) indicate that the capacitance influenced by this perturbation can be modeled surprisingly well as a single element located upstream of the major portion of coronary resistance. Absolute values are consistent with the presumed precapillary location. These values depend on distending pressure, vasomotor tone and viscoelastic effects. Their magnitude varies inversely with distending pressure, changing approximately three-fold over the range of pressures ordinarily encountered during a long diastole. Values at any given pressure are approximately twice as large in the maximally vasodilated bed as in the normally autoregulating bed, i.e., the bed with "tone intact". Viscoelastic effects relating to the rate at which the artery is distended or relaxes are quantitatively less important; capacitance decreases as the vessel is distended more rapidly.

During consideration of possible effects of coronary capacitance on diastolic pressure-flow relationships, attention has also focused on an "intramyocardial" capacitance of larger magnitude than thusfar identified by perturbations of inflow pressure. Spaan (7) has postulated that systole causes a capacitive discharge which can produce backflow in coronary arteries as well as augmented systolic venous outflow. The location and magnitude of the capacitive elements involved in these effects of systolic contraction remain to be defined. Spaan's estimate of "intramyocardial" capacitance of 0.07 ml/mm Hg/100 g was based on a time-constant derived from the pattern of arterial pressure decay following inflow occlusion in a bed with vasomotor tone intact. Since autoregulatory vasodilation no doubt occurred during the pressure decay, the reported time constant probably reflected variations in resistance as well as capacitive effects. While the capacitance value reported by Spaan is consistent with earlier estimates of intramyocardial blood pressure-volume relationships, the question again is what portion of total capacitance influences pressure-flow relations during long diastoles. Inflow recordings following a step-change in inflow pressure in the vasodilated bed in our own laboratory (Figure 1) and that of Downey (8) show capacitive time constants of ~100 msec and indicate absolute values of capacitance which are an order of magnitude less than estimated by Spaan. The longer time constants observed following a step change in inflow pressure in the non-vasodilated bed are influenced by autoregulation as well as capacitance and are therefore more difficult to interpret.

While dealing with capacitive effects during long diastoles, we need to recall that capacitive flow (CF) depends on two factors, the absolute value of capacitance (C) and the instantaneous rate at which transmural pressure is changing, i.e., $CF = C \times dP/dt$. Variations in the magnitude of capacitive effects in different studies of diastolic pressure-flow relationships may relate to differences in the rate of change of inflow pressure during long diastoles. In studies in which aortic pressure decays spontaneously, dP/dt is relatively high in the early portion of the long diastole but can fall to nearly negligible levels by the time inflow ceases. For example, in Bellamy's published record of a long diastole lasting ~2.5 seconds (1, figure 1) the rate of decrease of coronary inflow pressure was ~60 mm Hg/sec at the onset of diastole but had fallen to ~3 mm/sec at the point at which $P_{f=0}$ was recorded. Thus, although absolute values of capacitance increase 2-3 fold over the range of spontaneous pressure decay during a typical long diastole, capacitive flow may be an order of magnitude less at the time of $P_{f=0}$ than at the onset of diastole because of large reductions in dP/dt as diastole proceeds. This line of reasoning is consistent with the view that capacitive effects on $P_{f=\emptyset}$ may be less important than capacitive effects on the shape of the pressure-flow relationship in studies in which coronary inflow is allowed to decrease spontaneously, in tandem with aortic pressure, during long diastoles.

CAPACITANCE-FREE RELATIONSHIPS DERIVED FROM CONSTANT-PRESSURE PERFUSION DURING SEVERAL LONG DIASTOLES

Because of the potential importance of capacitive effects when changing pressure and flow are used to construct diastolic pressure-flow relationships, experimental approaches which can obviate capacitive flow have been of interest. If the coronary artery in a vasodilated bed is perfused at constant pressure during a long diastole, reactive effects should disappear after an initial transient, with the steady-state flow level representing the purely resistive component of impedance. Flow during later stages of a long diastole in an autoregulating bed should be free of reactive effects if the time constant for the initial transient is short in relation to the time constant for autoregulation. If flows are measured during several diastoles in which levels of constant pressure are varied, data from the several diastoles can be combined to obtain a capacitance- and inertia-free pressure-flow relationship. At least four laboratories have now reported comparisons of pressure-flow relationships constructed in this fashion with those obtained during declining inflow pressure. All agree that coronary capacitance results in an overestimate of $P_{f=\emptyset}$ during declining inflow pressure measurements. Variations in the magnitude of this overestimate are no doubt related, at least in part, to variations in experimental preparations and protocols:

[1] Our laboratory (9) studied the cannulated circumflex bed of open-chest heart blocked dogs anesthetized with pentobarbital and paced at 100 bpm. During constant pressure runs flows were measured 1-4 seconds after the concurrent cessation of pacing and onset of perfusion from a constant-pressure reservoir. During declining pressure runs, the circumflex artery was perfused from the aorta, with the latter being vented when pacing was terminated so that

circumflex inflow ceased before ventricular escape (2-8 seconds).
With vasomotor tone intact, zero-flow pressure averaged 22 mm Hg
during constant-pressure perfusion, as opposed to 28 mm Hg with
declining pressure. During vasodilation, $P_{f=0}$ was 11 mm Hg with
constant-pressure perfusion and 13 mm Hg with declining pressure.
In both situations, capacitance-free values of $P_{f=0}$ were systematically greater than right atrial or left ventricular diastolic
pressure. Additional points of interest were [1] that pressure-
flow relationships were curvilinear and better fit by a second-
order polynomial than a linear fit despite high correlation coefficients, and [2] that values of $P_{f=0}$ with vasomotor tone intact
varied directly with the level of diastolic pressure immediately
prior to long diastoles.

[2] Dole and Bishop (10) cannulated the left circumflex artery
of closed-chest dogs under alpha chloralose anesthesia and produced
long diastoles by vagal stimulation following intracoronary atropine. Pre-arrest heart rates averaged 112 bpm. Dynamic pressure-
flow relationships were obtained by decreasing coronary pressure at
a nominal decay rate of 40 mm Hg/sec; constant-pressure relationships were constructed by producing a step change in coronary
pressure several seconds after the onset of diastolic arrest, with
steady-state pressure and flow points taken 500 msec later. With
coronary tone intact and pre-arrest coronary pressure held at 125
mm Hg, $P_{f=0}$ was 37 mm Hg during constant-pressure perfusion, as
opposed to 48 mm Hg with declining pressure. At a pre-arrest
coronary pressure of 75 mm Hg, $P_{f=0}$ fell to 21 mm Hg during
constant-pressure perfusion, and to 34 mm Hg with declining pressure. During adenosine-induced vasodilation, $P_{f=0}$ was 15 mm Hg
during constant-pressure perfusion and 24 mm Hg with declining
pressure.

[3] Eng, Jentzer and Kirk (3) perfused the left main coronary
artery of open-chest pentobarbital-anesthetized heart blocked dogs
paced at a rate of 130 beats per minute. Constant-pressure flow
values were obtained by simultaneously discontinuing pacing and
switching to reservoir perfusion. In cases in which autoregulatory
flow reductions were noted during the long diastole, flow values
were taken immediately after induction of diastole (within 200

msec). With coronary tone intact, $P_{f=0}$ was 11 mm Hg during constant-pressure perfusion, as opposed to 25 mm Hg with declining pressure. During vasodilation, $P_{f=0}$ was 11 mm Hg during constant-pressure perfusion and 14 mm Hg with declining pressure. Similar findings were obtained in four animals in which flow in the circumflex artery was measured at constant pressure using a reservoir connected to one arm of a T-tube inserted into the thoracic aorta. Thus, although $P_{f=0}$ was systematically greater than left atrial and coronary venous pressure with and without vasodilation, values during constant-pressure perfusion were felt to be independent of vasomotor tone. Coronary pressures prior to long diastoles, and rates of coronary pressure decay during long diastoles, were not specified. It also seems possible that data taken within 200 msec of the onset of diastole during constant-pressure perfusion were influenced by inadvertent inclusion of capacitive flow related to refilling of an intramyocardial capacitance emptied during the preceding systole.

[4] Downey, Lee and Chambers (11) used a left main preparation to study differences between constant- and declining-pressure relationships with vasomotor tone operative. A step change in pressure was produced shortly after the onset of a long diastole and flow was measured 200 msec after this transition. Coronary pressure immediately prior to long diastoles varied from 130 mm Hg to 50 mm Hg. For a pre-arrest coronary pressure of 130 mm Hg, $P_{f=0}$ was 27 mm Hg during constant-pressure coronary perfusion and 39 mm Hg with declining pressure. For a pre-arrest coronary pressure of 50 mm Hg, $P_{f=0}$ fell to 18 mm Hg during constant-pressure perfusion and to 23 mm Hg with declining pressure.

All four of these studies agree that there is a back pressure to coronary flow which is systematically greater than coronary venous or left atrial pressure. Our laboratory (9), Dole and Bishop (10) and Downey, Lee and Chambers (11) find that the magnitude of $P_{f=0}$ is influenced by vasomotor tone as well as non-tone-dependent factors, and that $P_{f=0}$ varies directly with coronary pressure prior to diastolic arrest when tone is operative. The absence of a significant influence of vasomotor tone on $P_{f=0}$ in the study of Eng, Jentzer and Kirk may relate to some of the experimental conditions noted above.

POSSIBLE EFFECTS OF COLLATERAL FLOW

Studies in which diastolic pressure-flow relationships are determined in a cannulated portion of, as opposed to the total, left coronary bed are potentially subject to effects of collateral flow. In such a preparation, a pressure gradient often exists between the artery supplying the test portion of the bed and the arteries perfusing the remainder of the heart. Studies of Messina, et al., (12, personal communication) indicate that this gradient must be at least 40 mm Hg for measurable collateral flow to occur.

In studies employing constant-pressure perfusion during long diastoles, gradients between a cannulated coronary artery and coronary arteries perfused from the aorta vary during the long diastole. When pressure in the cannulated artery is higher than aortic pressure, collateral flow from the cannulated bed to the non-cannulated bed is possible. This flow will be included in the measured value of inflow into the cannulated bed. Its magnitude should vary with the level of constant pressure and, at any given pressure, should increase with time as aortic pressure falls. When pressure in the cannulated artery is less than aortic pressure (but greater than $P_{f=0}$), there may be collateral flow into the cannulated bed. This flow will not be included in the measured value of inflow. Its magnitude is expected to decrease with time as aortic pressure falls; measured inflow should increase correspondingly, to maintain pressure in the cannulated artery at the pre-set level.

The point of primary concern is whether values of $P_{f=0}$ derived from constant-pressure perfusion studies could be artifactually high because of unappreciated collateral flow. Among the four studies employing constant-pressure perfusion cited above, only those from our laboratory (9) and Dole and Bishop (10) are potentially subject to effects of collateral flow. As noted above, all four reports agree there is a back pressure to flow in the vasodilated bed which exceeds coronary venous and/or left ventricular intracavitary pressure. The agreement of Downey, Lee and Chambers' findings in a left main preparation (11) with those of ourselves and Dole and Bishop argues against the possibility that the higher values of $P_{f=0}$

observed with vasomotor tone intact in these three studies are an artifact of collateral flow. Potential effects of collateral flow on measured values of $P_{f=0}$ in cannulated preparations may be minimized by the decline in aortic pressure (and corresponding reduction in pressure gradient between the non-cannulated and cannulated beds) which occurs as diastole proceeds. If a finite time is required for pre-existent collateral channels to open when an appropriate pressure gradient is established (13), this factor could also minimize effects of collateral flow on $P_{f=0}$ (which is usually measured within a few seconds after establishment of the gradient).

CAPACITANCE-FREE PRESSURE-FLOW RELATIONSHIPS DURING SINGLE LONG DIASTOLES IN THE VASODILATED BED

Capacitive effects seem sufficiently important to limit the amount of new information which can be gained from studies in which

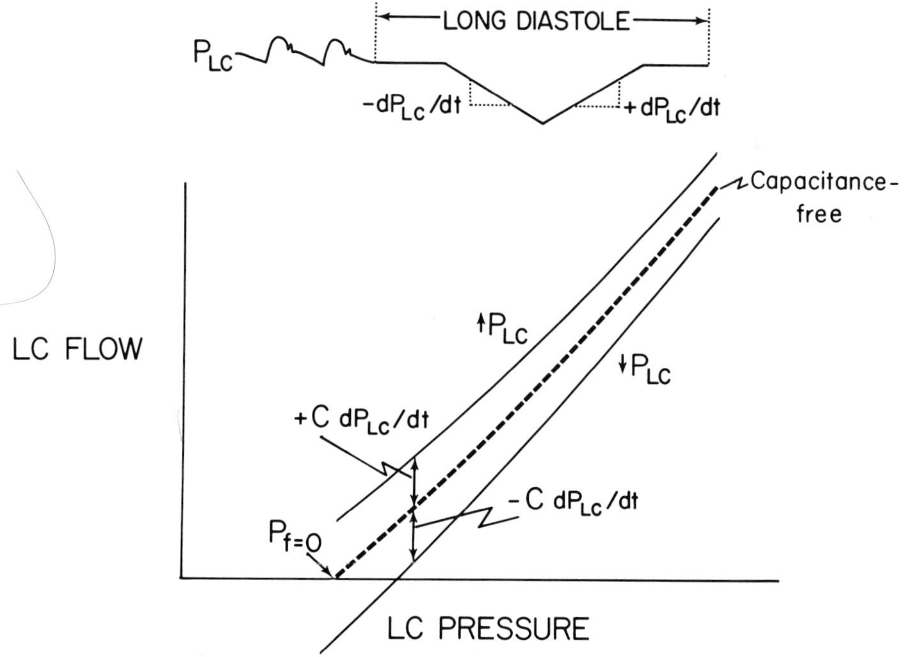

FIGURE 3. Experimental approach for obtaining capacitance-free pressure-flow relationships during single long diastoles. See text for details.

coronary pressure is allowed to change in an uncontrolled fashion. While it remains reasonable to construct a pressure-flow relationship from several long diastoles employing constant-pressure perfusion, this is a rather time-consuming process in which control of pertinent hemodynamic variables can be difficult. An alternate approach which we regard as promising in the vasodilated bed is shown in Figure 3. A servovalve capable of perfusing a cannulated coronary bed with any desired pressure wave form (2) is used to manipulate coronary inflow pressure (P_{LC}) during a long diastole. During the initial portion of the diastole, circumflex pressure is decreased at a constant rate ($-dP_{LC}/dt$) producing the conventional pressure-flow relationship labeled $\downarrow P_{LC}$. The direction of the linear pressure ramp is then reversed, so that a second pressure-flow relationship, labeled $\uparrow P_{LC}$, is recorded while pressure is increasing at the same magnitude ($+dP_{LC}/dt$). Because of coronary capacitance, measured inflow underestimates flow at the capillary level during the down ramp and overestimates it during the up ramp. The capacitance-free pressure-flow relationship is expected to lie between the bounds defined by the down and up ramp data. In order to account for capacitance quantitatively, we have initially employed the parallel RC model mentioned above. In this model, capacitive flow at any given pressure ($C \cdot dP_{LC}/dt$) is equal in magnitude but opposite in direction during the down and up ramps. The capacitance-free relationship therefore lies midway between the down and up ramp curves on the flow axis. Since the magnitude of capacitive flow varies directly with the magnitude of dP/dt, the separation between down and up ramp curves can be minimized by using slow rates of pressure change. Capacitance-free relationships derived from down and up ramps have been consistently curvilinear (14) and have corresponded closely to relationships derived from constant-pressure perfusion during several long diastoles (15). Using the down and up ramp approach, increases in preload have been found to alter capacitance-free diastolic pressure-flow relationships substantially in the vasodilated bed (14).

LONG DIASTOLES VS. NORMAL CARDIAC CYCLES

Extension of findings during long diastoles to normal cardiac cycles involves additional issues not yet clarified. Since the major

portion of coronary inflow occurs during diastole, initial attempts
to quantify pressure-flow behavior have understandably focused on
this period. The ability to produce long diastoles experimentally
has provided a convenient method for generating a prolonged quasi-
steady state in which pressure-flow relationships can be studied,
with separation of resistive components of impedance from reactive
ones.

While systolic flow is ordinarily small, the interaction between
systole and diastole may play a significant role in the magnitude and
distribution of total coronary flow, as suggested by Hoffman (16).
Since venous outflow occurs primarily during systole, refilling of
vessels emptied during systole must occur at least during the early
stages of diastole. Spaan (7) has suggested the concept of an intramyocardial pump coupled to a large capacitance to explain the

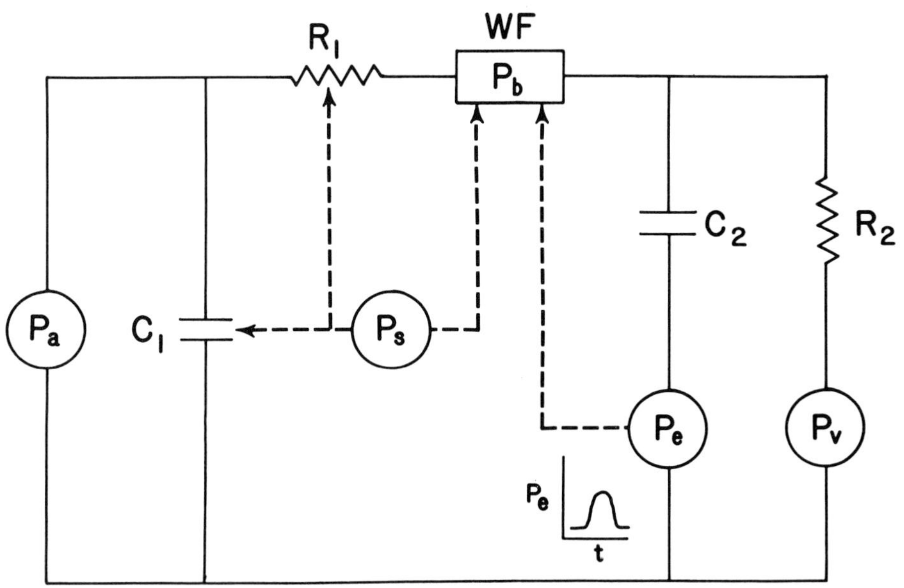

FIGURE 4. Modified waterfall model of the coronary bed. See text
for details.

difference between phasic coronary inflow and outflow. He also
pointed out that the vascular waterfall model suggested by Downey and
Kirk (17) cannot explain retrograde systolic flow observed at low
perfusion pressures. Downey and Kirk's original electrical analog
contained diodes to prevent backflow. The concept of a waterfall is
consistent with the observed pressure-flow behavior observed in long
diastoles. A modified description of the waterfall, in a model in-
corporating Spaan's intramyocardial pump, is one possible explanation
for the observed pressure-flow relationships. Such a model is shown
in Figure 4. In this model P_a represents aortic pressure and P_v
coronary venous pressure, P_e the extravascular or intramyocardial
pressure, and P_s an effective extravascular pressure due to smooth
muscle tone. Two resistive and two capacitive elements are shown as
suggested by Spaan. The waterfall (WF) in the model is a pressure
regulator. Pressure at this point in the circulation is prevented
from falling below an effective back pressure, determined by P_e and
P_s, by partial collapse of the vessel. However, if pressure distal
to the waterfall is greater than the proximal pressure and the
regulated value, retrograde flow can occur.

Since phasic pressure and flow can be measured only at the inlet
(coronary artery) and outlet (coronary sinus) it is not possible to
establish unequivocally the anatomic location of the elements in such
a model. In perturbing inlet pressure and flow with a sine wave as
described earlier (6), we were unable to identify two capacitive
elements. This suggests that the capacitance C_2, and therefore the
intramyocardial pump, lies distal to a major portion of the microcirculatory resistance. Spaan estimated the resistance R_1 to constitute 63% of total resistance. It therefore seems unlikely that the
intramyocardial capacitance plays a crucial role in controlling diastolic inflow. However, during a normal diastole, systolic emptying
of vessels may alter initial diastolic impedance to flow, as the ca-
pacitor C_2 is recharged. As discussed previously, it appears that
the waterfall is affected by smooth muscle tone P_s as well as precapillary capacitance C_1 and the resistance R_1. These relationships
are indicated by dotted lines in the figure.

The time course of the extravascular pressure P_e has not been
studied in detail. Spaan suggested that it is proportional to left

ventricular pressure. Bellamy's observation that apparent diastolic back pressure to flow is influenced by coronary sinus pressure (18) suggests that the blood content of the myocardium may play a role in regulating extravascular pressure, as expanding blood vessels compress surrounding tissue. Figure 5 shows schematically a possible time course of extravascular pressure P_e compared to left ventricular pressure P_{LV} and aortic pressure P_{AO}. P_e is assumed to rise in early systole as P_{LV} rises. The peak systolic value of P_e is shown as lower than P_{LV}. P_e probably varies across the ventricular wall and the model in Figure 5 represents only a lumped average. Extravascular pressure may approach ventricular pressure at the subendocardium. During systole, the average blood volume in the myocardium decreases as blood is expelled. If P_e is dependent on blood volume, its average value may be lower than P_{LV} during early diastole, and may rise

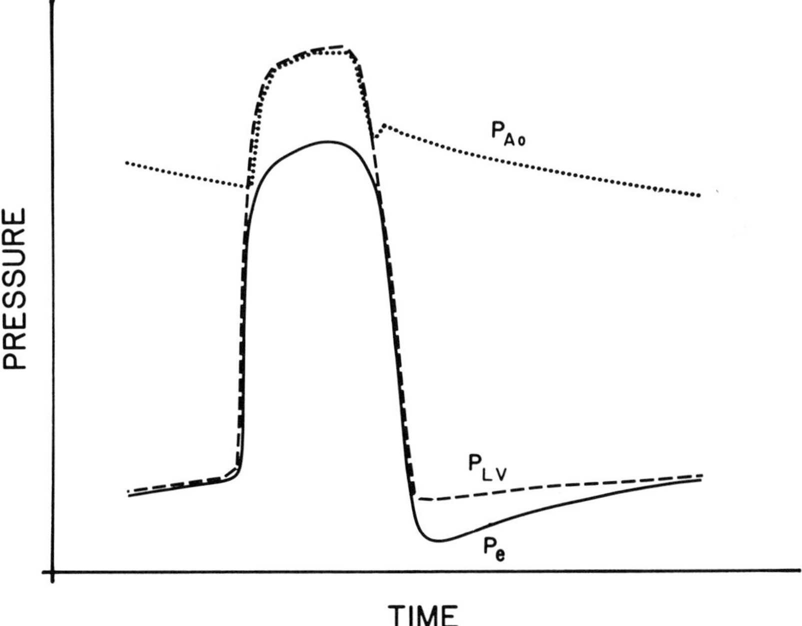

FIGURE 5. Hypothetical representation of a possible time-course of extravascular pressure (Pe) compared to left ventricular pressure (P_{LV}) and aortic pressure (P_{AO}) during a cardiac cycle.

more rapidly than P_{LV} as myocardial blood volume increases with
coronary inflow. Thus, the driving pressure for coronary flow could
be higher in early diastole, both because arterial pressure is high
and back pressure is low. The phenomenon might not be detected in
long diastoles unless measurements were made very early in diastole.
In addition, systolic compression may contribute to a redistribution of
flow across the myocardial wall. Thus, studies conducted during a
long diastole provide important information about impedance to diastolic inflow, but need to be supplemented by information not pres-
ently available concerning the interactions between systole and
diastole.

In the hope of avoiding reactive effects, calculations of diastolic coronary resistance have sometimes been based on the ratio of
end-diastolic pressure to end-diastolic flow rather than the ratio of

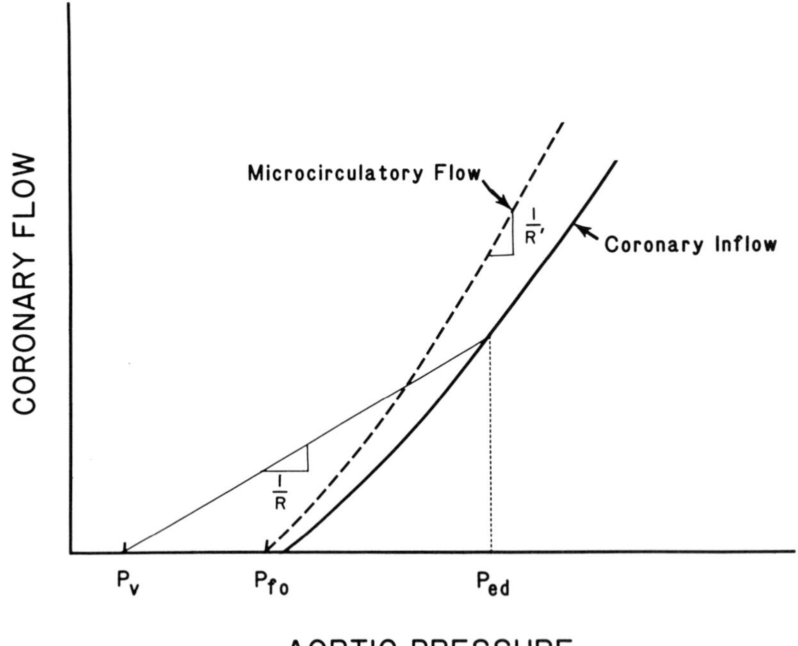

FIGURE 6. Complexities of attempts to quantify resistance from measurements of arterial pressure and coronary inflow. See text for
details.

mean diastolic pressure and flow. As the preceeding discussion has indicated, input impedance is a complicated quantity. Some of these complexities are indicated in Figure 6. The heavy solid line represents coronary inflow as a function of aortic pressure, determined while pressure is decreasing. Flow in the microcirculation, shown by the dashed line, will be higher due to capacitive discharge. Pressure at the end of a normal diastole is shown as P_{ed}, coronary venous pressure as P_v, and capacitance-free zero-flow pressure as P_{f0}. The traditional end-diastolic resistance is shown as R. The actual resistance of the bed at end-diastole is R'. R and R' differ for several reasons. First, the back pressure to flow is higher than venous pressure. Second, measured inflow is less than microcirculatory flow because of capacitive effects. Finally, conductance of the bed varies as a function of pressure, as reflected in the curvature of the pressure-flow relationship. Thus, the calculated resistance R may bear little relation to the actual resistance R'. Vlahakes and colleagues (19) have suggested that effects of capacitance may be cancelled by calculating a resistance based on the full-cycle mean pressure – mean flow relationship. Interpretation of such a resistance is still complicated by the effects of back pressure and curvature of the pressure-flow relationship, and by the likelihood that back pressure and conductance at any given pressure differ in systole and diastole. Thus, it seems increasingly clear that attempts to estimate inflow impedance from any single calculation of resistance have limited value.

REFERENCES

1. Bellamy RF: Diastolic coronary artery pressure-flow relations in the dog. Circ Res (43):92-101, 1978.

2. Canty JM, Mates RE: A programmable pressure control system for coronary flow studies. Am J Physiol (243)[Heart Circ Physiol(12)]: H796-H802, 1982.

3. Eng C, Jentzer JH, Kirk ES: The effects of the coronary capacitance on the interpretation of diastolic pressure-flow relationships. Circ Res (50):334-341, 1982.

4. Chilian WP, Bohling BA, Marcus ML: Interpretations of zero-flow pressures in the coronary circulation. Circ (66):II-43, 1982 (abstract).

5. Bellamy RF, O'Benar JD: Pressure-flow hysteresis loops in the

coronary circulation. Fed Proc (41):1097, 1982 (abstract).

6. Canty JM Jr, Klocke FJ, Mates RE: Pressure and tone dependence of coronary diastolic input impedance and capacitance. Submitted for publication. [Work in this paper has been reported in preliminary form in Fed Proc (41):1097, 1982 and Circ (66):II-42, 1982.]

7. Spaan JAE, Breuls NPW, Laird JD: Diastolic-systolic coronary flow differences are caused by intramyocardial pump action in the anesthetized dog. Circ Res (49):584-593, 1981.

8. Downey J, Lee J, Chambers D: Capacitive time constant of the coronary artery. Circ (66):II-42, 1982 (abstract).

9. Klocke FJ, Weinstein IR, Klocke JF, Ellis AK, Kraus DR, Mates RE, Canty JM, Anbar RD, Romanowski RR, Wallmeyer KW, Echt MP: Zero-flow pressures and pressure-flow relationships during single long diastoles in the canine coronary bed before and after maximum vasodilation. J Clin Invest (68):970-980, 1981.

10. Dole WP, Bishop VS: Influence of autoregulation and capacitance on diastolic coronary artery pressure-flow relationships in the dog. Circ Res (51):261-270, 1982.

11. Downey J, Lee J, Chambers D: Coronary critical closing pressure corrected for coronary capacitance effects. Physiologist (24):26, 1981 (abstract).

12. Messina LM, Hanley FL, Hoffman JIE: Comparison of left main and circumflex coronary artery pressure-flow relations. Fed Proc (42):1092, 1983 (abstract).

13. Khouri EM, Gregg DE, McGranahan GM Jr: Regression and reappearance of coronary collaterals. Am J Physiol (220):655-661, 1971.

14. Aversano T, Klocke FJ, Mates RE, Canty JM: Preload-induced alterations in capacitance-free diastolic pressure-flow relationships. Am J Physiol [Heart Circ Physiol], in press.

15. Canty JM Jr, Mates RE, Klocke FJ: Rapid determination of capacitance-free pressure-flow relationships during single diastoles. Fed Proc (42):1092, 1983 (abstract).

16. Hoffman JIE, Baer RW, Hanley FL, Messina LM, Grattan MT: Regulation of transmural myocardial blood flow. In: Mates RE, Nerem RM, Stein PD (ed) Mechanics of the Coronary Circulation. American Society of Mechanical Engineers, New York, 1983, pp. 1-17.

17. Downey JM, Kirk ES: Inhibition of coronary blood flow by a vascular waterfall mechanism. Circ Res (36):753-760, 1975.

18. Bellamy RF, Lowensohn HS, Ehrlich W, Baer RW: Effect of coronary sinus occlusion on coronary pressure-flow relations. Am J Physiol (239) [Heart Circ Physiol (8)]:H57-H64, 1980.

19. Vlahakes GJ, Baer RW, Uhlig PN, Verrier ED, Bristow JD, Hoffman JIE: Adrenergic influence in the coronary circulation of conscious dogs during maximal vasodilation with adenosine. Circ Res (51):371-384, 1982.

4

TRANSMURAL FLOW DURING PHYSIOLOGICAL VASODILATION

H. FRED DOWNEY

It is well established that coronary blood flow is influenced by 1) metabolic activity of the myocardium and 2) by mechanical forces generated by contracting cardiac muscle. Of course, these factors are interrelated. Usually they are positively correlated with increases in cardiac function associated with increases in myocardial metabolism and with increases in coronary blood flow (1,2,3). On the other hand, cardiac function directly influences coronary blood flow, and this direct effect may oppose that caused indirectly by associated changes in myocardial metabolism. Thus, it is appropriate for this symposium to address the question of metabolic versus mechanical control of the coronary circulation.

With the advent of high fidelity measurements of coronary blood flow, it was evident that cardiac systole impeded coronary blood flow, particularly into left ventricular myocardium. Such records led investigators to proclaim that the beating heart inhibits its own blood supply. Cardiac contraction does not only cause phasic changes in coronary flow during the cardiac cycle, but the beating heart also generates a component of extravascular resistance which limits diastolic as well as systolic flow. This was demonstrated by Gregg and Sabiston (4), who caused asystole by vagal stimulation and observed that coronary flow increased abruptly upon cessation of cardiac contraction. Since the increase in coronary flow following asystole was modest, the extravascular component of coronary resistance was small compared to the resistance due to normal vascular tone. With such a large ratio of vascular to extravascular resistance under normal conditions, changes in vascular tone can readily compensate for changes in extravascular resistance due to altered cardiac function. However, this might not be the case when coronary vascular resistance is significantly decreased. Thus, I will discuss findings from our investigations of transmural blood flow during coronary vasodilation.

Downey and Kirk (5) demonstrated that systolic coronary flow is distributed subepicardially, although the left ventricular free wall is normally perfused uniformily (6,7). To accomplish this, diastolic flow must be distributed preferentially to the subendocardium. Moir and DeBra (6) postulated that an autoregulatory adjustment of vascular tone, i.e., greater constriction of subepicardial arterioles compared to subendocardial arterioles, was responsible for maintaining uniform transmural perfusion. If, however, metabolically-coupled autoregulation is the only mechanism available to adjust blood flow to regional requirements, dilation of the subepicardial coronary vasculature would result in relative underperfusion of the subendocardium. We investigated this possibility in anesthetized, open-chest dogs whose coronary vasculature was dilated physiologically by 90 sec of ischemia or pharmacologically by intra-coronary infusion of papaverine or adenosine (7). Regional coronary flow was measured with 8-10 micron radioactive microspheres.

The duration of the ischemic period and the dosage of the dilator agents were adjusted to cause maximal coronary vasodilation. Figure 1 demonstrates that left ventricular perfusion remained uniform even though coronary flow increased by more than 500%. Since the coronary vasculature was maximally dilated, some mechanism other than a transmural gradient of vascular tone must have been responsible for preferential subendocardial perfusion during diastole to compensate for underperfusion of this region during systole.

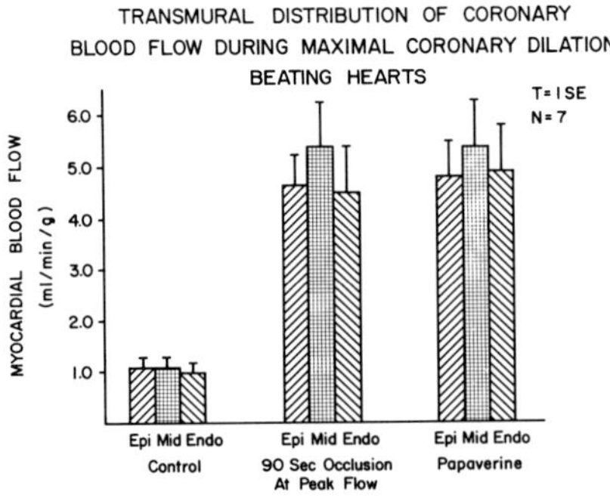

FIGURE 1. Transmural blood flow under control conditions at peak reactive hyperemia following 90-sec coronary artery occlusion, and during maximal coronary vasodilation induced by intracoronary infusion of papaverine.

To demonstrate this other mechanism, we examined the transmural flow distribution in the absence of rhythmic cardiac contraction (7). _In situ_

canine hearts were fibrillated, and their coronary circulations were retro-
perfused with venous blood containing papaverine or adenosine. Figure 2
shows transmural flow distributions in these weakly fibrillating hearts.
Again, coronary flow was markedly increased, but now in the absence of
rhythmic cardiac contraction, left ventricular blood flow was distributed
preferentially toward the subendocardium. There, subendocardial flow exceeded subepicardial flow by 36%. In the absence of transmural gradients
of vascular tone or extravascular compression, this flow distribution should
reflect the hydraulic conductivity of the left ventricular coronary vasculature. Thus, this flow gradient favoring the subendocardium is consistent
with a gradient of vascularity favoring the subendocardium. This gradient
of vascularity may result from either a greater number of vessels in the
subendocardial region or slightly larger arterioles supplying that region.
We have found confirmatory evidence of this gradient of vascularity in an
investigation of small vessel blood volume across the left ventricular free
wall (8). In that study, small vessel blood volume was consistently greater
in the subendocardial region than in the subepicardial region.

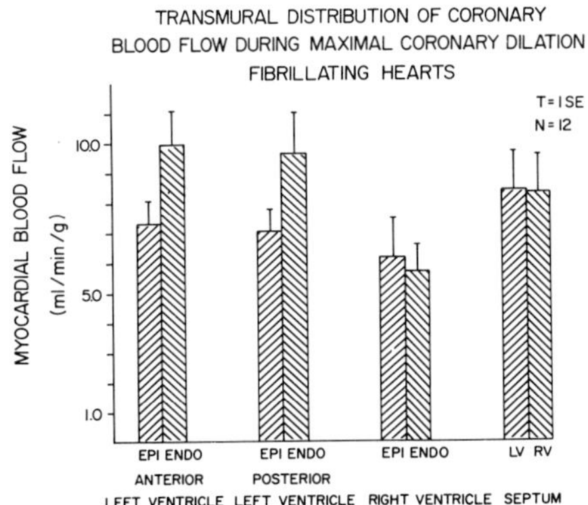

FIGURE 2. Regional myocardial vasodilation in weakly fibrillating hearts.

Transmural flow gradients were not detected in the right ventricular
free wall or in the interventricular septum of fibrillating hearts during
maximal coronary dilation. This fact may reflect the smaller transmural
pressure gradients experienced by these regions during systole and, thus,
the lesser need for these regions to have an increased subendocardial vascularity in order to ensure adequate perfusion during maximal coronary vasodilation.

Although we observed uniform transmural blood flow when maximal vasodilation was induced by either brief coronary occlusion or by pharmacological
mechanisms, Warltier _et al_. (9) recently reported that residual subepicardial
vascular tone caused peak reactive hyperemic flow to be preferentially distributed toward the subendocardium, and on the basis of this finding, challenged
the widely held view that myocardial ischemia causes maximal coronary vasodilation (7,10,11). In search of a reason for the discrepancy between our
findings and those of Warltier _et al_., we conducted additional experiments
to examine more closely the transmural distribution of flow in the left
ventricular free wall throughout the coronary reactive hyperemic response
(12).

After exposure of the heart through a thoracotomy in the fourth left
intercostal space, the left anterior descending coronary artery (LAD) was
isolated beyond its first major branch and an electromagnetic flow transducer was positioned at that point. A silk snare was placed around the LAD
distal to the flow transducer, so that the LAD could be abruptly occluded
for 90 sec. This period of occlusion was chosen because we (7) and others
(9) have found that longer occlusions do not result in greater peak reactive
hyperemia. Also, the reactive hyperemic response following 90 sec of ischemia
is sufficiently prolonged to allow multiple determinations of regional flow.

Regional myocardial blood flow was measured under control conditions
and during the reactive hyperemic response following abrupt release of a
90 sec LAD occlusion. These flow measurements were made by injecting sequen-
tially into the left atrium microspheres (8-10 micron) labeled with gamma
emitting radionuclides. Doses of microspheres were injected as a bolus in
less than 2 sec, and regional myocardial blood flow was computed from radioactivity trapped in different layers of the left ventricular free wall.
Transmural variations in myocardial blood flow were examined by computing
endocardial/epicardial flow ratios from flows measured in the inner and outer
thirds of the left ventricular free wall.

The 90-sec LAD occlusion caused a slight fall in systemic arterial blood
pressure and in left ventricular dP/dt_{max} and a modest elevation in left
atrial blood pressure, but these parameters quickly returned to normal following release of the coronary occlusion. Mean LAD blood flow rose for about
15 sec following release and then was essentially constant for approximately
30 sec before beginning to decline.

Figure 3 shows mean endocardial/epicardial flow ratios for control con-

ditions and during various phases of the hyperemic response. This figure
demonstrates that 1) the endo/epi flow ratio was significantly less than
control during the rising phase, 2) this ratio then increased to 1.08,
significantly greater than that during the rising phase, and 3) for a sustained period during the recovery phase, the endocardial/epicardial flow
ratio was significantly greater than both the control and the pre-peak
value.

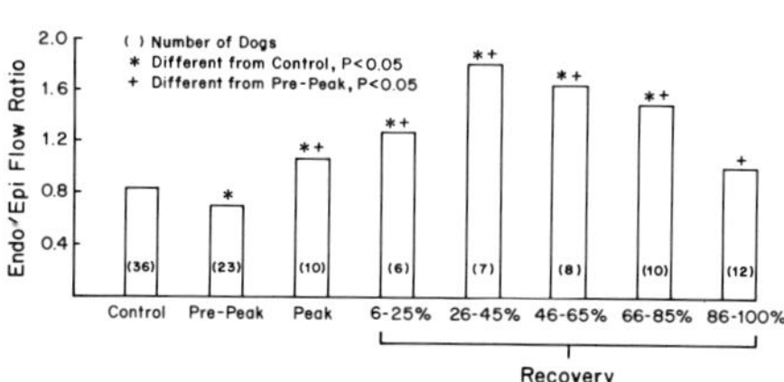

FIGURE 3. Endocardial/epi-
cardial flow ratios under
control conditions and during
the hyperemic response to a
90-sec occlusion of the left
anterior descending coronary
artery. Published with
permission of the British
Medical Association.

Early preferential flow to subepicardium and late preferential flow to
subendocardium suggested that peak flow to these regions might have been
asynchronous and, therefore, that dynamic transmural variations in flow
contributed to the relatively prolonged duration of peak mean coronary
flow. Further analsyis of the transmural distribution of microspheres
injected during the plateau phase of the reactive hyperemia revealed that
those injected early were distributed toward the epicardium, whereas microspheres injected during the mid and later portion of the plateau were
distributed preferentially toward the endocardium.

Figure 4 shows a schematic representation of the time-dependent differences in subepicardial and subendocardial reactive hyperemia. Regional
peak flows are asynchronous and both exceed maximal coronary artery flow.
These asynchronous regional flow distributions account for the prolonged
plateau phase of maximal coronary artery blood flow. This figure also demonstrates how asynchronous regional peak hyperemic flows pose problems for
investigators seeking to compare peak coronary flow during this response
with maximal steady-state flow induced by pharmacological coronary vaso-

dilators. At any point during the peak coronary reactive hyperemia, flow measured by a transducer on a coronary artery would be less than asynchronous regional peak flows. Pharmacological vasodilators, on the other hand, would synchronously dilate subepicardial and subendocardial vessels and result in greater flows measured by a transducer on the coronary artery or by microspheres injected during the steady-state vasodilation.

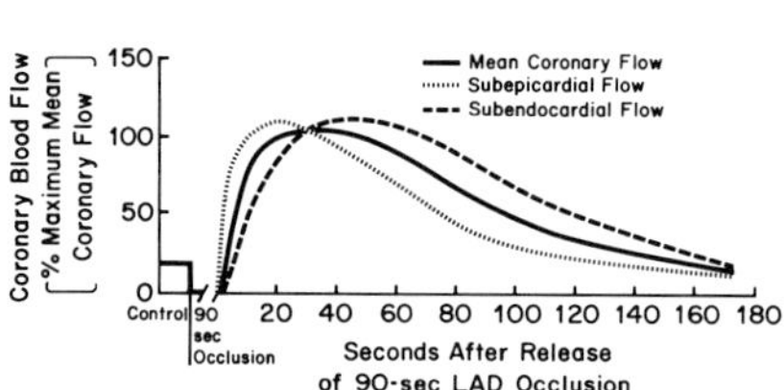

FIGURE 4. Illustration of time-dependent differences in subepicardial and subendocardial reactive hyperemia. Regional peak flows are asynchronous and exceed maximal coronary artery flow. The asynchronous regional flow distributions account for the plateau phase of maximum coronary artery flow. Published with permission of the British Medical Association.

The dynamic changes in transmural blood flow during reactive hyperemia are likely due to interactions between mechanical forces tending to restrict coronary flow and metabolic factors which act to dilate the coronary vessels. Since the ischemic insult caused by the 90-sec coronary occlusion resulted in ultimate maximal vasodilation of both subendocardial and subepicardial vessels, the delay in reaching peak flow to these regions must be the result of mechanical properties of the coronary vessels or the result of mechanical forces imposed on these vessels by the myocardium. Two different mechanisms have been proposed to account for the delay in reaching peak coronary reactive hyperemia: 1) time-dependent stretching of viscoelastic elements of the vessel wall (11); and 2) time-dependent reopening of coronary vessels compressed by ischemic myocardium, whose relaxation has been impaired by ischemia (13). The greater impediment to reperfusion of the subendocardium is consistent with the second mechanism, since coronary occlusion results in more severe ischemia in that region (14,15). In addition, left ventricular diastolic pressures were elevated by the 90-sec LAD occlusion, and the resulting increase in myocardial tissue pressure may have contributed to delayed recovery of subendocardial flow.

In as much as the coronary reactive hyperemic response is a function
of the coronary flow deficit incurred during the occlusion (10,11), it is
not surprising that recovery of normal coronary tone takes place at a slower
pace in the initially more ischemic subendocardium. This delay in recovery
of subendocardium tone is also in agreement with the finding of Dunn _et al._
(16) that return of lactate concentrations to control levels occurred more
slowly in subendocardium.

To further explore the effects of coronary vasodilation on transmural
myocardial blood flow we have devised a model of regional non-ischemic, myocardial hypoxia (17). Figure 5 illustrates the perfusion system used for
this model. After left thoracotomy and artificial ventilation, the left
anterior descending coronary artery was cannulated and perfused at constant
pressure with either arterial blood or hypoxic blood. Hypoxic blood was
obtained by pumping venous blood through an extracorporeal canine lung which
was ventilated with 4% carbon dioxide, 96% nitrogen. Thus, it was possible
to reduce the PO_2 of the LAD perfusate to 8 to 16 mmHg while keeping PCO_2
and pH normal. Perfusion flow rate was measured with an electromagnetic
flow transducer, and the perfusion pressure was measured with a transducer
attached to a small diameter tube advanced to the orifice of the perfusion

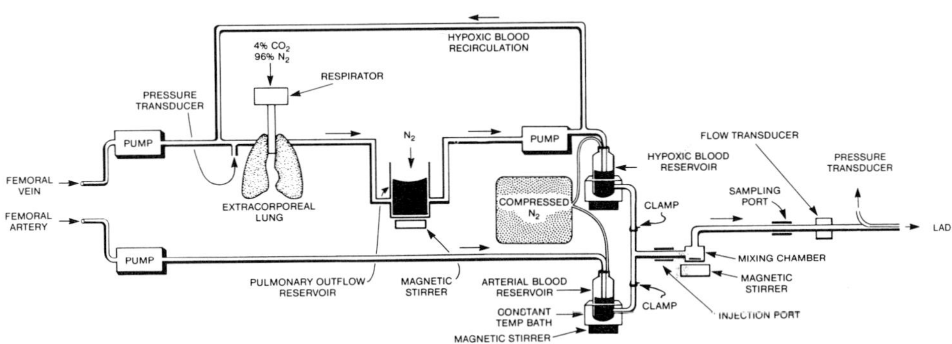

FIGURE 5. Extracorporeal system for perfusion of the left anterior descending
coronary artery (LAD) at constant pressure with blood of controlled oxygen
content.

cannula. LAD perfusion pressure was maintained similar to mean aortic pressure throughout the experiment. Radioactive microspheres were injected into the perfusion line to measure regional myocardial blood flow. A mixing chamber in the perfusion line ensured their uniform distribution in the LAD perfusate.

Figure 6 illustrates the coronary flow response to brief, 15 sec, and to more prolonged, 3+ min, hypoxia. Fifteen seconds of hypoxia caused only a small increase in coronary flow. This increase was much less than that following 15 sec of ischemia. Kelley and Gould (18) recently reported similar observations and concluded that rapid changes in intravascular pressure were responsible for the greater dilation during reactive hyperemia. Washout of vasoactive metabolites during hypoxic perfusion might also have prevented the marked dilation they observed after a similar period of ischemia. Note, however, that prolonged hypoxic perfusion resulted in a marked hyperemia that clearly exceeded the reactive hyperemia following 15 sec of coronary occlusion.

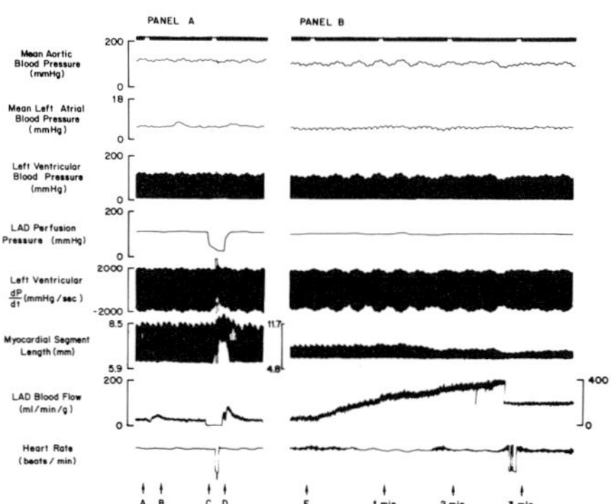

FIGURE 6. Effects of brief (15 sec A to B) and prolonged (3 + min, begun at E) perfusion of the LAD with hypoxic blood (PO$_2$ = 15 mmHg). Brief hypoxic perfusion resulted in less dilation than did 15 sec of ischemia (C to D), but prolonged hypoxic perfusion resulted in maximal coronary dilation. LAD flow record was attenuated by 50% at approximately 3 min (note new scale at right).

In 7 animals we compared the vasodilatory potency of 3 min of myocardial ischemia with 3 min of hypoxia. Peak LAD flow after release of a 3-min occlusion was 5.0±0.7 ml/min/g and 5.8±0.7 ml/min/g after 3 min of hypoxia. Thus, we concluded that the 3-min hypoxic perfusion resulted in maximal coronary vasodilation. Although the difference in flows observed at peak reactive hyperemia and during hypoxic perfusion was not statistically significant in this group of 7 dogs, the tendency toward a greater flow during hypoxia is consistent with our previous report of asynchronous regional flow during the

peak hyperemic response, which results in underestimation of maximal coronary
flow from records of coronary reactive hyperemia.

Figure 7 shows regional myocardial blood flow in 3 layers of the left
ventricular free wall during control conditions and at 3 min of hypoxic
perfusion of the LAD. Blood flow was distributed uniformly under control
conditions and also during hypoxic perfusion (19). This uniformity of transmural flow is consistent with our earlier findings of uniform transmural
perfusion when coronary vasodilation was caused by ischemia or by pharmacological agents, adenosine or papaverine, and is consistent with our proposal
of a transmural gradient of vascularity favoring the subendocardium.

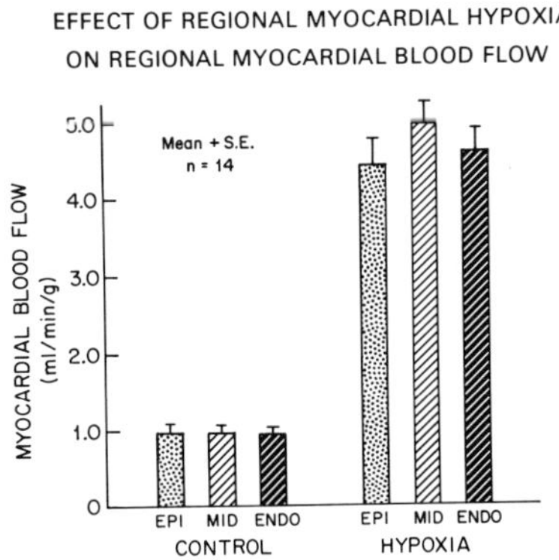

FIGURE 7. Distribution of myocardial blood flow in left ventricular myocardium during control conditions and during hypoxic perfusion of the left anterior descending coronary artery (LAD).

We have also utilized the hypoxic perfusion model to examine coronary
effects of altered regional cardiac function. Figure 8 shows results of
such an experiment. While the LAD was perfused with hypoxic blood, a large
dose of isoproterenol was administered intravenously. Isoproterenol reached
the normally perfused myocardium much sooner than the hypoxic perfused region
due to its delay in the perfusion system. As expected, isoproterenol caused
pronounced increases in left ventricular pressure and dP/dt of the normally
perfused region. However, these mechanical changes had very little effect
on blood flow through the maximally dilated, hypoxic LAD region. Later,
when isoproterenol reached the LAD region, a pronounced increase in myocardial
contractility was observed. Concurrently, LAD blood flow fell precipitously
as the enhanced contraction of this region mechanically impaired its blood
flow. This attenuation of flow by enhanced contractility is consistent with

a recent report of Marsilli _et al_. (20). They measured regional myocardial
blood flow during intracoronary infusion of either isoproterenol to stimulate
contractility or lidocaine to depress contractility of hearts whose coronary
circulations were maximally dilated with adenosine. Isoproterenol concurrently enhanced myocardial contraction and significantly reduced myocardial
blood flow from 6.4 to 4.2 ml/min/g. It is of interest that the mean flow
during isoproterenol infusion agreed closely with flows reported for canine
heart during strenuous exercise, a topic I will address shortly. The impediment of flow was more severe in the subendocardial region as reflected by
a decrease in the endocardial/epicardial flow ratio from 1.08 to 0.75. On
the other hand, when myocardial contractility was attenuated by lidocaine,
coronary flow through these maximally dilated vessels increased from 6.2 to
9.4 ml/min/g and the endocardial/epicardial flow ratio increased from 1.02
to 1.28. These findings are similar to our measurements of regional flow
in maximally dilated coronary circulations of weakly fibrillating hearts (7).
Thus, in the absence of coronary vascular tone, the mechanical action of the
heart becomes a controlling influence on coronary blood flow.

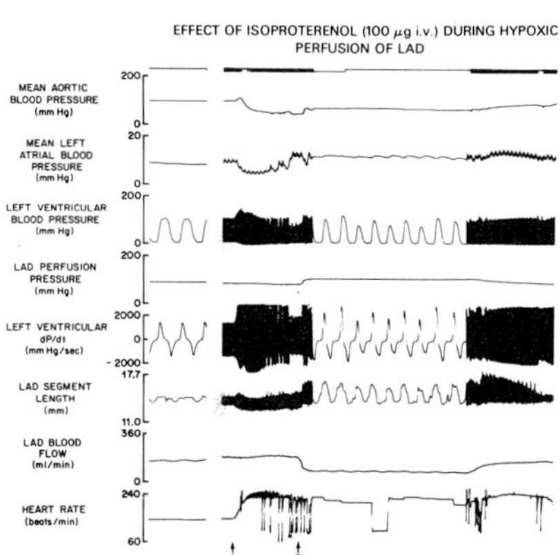

FIGURE 8. Effect of intravenous isoproterenol during
hypoxic perfusion of the left
anterior descending coronary
artery (LAD). Isoproterenol
reached the normally-perfused
myocardium (A) before reaching
the hypoxic region (B) due to
delay in the perfusion system.
Initial stimulation of mechanical function in normally perfused myocardium had no effect
on blood flow in the hypoxic
region. Isoproterenol subsequently also increased function in the hypoxic LAD region,
and this caused a marked
decrease in LAD blood flow.

Are there physiological situations where, in the absence of coronary
artery obstruction, coronary perfusion is limited by mechanical forces?
I suggest that this is an important area for future investigation.

Although physiological conditions which caused pronounced coronary
vasodilation have been studied extensively, little attention has been given
to the possibility that coronary blood flow may be limited mechanically.

Consider, for example, strenuous exercise, where heart rate as well as left ventricular systolic and diastolic pressures are markedly elevated (21,22). These mechanical changes would impede both systolic and diastolic coronary flow (20,23) in any region where coronary tone was exhausted. Furthermore, myocardial blood flow does not increase in proportion to myocardial oxygen demands during strenuous exercise since coronary venous oxygen saturation decreases (3). While a decrease in coronary venous oxygen may, to some extent, reflect improved gas exchange between blood and tissue brought about by the opening of additional capillaries, it may also reflect inappropriate coronary constriction in the face of increased myocardial oxygen requirements.

Is there significant transmural vasomotor tone during strenuous exercise? Several lines of evidence bear on this question. 1) Coronary flow measured during strenuous exercise is consistently less than that measured in the resting heart during maximal coronary vasodilation, even if the heart is paced at comparable rates (21,22). 2) Increases in coronary flow are not sufficient to meet myocardial oxygen requirements without a marked increase in myocardial oxygen extraction. For example, in the study of von Restorff et al. (3), coronary sinus oxygen saturation fell from 24 to 9% while coronary flow increased to 2.6 ml/min/g, less than one-half of the flow which the coronary circulation is capable of delivering. Under more moderate stresses, metabolically-linked vasodilation of coronary vessels prevent such pronounced decreases in venous oxygen saturation (2). 3) Experiments designed to directly demonstrate vasomotor tone during strenuous exercise have been few and are subject to problems of interpretation. For example, von Restorff et al. (3) reported that a reactive hyperemic response could be elicited after an unspecified period of coronary occlusion in strenuously exercising dogs. Since ischemia attenuates cardiac function, the hyperemia could have resulted from a reduction of regional contractility (20) instead of a further reduction in vasomotor tone. In another evaluation of vasomotor tone during exercise, Barnard et al. (24) administered dipyridamole intravenously to exercising dogs and observed an increase in coronary blood flow. However, no data was provided on hemodynamic or coronary sinus oxygen parameters before and after systemic administration of this vasodilator. Problems arise also in interpreting the results of experiments where alpha receptor antagonists were administered to block alpha mediated coronary constriction (21,22) because of altered metabolic and mechanical parameters. While alpha adrenergic blockade does result in increased coronary flow during strenuous exercise (21,22), proof that this intervention functions solely by eliminating inappropriate vasomotor tone awaits further experiments where both metabolic and mechanical parameters are maintained constant independent of the blockade.

SUMMARY

1) We have demonstrated that coronary blood flow in the left ventricular free wall of the anesthetized dog's heart is distributed uniformly during maximal coronary vasodilation as well as under control conditions. A gradient of vascularity favoring the subendocardium compensates for systolic limitation of flow to subendocardium.

2) We have shown that the peak reactive hyperemic response following a 90-sec coronary occlusion occurs asynchronously. Subepicardial flow rises faster, reaches its peak earlier, and falls faster than does subendocardial flow. Asynchronous hyperemias account for the plateau phase of maximum coronary artery flow.

3) Myocardial hypoxia causes maximal coronary vasodilation. The left ventricular free wall is perfused uniformly during hypoxia-induced maximal coronary vasodilation.

4) Increased myocardial contractility in normally perfused regions has little effect on flow in maximally dilated vessels in adjacent, hypoxic myocardium if contractility of the hypoxic region is not altered. Increased mechanical function of either normal or hypoxic myocardium impedes flow through its maximally dilated coronary vessels.

5) The possibility of mechanical limitation of coronary flow under stressful conditions which result in maximal coronary dilation merits further investigation.

ACKNOWLEDGEMENTS

The author acknowledges the professional contributions of his colleagues, Drs. G. J. Crystal, P. E. Parker, R. B. Boatwright, and F. A. Bashour, who were associated with one or more of the investigations described in this report. Expert technical assistance for these investigations was provided by Mr. A. G. Williams, Mrs. B. Alferez Oberholtzer and Mrs. R. Holton Stevens. Excellent secretarial assistance of Mrs. O. Fagala and Ms. L. Barnes is also gratefully acknowledged. The author's research described in this report was sponsored in part by National Heart, Lung, and Blood Institute grant HL-21657, a grant from the American Heart Association, Texas Affiliate, and by the Cardiology Fund.

REFERENCES

1. Braunwald E: Control of myocardial oxygen consumption. Physiologic and clinical considerations. Am J Cardiol (27): 416-432, 1971.
2. Rubio R, Berne RM: Regulation of coronary blood flow. Progr Cardio-vascular Diseases (18): 105-122, 1975.
3. von Restorff W, Holtz J, Bassenge E: Exercise induced augmentation of myocardial oxygen extraction in spite of normal coronary dilatory capacity in dogs. Pflugers Archiv (372): 181-185, 1977.
4. Gregg DE, Sabiston DC: Current research and problems of the coronary circu-lation. Circulation (13): 916-927, 1956.
5. Downey JM, Kirk ES: Distribution of coronary blood flow across the canine heart wall during systole. Circ Res (34): 251-257, 1974.
6. Moir TW, DeBra DW: Effect of left ventricular hypertension, ischemia and vasoactive drugs on the myocardial distribution of coronary flow. Circ. Res (21): 65-74, 1967.
7. Downey HF, Bashour FA, Boatwright RB, Parker PE, Kechejian SJ: Uniformity of transmural perfusion in anesthetized dogs with maximally dilated coro-nary circulations. Circ Res (37): 111-117, 1975.
8. Crystal GJ, Downey HF, Bashour FA: Small vessel and total coronary blood volume during intracoronary adenosine. Am J Physiol 241 (Heart Circ Physiol 10): H194-H201, 1981.
9. Warltier DC, Gross GJ, Brooks HL: Pharmacologic- vs ischemia-induced coronary artery vasodilation. Am J Physiol (Heart Circ Physiol 240): H767-H774, 1981.
10. Coffman, JD, Gregg DE: Reactive hyperemia characteristics of the myocar-dium. Am J Physiol (199): 1143-1149, 1960.
11. Olsson RA: Myocardial reactive hyperemia. Circ Res (37): 263-270, 1970.
12. Downey HF, Crystal GJ, Bashour FA: Asynchronous transmural perfusion during coronary reactive hyperaemia. Cardiovasc Res (27): 200-206, 1983.
13. Murthy VS, Lee PL: Effect of left ventricular relaxation on diastolic coronary blood flow during maximal vasodilation of reactive hyperemia. Fed Proc (35): 349, 1976.
14. Dunn RB, Griggs DM Jr: Transmural gradients in ventricular tissue metab-olites produced by stopping coronary blood flow in the dog. Circ Res (37): 438-445, 1975.
15. Weiss HR, Neubauer JA, Lipp JA, Sinha AK: Quantitative determination of regional oxygen consumption in the dog heart. Circ Res (42): 394-401, 1978.
16. Dunn RB, McDonough KM, Griggs DM Jr: High energy phosphate stores and lactate levels in different layers of the canine left ventricle during reactive hyperemia. Circ Res (44): 788-795, 1979.
17. Downey HF, Crystal GJ, Bockman EL, Bashour FA: Nonischemic myocardial hypoxia: coronary dilation without increased tissue adenosine. Am J Physiol 243 (Heart Circ Physiol 12): H512-H516, 1982
18. Kelley KO, Gould KL: Coronary reactive hyperaemia after brief occlusion and after deoxygenated perfusion. Cardiovasc Res (15): 615-622, 1981.
19. Downey HF, Crystal GJ, Williams AG, Bashour FA: Transmural uniformity of coronary blood flow in hypoxic, non-ischemic left ventricular myocardium. Physiologist (26): A43, 1983.
20. Marzilli M, Goldstein S, Sabbah HN, Lee T, Stein PD: Modulating effect of regional myocardial performance on local myocardial perfusion in the dog. Circ Res (45): 634-641, 1979.

21. Gwirtz PA, Stone HL: Coronary blood flow and myocardial oxygen consumption alter alpha adrenergic blockade during submaximal exercise. J. Pharmacol Exp Ther (217): 92-98, 1981.
22. Murray PA, Vatner SF: Alpha-adrenergic attenuation of the coronary vascular responses to severe exercise in the conscious dog. Circ Res (45): 654-660, 1979.
23. Raff WK, Kosche F, Lochner W: Extravascular coronary resistance and its relation to microcirculation. Am J Cardiol (29): 598-603, 1972.
24. Barnard RJ, Duncan HW, Livesay JJ, Buckberg GD: Coronary vasodilator reserve and flow distribution during near-maximal exercise in dogs. J Appl Physiol: Respirat Environ Exercise Physiol (43): 988-992, 1977.

5

REGULATION OF CORONARY BLOOD FLOW IN THE
UNDERPERFUSED VENTRICLE

Douglas M. Griggs, Jr.

The role of mechanical factors in the regulation of coronary
blood flow and its transmural distribution takes on special
significance under conditions in which autoregulation is
eliminated. For instance, when coronary artery pressure is
reduced below the autoregulatory range, coronary blood flow
becomes directly dependent on coronary driving pressure, or the
difference between coronary input pressure and the effective
coronary back pressure. In this setting, intramyocardial tissue
pressure, which influences the effective coronary back pressure,
assumes major importance as a determinant of coronary blood
flow. Because of transmural variations in intramyocardial tissue
pressure, myocardial blood flow distribution may be altered.

In this presentation I would like to review some studies from
my laboratory which I believe demonstrate the importance of
mechanical factors in the regulation of myocardial blood flow when
coronary artery pressure is independently reduced below the
autoregulatory range.

The first study to be described is one performed a number of
years ago (1) in which we determined the effect of progressively
lowering left main coronary artery pressure in the open chest dog
on the transmural distribution of a highly diffusible, and thus
flow dependent, indicator, I-131-iodoantipyrine. In this study we
employed a self perfusing coronary cannula which received blood
from the root of the aorta through a sidehole in one barrel of the
cannula, passed the blood through an extracorporeal loop which
contained an electromagnetic flowmeter, and then returned it to
the isolated main left coronary artery through a second barrel in
the cannula. The cannula circuit contained a short section of
rubber tubing that could be constricted to reduce coronary artery
pressure. The indicator was infused directly into the coronary

cannula for 1 minute, after which time the heart was arrested, rapidly excised, and then divided into multiple sections for isotope analysis.

We noted that when coronary artery pressure was lowered in a stepwise manner by constricting the tubing, there was at first no change in the transmural distribution of indicator uptake, but after the coronary artery pressure was reduced beyond a certain point, there began a redistribution of indicator uptake away from the inner or endocardial region of the ventricle. In correlating the inner to outer wall isotope ratio with various hemodynamic variables measured at the time, we found the best correlation with a pressure index derived from the areas under the coronary artery and ventricular pressure curves, called the coronary-ventricular pressure index.

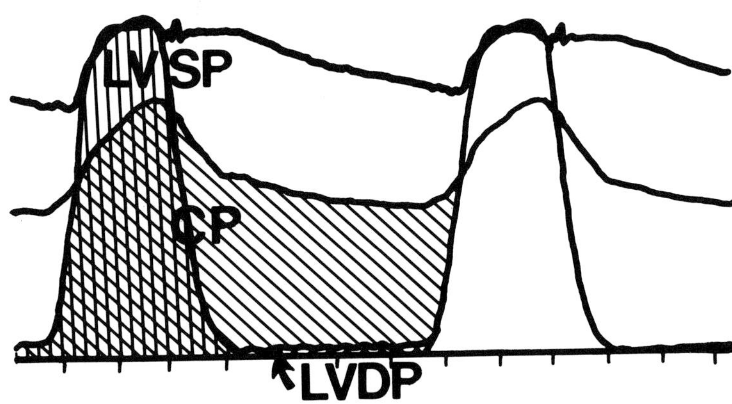

$$\text{C-VPI} = \frac{\text{CP} - \text{LVDP}}{\text{LVSP}}$$

FIGURE 1. C-VPI = Coronary ventricular pressure index CP = coronary artery pressure area for cardiac cycle. LVSP = left ventricular systolic pressure area. LVDP = left ventricular diastolic pressure area.

The coronary-ventricular pressure index and its method of
calculation are shown in Figure 1. The pressure curves shown are
left ventricular pressure, aortic pressure, and left coronary
artery pressure, which is reduced due to constriction of the
coronary cannula tubing. The index is calculated by subtracting
the area under the diastolic portion of the left ventricular
pressure curve from the area under the coronary artery pressure
curve in systole and diastole and dividing this difference by the
area under the left ventricular pressure curve during systole.
The upper term is an index of coronary driving pressure and the
lower term is an index of intramyocardial tissue pressure during
systole. A similar index based on a somewhat different conceptual
approach was later developed in Hoffman's laboratory (2).

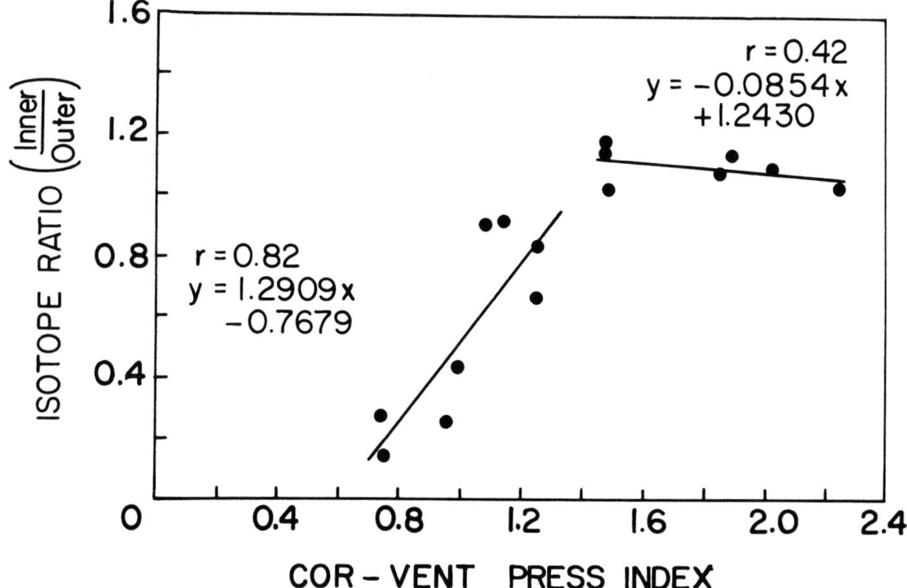

FIGURE 2. Plot of inner to outer ventricular wall ratio of I-131
iodoantipyrine against the coronary ventricular pressure index of
individual animals subjected to different degrees of coronary
constriction.

The relationship between our coronary-ventricular pressure index and the inner to outer wall isotope ratio obtained in 15 animals with varying degrees of coronary artery pressure reduction is shown in Figure 2. Below an index value of 1.3, there was a decrease in the inner to outer wall isotope ratio which correlated well with a decrease in the coronary-ventricular pressure index. We interpreted these findings as evidence that regulation of isotope distribution, and thus flow, underwent a transition from that of active vasomotor control under normal conditions to that of passive dependence on intra- and extravascular pressure phenomena within the ventricle under conditions of reduced coronary artery pressure.

This analysis was consistent with the concept advanced at that time by Moir (3) that a nonuniform compressive stress causes a transmural gradient in myocardial blood flow during systole which is compensated for by a reciprocal gradient in coronary vasomotor tone under normal conditions, but not under conditions of maximal coronary vasodilation induced by a reduction in coronary artery pressure. Subsequent studies by Downey, et al. (4) and L'Abbate, et al. (5) suggested that this compensation could be partly accounted for by a gradient in coronary vascularity, increasing from epicardium to endocardium. Also, further consideration by Downey and Kirk (6) of the role of intramyocardial tissue pressure led to the concept that myocardial blood flow distribution during systole is regulated by a systolic vascular waterfall mechanism.

More recently, attention has been focused on the role of diastolic intramyocardial tissue pressure and the possible role of a diastolic vascular waterfall mechanism in the regulation of coronary blood flow. From studies on diastolic coronary artery pressure-flow relations (7-9), evidence has been obtained that neither coronary venous pressure nor ventricular filling pressure serve as the effective coronary back pressure in the well perfused canine left ventricle. Critical pressures for flow ranging between 11 and 20 mmHg have usually been reported in the maximally vasodilated ventricle with a filling pressure of only a few millimeters of mercury.

These recent findings have important implications for the underperfused, ischemic ventricle in which ventricular filling pressure, and presumably diastolic intramyocardial tissue pressure, may rise. Under these conditions myocardial blood flow is regulated by coronary driving pressure, and the importance of the effective coronary back pressure as a determinant of myocardial blood flow is greatly augmented. Any increase in the effective coronary back pressure adversely affects coronary blood flow by encroaching on the coronary driving pressure. Moreover, data obtained in the well perfused ventricle by Ellis and Klocke (8) have suggested that the effective diastolic coronary back pressure is slightly higher in the endocardium than in the epicardium, and that this difference is accentuated by an increase in ventricular preload. This could have an important effect on the transmural distribution of myocardial blood flow in the underperfused ventricle with a spontaneously rising filling pressure due to ischemia.

The role of ventricular filling pressure as a determinant of coronary blood flow in the underperfused, acutely ischemic ventricle was examined in my laboratory under conditions of a reduced, constant coronary artery pressure (10). A diagram of the experimental set up is shown in Figure 3. The left main coronary artery of the open chest dog was cannulated with the previously described self-perfusing coronary cannula. Attached to the cannula circuit were one or more pressurized reservoirs containing arterial blood. By clamping the normal cannula circuit between the aorta and the coronary artery and unclamping the tubing from a reservoir, the coronary artery could be perfused at a constant pressure for a short period of time while an equal quantity of blood was pumped from the animal into a graduated cylinder through a connection to the occluded side of the cannula circuit. Reservoir pressure could be preset to any desired level using a compressed gas system. Total left coronary blood flow was measured with an electromagnetic flowmeter incorporated into the

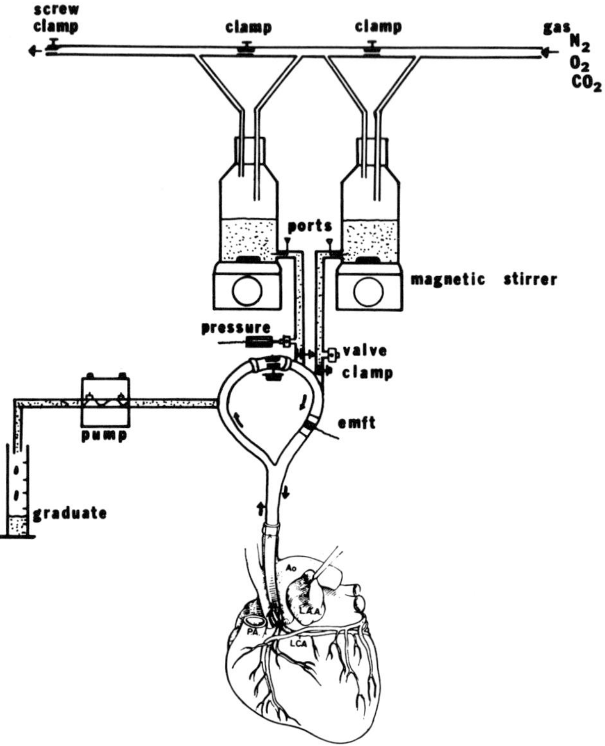

FIGURE 3. Diagram of preparation. See text.

cannula circuit. The transmural distribution of blood flow in the ventricle was determined by introducing radioactively labeled 8-10 micron diameter microspheres into the reservoir and then counting tissue radioactivity after perfusing the coronary cannula from the reservoirs.

Results were obtained in control animals perfused at a coronary artery pressure within the autoregulatory range and in experimental animals perfused at a pressure well below the autoregulatory range. These experimental animals were divided

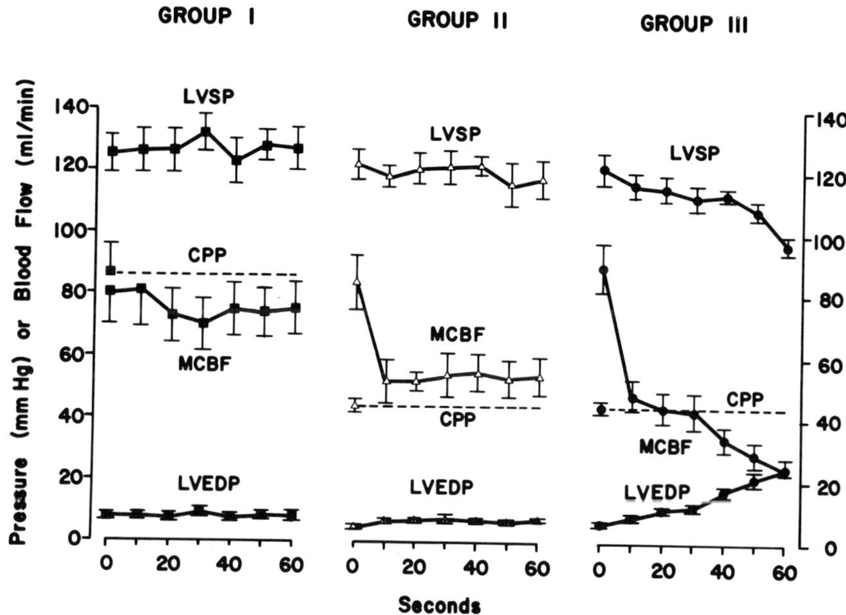

FIGURE 4. Hemodynamic data. LVSP = left ventricular systolic pressure CPP = coronary (reservoir) perfusion pressure: MCBF = mean coronary blood flow. LVEDP = left ventricular end-diastolic pressure. Bars denote SE.

into two groups for purposes of analysis, depending upon whether left ventricular filling pressure remained within normal limits or rose to an abnormal level during the period of reservoir perfusion.

Figure 4 contains the hemodynamic data obtained in the control animals (Group I) and the two groups of experimental animals (Groups II and III). Data points are shown before switching to a constant coronary perfusion pressure and at 10 second intervals for the 60 second period of reservoir perfusion. In Group I coronary perfusion pressure was set at a mean value of 85 mmHg, well within the autoregulatory range. Under these conditions mean coronary blood flow did not decrease significantly and left ventricular systolic and diastolic pressures remained within normal limits. In Group II coronary perfusion pressure was set at a mean value of 45 mmHg. Coronary

blood flow promptly decreased to 63% of the control value and
remained relatively constant. Left ventricular filling pressure
remained within normal limits during the 60 second reservoir

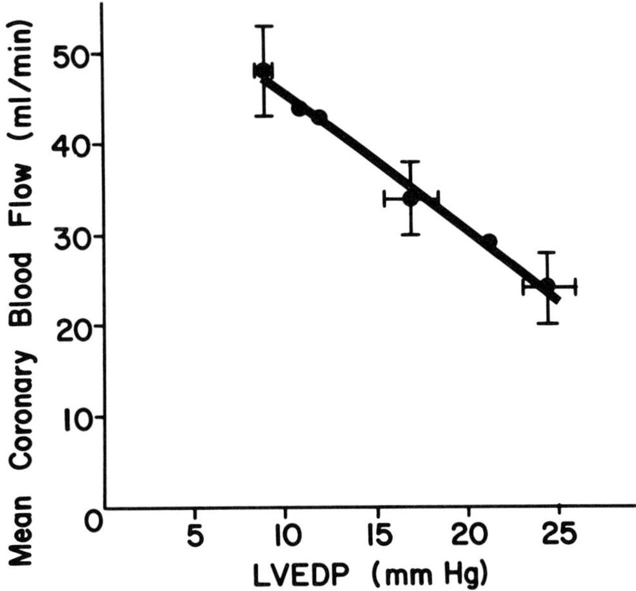

FIGURE 5. Relationship between left ventricular end diastolic
pressure (LVEDP) and mean coronary blood flow for all Group III
animals. Bars denote SE.

perfusion period. In Group III coronary perfusion pressure was
also set at a mean value of 45 mmHg. In this group coronary blood
flow decreased to 54% of the control value and then progressively
declined despite the presence of a constant coronary perfusion
pressure. Left ventricular filling pressure rose progressively
from normal to abnormal values during the 60 second reservoir
perfusion period. No reason could be found for the greater effect
of reducing coronary perfusion pressure in Group III, but the
results suggest the possibility of an innately higher effective
coronary back pressure in this group.

Shown in Figure 5 is the quantitative relationship between
ventricular filling pressure (end diastolic pressure) and mean

coronary blood flow in Group III. As filling pressure rose from 6 to 25 mmHg, mean coronary blood flow declined from 50 to 25 ml/100 g/min. The relationship proved to be an inverse, linear one with a correlation coefficient of 0.99. The linearity of this relationship indicates that coronary blood flow is equally sensitive to changes in filling pressure below and above previously established values for the effective coronary back pressure in the well perfused ventricle. This suggests that the effective coronary back pressure in the acutely ischemic ventricle is a direct function of ventricular filling pressure irrespective of evidence that the two variables are not equal in the well perfused ventricle.

Data on the transmural distribution of myocardial blood flow in all three groups of animals are shown in Figure 6. The amount of blood delivered to the epi, mid, and endocardial regions of the ventricle during reservoir perfusion is shown on the left and the corresponding endo to epi ratio of delivered blood is shown on the right. Results in Group I were similar to steady state values for blood flow and endo to epi blood flow ratios obtained by others in normal animals (11). In Group II, the amount of blood delivered to all three regions was less than that in Group I, with the greatest difference being in the endo region. The endo to epi ratio of 0.85 in Group II was significantly lower than the 1.23 value obtained in Group I.

The lower than normal endo to epi ratio in Group II was obtained under conditions in which ventricular filling pressure remained low throughout the reservoir perfusion period. Thus, the results are explainable on the basis of a systolic vascular waterfall mechanism which is not adequately compensated for during diastole due to loss of autoregulation and a low diastolic coronary driving pressure.

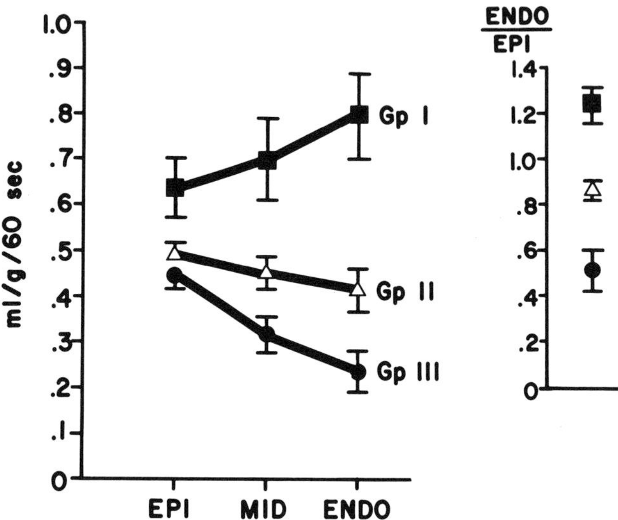

FIGURE 6. Data on the amount of blood delivered to different
layers of ventricle (left) and on the endocardial-to-epicardial
ratio of delivered blood (right) during reservoir perfusion period
in different animals groups. EPI = epicardial region; MID =
midmyocardial region, ENDO = endocardial region. Bars denote SE.

Returning to Figure 6, the values for delivered blood were
further reduced in Group III, particularly in the endocardial
region, and the endo to epi ratio of 0.53 was significantly lower
than that in Group II. These findings indicate that an increase
in filling pressure contributes to the preferential decrease in
endocardial blood flow seen in the underperfused ventricle. The
results support the concept that blood flow in the ischemic
ventricle is regulated by a pre-load dependent transmural gradient
in coronary driving pressure as described in the well perfused
ventricle by Ellis and Klocke (8). Although explainable on the

basis of a diastolic vascular waterfall mechanism, the results are
also consistent with the concept that distention of the ventricle
results in deformation of coronary resistance vessels and an
uneven increase in coronary vascular resistance across the
ventricular wall despite metabolically induced maximal coronary
vasodilation. The present study did not allow a distinction
between the two mechanisms.

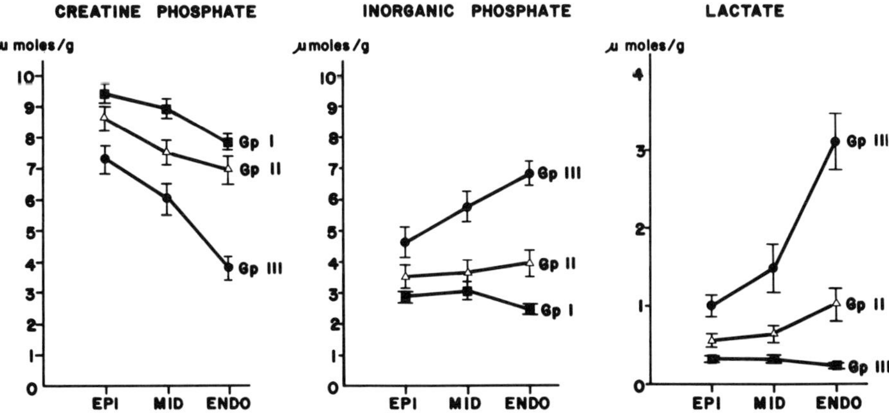

FIGURE 7. Data on regional myocardial tissue metabolite levels at
end of reservoir perfusion period in different animal groups.
Bars denote SE.

As a means of verifying and assessing the degree of
myocardial ischemia present in Groups II and III, transmural
myocardial tissue samples were obtained at the end of the
reservoir perfusion period in all animals for determination of the
tissue levels of several oxygen sensitive metabolites in different
layers of the ventricle. A rapid (less than 2 seconds) tissue
sampling and freezing technique previously developed in my
laboratory was used (12).

Figure 7 contains data on the myocardial tissue levels of creatine phosphate, inorganic phosphate, and lactate in epi, mid, and endo regions of the ventricle in all three animal groups. Results in Group I were similar to those previously obtained in my laboratory under control experimental conditions in non-cannulated animals (12). In Group II, statistically significant alterations were noted in midmyocardial creatine phosphate, endocardial inorganic phosphate, and endocardial lactate. In Group III, on the other hand, there were significant changes in all metabolite levels and evidence of a steep transmural gradient in ischemic metabolic changes, increasing from epicardium to endocardium. Thus, these metabolic findings verify that the ventricle was indeed ischemic and they demonstrate by a completely independent method that an increase in ventricular filling pressure accentuates the degree of endocardial ischemia in the underperfused ventricle.

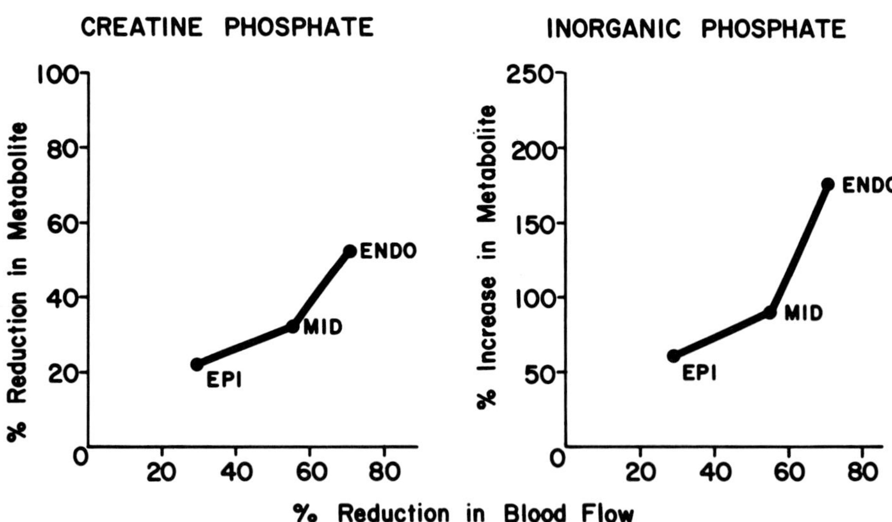

FIGURE 8. Relationship between reduction in blood flow and tissue creatine phosphate and inorganic phosphate changes in different layers of the left ventricle in Group III animals.

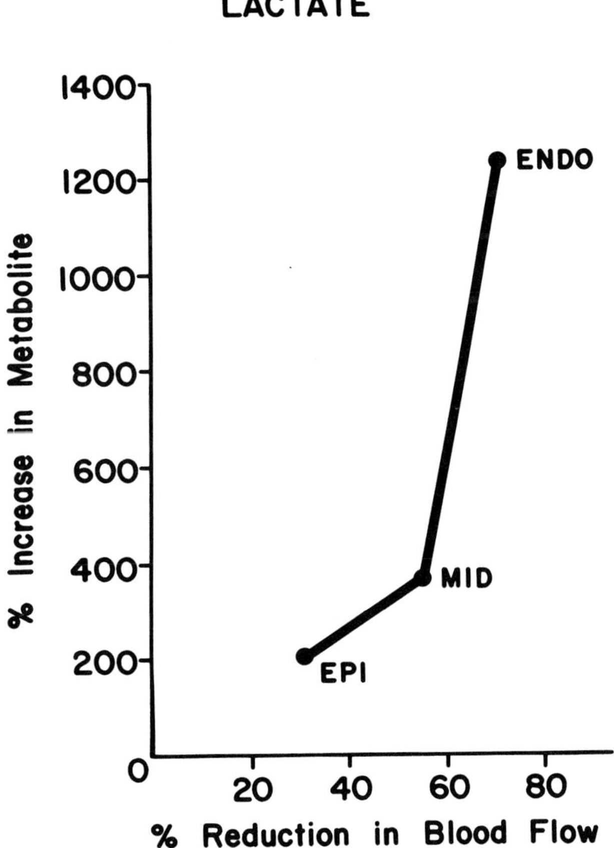

FIGURE 9. Relationship between reduction in blood flow and tissue
lactate changes in different layers of the left ventricle in Group
III animals.

An additional factor accounting for the more severe metabolic
changes in the endocardial region could be a greater energy need
in this region (12). This was suggested from a plot of the
relationship between metabolite changes and blood flow changes in
the epi, mid, and endo region of the Group III animals. As shown

in Figures 8 and 9, the transmural relationship between percent change in metabolite level and percent reduction in blood flow was curvilinear for all three metabolites with a disproportionately greater change in metabolite level in the endocardial region. One might envision that with an increase in ventricular diastolic radius during ischemia, the metabolic needs of the myocardium would be increased, contributing further to an imbalance between myocardial oxygen supply and demand, especially in the endocardial region.

The results of this study have considerable clinical relevance in terms of demonstrating a positive feedback mechanism for subendocardial ischemia that could be detrimental to patients with a flow limiting stenosis or occlusion of a proximal coronary vessel.

In summary, it has been shown that mechanical factors play an important role in the regulation of coronary blood flow and its transmural distribution in the left ventricle when coronary artery pressure is reduced below the autoregulatory level. A transmural gradient in coronary driving pressure which is dependent on ventricular filling pressure is unmasked in the acutely ischemic ventricle. An inverse, linear relationship exists between ventricular filling pressure and coronary blood flow as ventricular filling pressure rises from normal to abnormal values. This finding suggests that the effective coronary back pressure in the acutely ischemic ventricle is a direct function of ventricular filling pressure, irrespective of evidence that the two variables are not equal in the well perfused ventricle. Greater vulnerability of the subendocardium to ischemic injury is accentuated in the underperfused ventricle with a rising filling pressure secondary to a further reduction in subendocardial blood flow and to a greater energy need of the more distended ventricle.

References

1. Griggs DM Jr, Nakamura Y: Effect of coronary constriction on myocardial distribution of iodoantipyrine-^{131}I. Am J Physiol (215):1082-1088, 1968.

2. Buckberg GD, Fixler DE, Archie JP, Hoffman JIE: Experimental subendocardial ischemia in dogs with normal coronary arteries. Circ Res (30):67-81, 1972.

3. Moir TW: Brief reviews: Subendocardial distribution of coronary blood flow and the effect of antianginal drugs. Circ Res (30):621-627, 1972.

4. Downey HF, Bashour FA, Boatwright RB, Parker PE, Kechejian SJ: Uniformity of transmural perfusion in anesthetized dogs with maximally dilated coronary circulation. Circ Res (37):111-117, 1975.

5. L'Abbate A, Marzilli M, Ballestra AM, Camici P, Trivella MG, Pelosi G, Klassen G: Opposite transmural gradients of coronary resistance and extravascular pressure in the working dog's heart. Cardiovas Res (14):21-29, 1980.

6. Downey JM, Kirk ES: Inhibition of coronary blood flow by a vascular waterfall mechanism. Circ Res (36):753-760, 1975.

7. Bellamy RF: Diastolic coronary artery pressure-flow relations in the dog. Circ. Res (430:92-101, 1978.

8. Ellis AK, Locke FJ: Effect of preload on the transmural distribution of perfusion and pressure-flow relationships in the canine coronary vascular bed. Circ Res (46):68-77, 1980.

9. Eng CJ, Jentzer H, Kirk ES: The effects of coronary capacitance on the interpretation of diastolic pressure-flow relationships. Circ Res (50):334-341, 1982.

10. Dunn RB, Griggs DM Jr: Ventricular filling pressure as a determinant of coronary blood flow during ischemia. Am J Physiol (244):H429-H436, 1983.

11. Cobb FR, Bache RJ, Greenfield JC Jr: Regional myocardial blood flow in awake dogs. J Clin Invest (53):1618-1625, 1974.

12. Dunn RB, Griggs DM Jr: Transmural gradients in ventricular tissue metabolites produced by stopping coronary blood flow in the dog. Circ Res (37):438-445, 1975.

II
VASCULAR SMOOTH MUSCLE

Section II of this volume is devoted to a discussion of the factors that regulate the contraction of smooth muscle, particularly the role of sodium and calcium in controlling smooth muscle contractility. This is an area of great theoretical importance as well as directly related to the recent use of calcium blocking agents. Calcium in turn is also directly involved with the phosphorylation of myosin and the resultant responses to beta-adrenergic stimulation. The third paper in this section discusses this area. The last paper deals specifically with the responses of the coronary vasculature to autonomic nerve stimulation and relates this response to other vasoactive substances which may be released by platelet aggregation.

6

EXCITATION, CONTRACTION AND THE DISTRIBUTION OF CALCIUM AND SODIUM IN
SMOOTH MUSCLE.

A.P. SOMLYO, A.V. SOMLYO, M. BOND, T. KITAZAWA, H. SHUMAN and
A.J. WASSERMAN

Contraction of smooth muscles is mediated by the filamentous
proteins actin and myosin, and is activated by a rise in cytoplasmic
free Ca^{2+} (for review, 1,2). Ultrastructural methods have played a
major role in establishing the organization of the contractile and
cytoskeletal proteins (actin, myosin, desmin, vimentin and
alpha-actinin) and, more recently, the cellular concentrations and
subcellular localization of major cellular cations (3,5). We present
here 1., a brief summary of recent studies showing the ultrastructure
of the contractile apparatus in smooth muscle, 2., further evidence
that the sarcoplasmic reticulum is the major source (as well as sink)
of intracellular activator calcium in smooth muscle, 3., an estimate of
the total rise in cytoplasmic Ca associated with contraction and 4.,
electron probe analytic results demonstrating a previously unrecognized
component of cytoplasmic Na-efflux.

Contractile apparatus

The contractile unit of smooth muscle is a "mini-sarcomere-like"
structure consisting of a group (3-5 in rabbit portal anterior
mesenteric vein) of myosin filaments, associated actin filaments and
the dense bodies on which the latter insert (Fig. 1). The presence of
cross-bridges on the myosin filaments (3,6) together with the
mechanical properties (e.g. length-tension curve) of smooth muscle led
to the generally accepted conclusion that a sliding filament mechanism
of contraction based on cycling cross-bridges having ATPase activity
operates in smooth muscle. It is believed by most, though not all
investigators in this field, that for myosin ATPase to be activated by
actin, the light chains (LC_{20}) of myosin have to be phosphorylated
by a calcium-dependent light chain kinase (for review, 2,7,8). It is
important to note, however, that the organization of myosin into

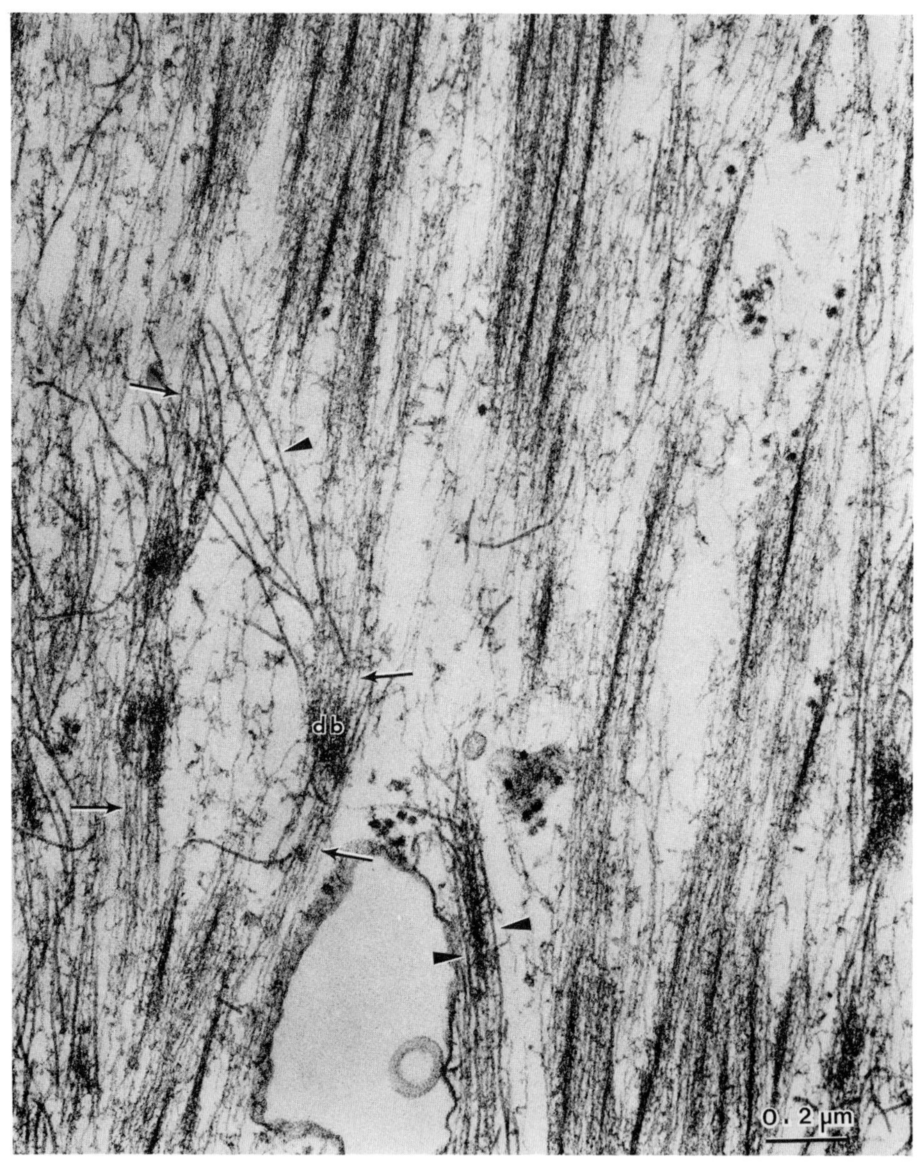

Fig. 1 Longitudinal section of a saponin-skinned PAMV smooth muscle cell.
The filaments are splayed out in some of the cells, as shown, which reveals
the relationship of the dense bodies with associated actin to the
neighboring myosin filaments. Thin filaments (indicated by arrows) which
emerge from cytoplasmic dense bodies (db) can be traced to the myosin
filaments on either side forming an I-band. The 10-nm filaments
(arrowheads) do not run parallel to the sarcomeres. Connections between
10-nm filaments and a cytoplasmic dense body occur at the lower center part
of the figure. x70,000. From Ref. 12.

filaments is <u>not</u> dependent on phosphorylation, and myosin filaments are present in smooth muscle regardless of whether LC_{20} is phosphorylated or not. These ultrastructural findings are consistent with observations showing the persistence of <u>maintained</u> (tonic) tension, at least in some smooth muscles, even after LC_{20} phosphorylation has declined or even returned to control (resting) levels (7,10).

Both types of dense bodies, either attached to the plasma membrane or those scattered throughout the interior of the cell, are attachment sites for actin filaments analogous to the Z-lines of striated muscle (3,11,12). When actin filaments are decorated with the S-1 subfragment of myosin, they show the proper arrowhead configuration (pointing away from either side of the dense body) consistent with functional actin attachment sites (12).

A third type of filament in smooth muscle is the intermediate filament (10nm diameter). These filaments are distinct from actin or myosin filaments, surround the dense bodies and appear to link them throughout the cell. Desmin and vimentin are the major constituent proteins of the intermediate filaments, and although one or the other protein may be exclusively present (Fig. 2) in certain types of smooth muscle (e.g., desmin in intestinal and vimentin in aorta), the presence of both types of protein in a single smooth muscle cell (Fig. 3) has also been observed (e.g. 13). In hypertrophied smooth muscle (14) abnormal proliferation of intermediate filaments (Fig. 4) is associated with an increase in the actin/myosin filament ratio.

Sources and sinks of activator calcium

The influx of calcium can be stimulated by a variety of excitatory agents, such as norepinephrine (for review, 1,15). Although initially disputed (16), the conclusion based on electrophysiological studies that norepinephrine induces Ca influx (17) was subsequently confirmed by ^{45}Ca flux studies (for review, 15). Given the occurrence of Ca influx, it is also clear that the maintenance of steady state in the long term requires the eventual efflux of Ca^{2+} against its electrochemical gradient (for review, 15; 18-20). However, the observation that contraction and even rhythmic activity of smooth muscle occurs in the absence of extracellular Ca^{2+} (21-24) and the

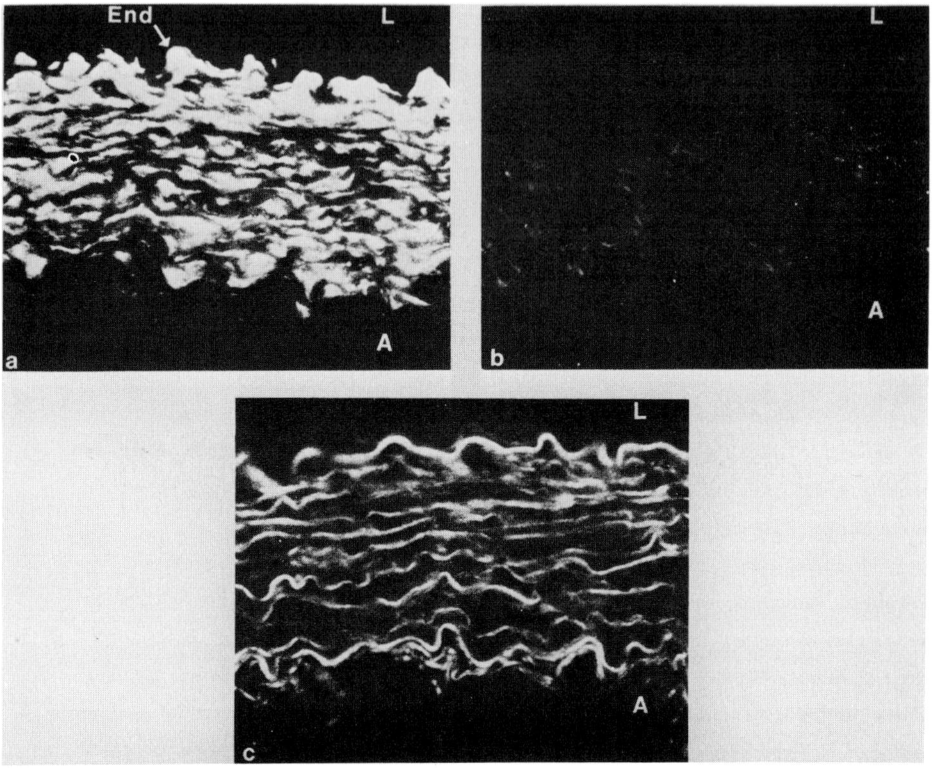

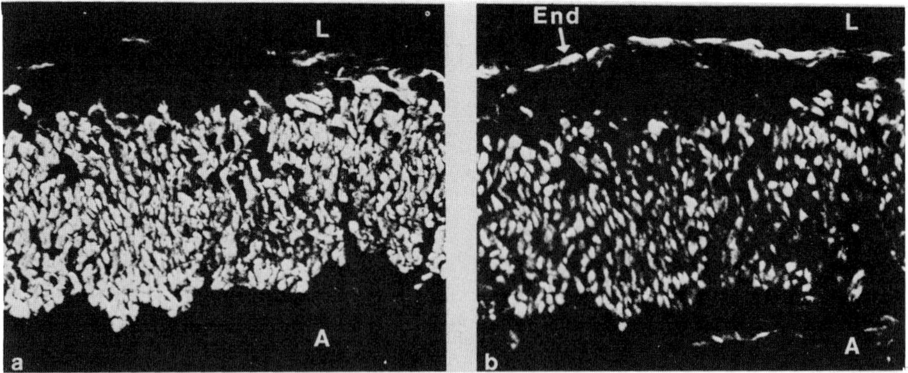

Fig. 2. Transverse sections of the abdominal aorta: (a) anti-hamster
vimentin staining showing luminal (L) and adventitial (A) areas and the
endothelium (End); (b) nonspecific goat IgG staining; (c) autofluorescence
of the internal elastic laminae. x340. From Ref. 13.

Fig. 3. Transverse sections of the PAMV: double immunofluorescence using the
anti-chick desmin antibody and rhodamine (a) and monoclonal anti-vimentin
and fluorescein (b) showing the luminal (L) and adventitial (A) areas with
the endothelium (End.) Modified from Ref. 13.

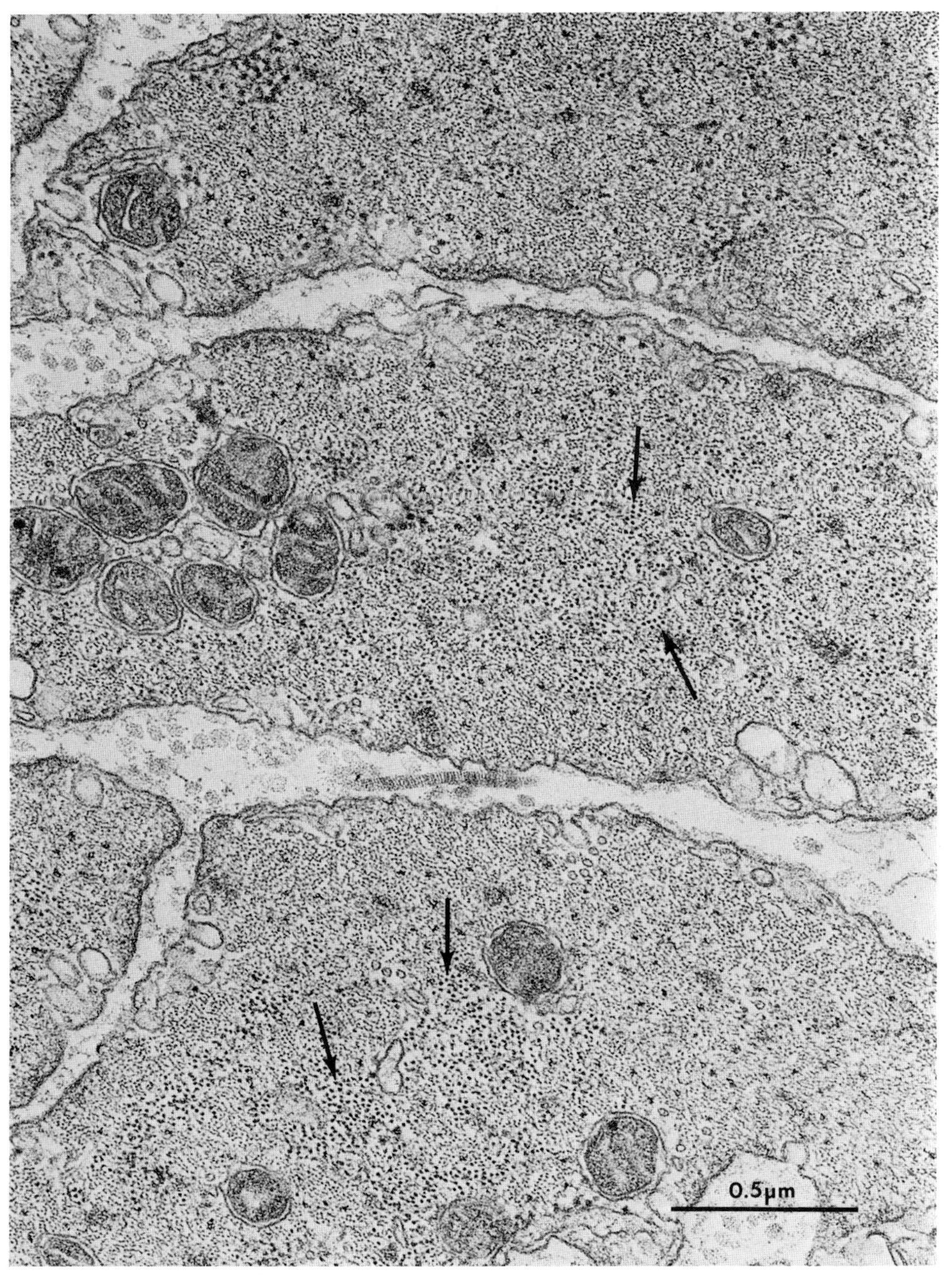

Fig. 4. Transverse section of a bundle of smooth muscle fibres from
hypertrophied PAMV showing the predominantly central location of the
abnormally increased number of intermediate filaments (arrows). Bar, 0.5μm.
x61,200. From Ref. 14.

general failure to correlate relaxation with ^{45}Ca efflux, indicate
the existence of intracellular organelles capable of releasing and
accumulating Ca. The demonstration of, first, strontium and, later,
calcium accumulation by the sarcoplasmic reticulum (SR) in situ
(25,26), and the eventual isolation of an active fragmented SR from
smooth muscle (27), suggested that the SR is a calcium sink in smooth
muscle. Subsequent studies on saponin-skinned smooth muscle in which
the cytoplasmic free Ca^{2+} could be controlled, demonstrated that
the SR can accumulate calcium at relatively low Ca (10^{-6}M) free Ca
concentrations (Fig. 5), concentrations that were too low to allow
mitochondrial Ca uptake (5). Mitochondria, in contrast, do not play a
physiological role in the control of cytoplasmic Ca, due to their low
apparent affinity for Ca^{2+}, as demonstrated in studies of
mitochondria isolated from vascular (28) and uterine smooth muscle (29),
and shown by the absence of mitochondrial calcium accumulation in
maximally contracting smooth muscle in situ (26). Mitochondria can
accumulate massive amounts of Ca when free-Ca^{2+} rises to 10^{-5}M
or higher (5,26). The abnormally high concentration of calcium in
mitochondria isolated from atherosclerotic (bovine) blood vessels
suggested that mitochondria may serve as pathological foci of vascular
(e.g.: coronary) calcification (30).

Contractions can be evoked repeatedly, in Ca-free solutions by
excitatory drugs (norepinephrine, cholinergic agents, caffeine), in
contrast to earlier observations that generally showed only a single
contraction when smooth muscles were stimulated in Ca-free solution.
The major difference in the recent studies (31) was that the excitatory
agonist was removed at the peak of tension development in Na-free,
lanthanum (La) containing solutions to reduce the loss of cellular Ca.
Under these conditions, repeatable contractions can be observed (Fig.
6) for up to half an hour in vascular (guinea pig portal vein) strips
less than 100μm in diameter, in the virtual absence of extracellular Ca
(Fig. 6). We interpret these findings to indicate the recycling of
calcium from an intracellular store: the sarcoplasmic reticulum.

To assay the release of calcium from the junctional sarcoplasmic
reticulum (3,23,32) we have measured with electron probe analysis
(33) the Ca concentration in submembranous micro regions of approximately 50-80nm diameter cell areas in guinea pig portal anterior

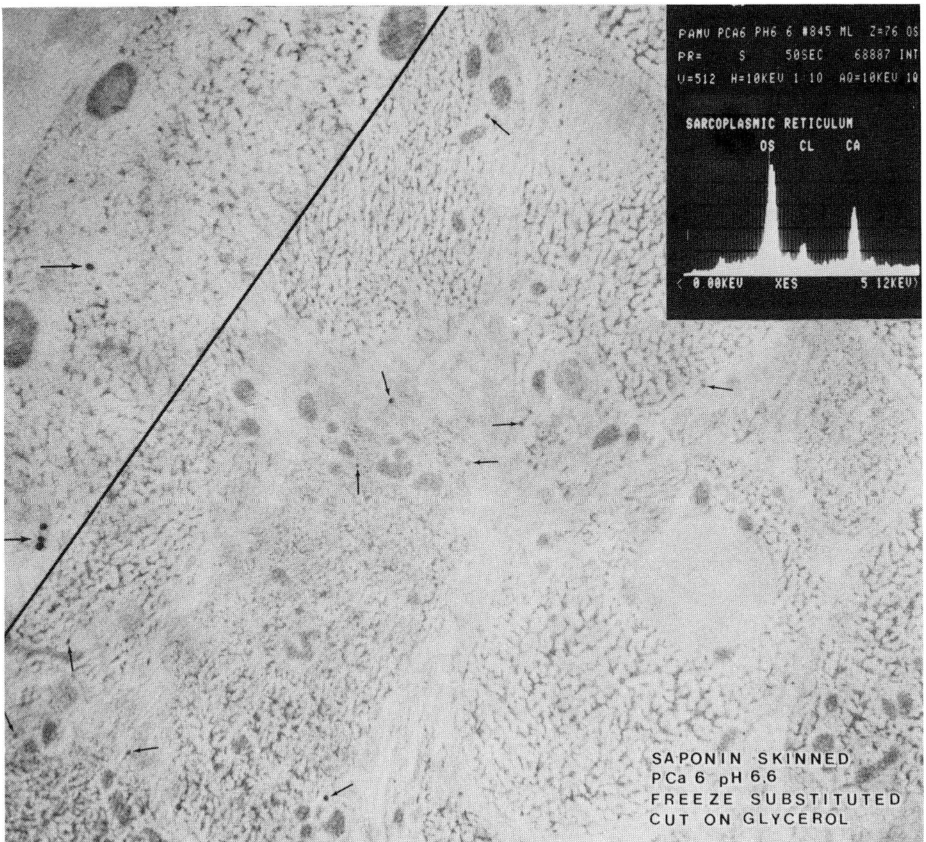

Fig. 5. Transverse section of saponin-skinned smooth muscle cells from rabbit portal vein. The skinned cells were exposed to a pCa 6 pH 6.6 EGTA buffer containing 2 mM free Mg for 30 min, were frozen, and were processed by freeze substitution. Deposits (arrows) of Ca associated with P in the SR are frequent at the periphery of the cells (shown at higher magnification at the upper left). Note the absence of mitochondrial loading. A typical spectrum from one of the SR deposits is shown. The osmium peak arises from the osmium included with the acetone to enhance contrast. Similar deposits were found in cryosections. m = mitochondrion. From Ref. 5.

mesenteric vein smooth muscles frozen either at rest or at the peak of a contraction. The solutions (including La) and experimental design for these experiments were identical to those in which the repeated contractions were demonstrated in the absence of external Ca. The presence of lanthanum in the bathing solution served as an extracellular marker in the cryosections (100nm thick) and allowed us to discriminate between caveolae and the sarcoplasmic reticulum in positioning the probe along the cell perimeter. The cytoplasm did not

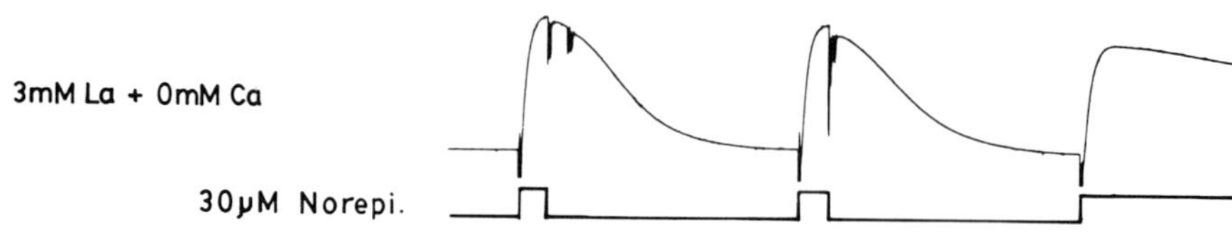

Fig. 6. Tension traces of a thin strip of guinea pig portal vein (50µm diameter). Following a contraction induced by high K+2mM Ca, there was a 2 min. incubation in high K, 0-Ca solution. After the addition of 3mM La in high K, a norepinephrine (NE)-induced contraction is elicited. This NE-induced contraction is of a similar magnitude as the high K-contracture, and can be repeated in the absence of Ca if the NE-induced contraction is interrupted (NE washed out) after 10 sec. Ion diffusion across the strip was ascertained in a separate experiment: guinea pig portal vein strips were frozen 2 min. after La^{3+} addition. La in the extracellular space was measured by EPMA in transverse cryosections across the smooth muscle bundle, and was found to be present in the extracellular space across the entire thickness of the strip. From Ref. 31.

contain lanthanum. These studies showed that the number of areas having high calcium content was 4-5/cell perimeter in relaxed smooth muscle; there was a marked reduction in the number of these "calcium hot spots" in muscles frozen at the peak (10 sec. after activation) of contraction. We conclude that sufficient calcium can be released from the junctional SR of smooth muscle to activate, in the absence of Ca-influx, a maximal or near maximal contraction. We believe that these findings render unnecessary some of the earlier speculations concerning an activator Ca compartment bound to the external plasma membrane in smooth muscle (e.g.: 34).

The second question concerning the activation of smooth muscle by intracellularly released calcium, and also bearing on the mechanism through which Ca^{2+} regulates contractile proteins, is the increase in free (35,36) and in <u>total</u> cytoplasmic calcium increases during contraction. Because electron probe analysis measures total cytoplasmic calcium, whether it is free or bound, these measurements provide information about the concentration of high affinity Ca binding proteins in smooth muscle. The absence of mitochondrial Ca uptake in normally contracting smooth muscle suggests that, even during a maximal contraction, free Ca^{2+} does not rise above 5×10^{-6}M (5).

Total cytoplasmic calcium was measured with small probes (to exclude overlap with elements of SR) in the central regions of portal vein smooth muscle cells in which elements of SR are extremely rare. Measurements were made in rabbit portal anterior mesenteric vein smooth muscle completely relaxed with isoproterenol ($0.2\mu g/ml$) and in paired strips maximally contracted with high K (in some experiments Rb was used) and norepinephrine ($30\mu M$), and frozen after a contraction maintained for 30 min. The cytoplasmic Ca concentration (mmol/kg dry wt) was 0.95 ± 0.17 in relaxed (N=224, 65 cells) and 1.9 ± 0.16 S.E.M. (N=289, 95 cells) in the contracted smooth muscles (P<0.0005). Therefore (assuming about 81% hydration of smooth muscle cells) total cytoplasmic Ca increases by approximately $300\mu mol/liter$ cell water during maximal contraction. Allowing for cumulative measurement errors due to occasional partial overlap of SR by the probe, contamination of carbon films, etc., our estimate of the lower limit of increase of total Ca $200\mu mol/kg$ cell water, is still highly significant (P<0.02). It is unlikely that the calcium binding sites (4/calmodulin) on calmodulin are sufficient to accommodate, in the presence of Mg, the entire rise in cytoplasmic Ca, even if cytoplasmic calmodulin concentration is as high as $40\mu M$ (37). It is possible that some of the calcium is bound to myosin (38) or to other cytoplasmic calcium binding proteins. The observed increase in cytoplasmic Ca concentration, while unexpectedly large, is still very much less than found in muscles containing parvalbumin: in frog muscle during tetanus the increase in cytoplasmic calcium in the I-band is approximately 3-4mmol/kg dry wt (39).

Sodium in normal and in hypertrophied smooth muscle

The accurate measurement of cellular sodium has presented one of the more vexing problems of smooth muscle physiology, and gained parti-cular importance with the recognition of the possibly major role of sodium in hypertension. Ion flux methods for measuring cytoplasmic Na have been specially designed in attempts to eliminate the contribution of extracellular Na to Na-fluxes, largely by conducting the initial part of [22]Na washout at low temperature and/or attempting to wash out extracellular Na with cold, Na free solutions (for review, see 15).

With electron probe analysis, it is possible to measure cytoplasmic Na under direct vision, by placing the electron probe on a selected region of the cell without interference by extracellular Na. As an initial investigation of the possible role of changes in cytoplasmic Na in hypertension, we attempted to determine whether changes in cytoplasmic Na occur as a consequence of increased distending pressure. We measured cell Na in rabbit portal anterior mesenteric vein smooth muscle subjected to distention hypertrophy (14,40). These experiments (41) showed no significant difference in the Na content or K : Na ratio of hypertrophied, sham operated and normal smooth muscles, but, like an earlier electron probe analytic study (26), revealed a significantly higher cell Na concentration than had been estimated from ion flux studies (15,42). Therefore, we were led to examine the concentration of normal cytoplasmic Na in smooth muscle and whether washout at low (2°C.) temperatures, used in ion flux studies, eliminates only the extracellular Na. Parallel studies have already shown that the high cytoplasmic Na values measured with electron probe analysis in rabbit portal anterior mesenteric vein were not an artifact of the preparatory or analytic techniques, because much lower Na concentrations were measured with electron probe analysis in frog skeletal muscle (39) and in guinea pig taenia coli (41).

The effect of washing smooth muscle in Na-free (Li) solution at 2°C. was determined in normal and Na-loaded rabbit portal anterior mesenteric vein and taenia coli. The amount of Na lost with cold Li wash was proportional to the initial cytoplasmic Na concentration: massive amounts (405mmol/kg dry wt.) of Na were lost from Na-loaded smooth muscle, and about 60% of the Na was lost from normal PAMV (a reduction from about 198mmol/kg dry wt to 74mm/kg dry wt). The reduction in cytoplasmic sodium with cold Na-free (Li wash) of normal rabbit portal vein did not further progress beyond the level reached at 30 min. washout, even when washout was followed for 2 hrs, and the already low Na content of the normal guinea pig taenia coli was not significantly reduced by lithium wash. On the basis of these findings, we concluded that there is in smooth muscle a relatively temperature insensitive Na-efflux system that, although having a lower affinity for Na than the Na,K ATPase Na pump, can lead to significant loss of cytoplasmic Na at low temperatures, and to underestimates of cytoplasmic Na measured with flux methods. An incidental finding in Na-loaded muscles was the appearance of two cell populations in cryosections: 1., light cells that were massively loaded with Na, contained abnormally high concentrations of Ca and low Mg, K and P and 2., a darker cell population in which Na gain was more moderate, cytoplasmic Mg and P were normal and the reduction in K more modest. These findings are in agreement with the interpretation that light and dark cells in conventionally fixed material reflect different degrees of cell hydration (26,32,43). Washout in Na-free solutions was followed by complete disappearance of massively Na-loaded cells, suggesting that these cells were extremely permeable, and lost all of their Na content during washout (41).

CONCLUSIONS

The sarcoplasmic reticulum is the physiological (intracellular) source and sink of activator calcium in smooth muscle, and the present studies have demonstrated directly the release of Ca from this site by norepinephrine. A rise in _total_ cytoplasmic Ca of approximately 200-300µM/liter cell water activates a sliding filament mechanism of contraction based on a contractile apparatus of myosin filaments that are assembled, regardless of their state of phosphorylation, and interact with actin filaments inserting on dense bodies. Electron probe analysis revealed the presence of a low affinity, relatively temperature insensitive, rapid component of Na-efflux in smooth muscle and the existence of a heterogeneous cell population following sodium-loading. No significant changes in K or Na content were found in hypertrophied vascular smooth muscle.

Supported by HL15835 to the Pennsylvania Muscle Institute, HL25348 and HL07499.

REFERENCES

1. Johansson B, Somlyo AP: Electrophysiology and excitation-contraction coupling. In: Bohr DF, Somlyo AP, Sparks HV (eds) The handbook of physiology. Vascular smooth muscle. Williams and Wilkins Co., Baltimore, MD, 1980, pp 301-324.
2. Hartshorne DJ: Biochemistry of the contractile process in smooth muscle. In: Johnson LR (ed) Physiology of the gastrointestinal tract. Raven Press, New York, pp 243-267.

3. Somlyo AV: Ultrastructure of vascular smooth muscle. In: Bohr DF, Somlyo AP, Sparks HV (eds) The handbook of physiology. Vascular smooth muscle. Williams and Wilkins Co., Baltimore, MD, 1980, pp 33-67.

4. Somlyo AP, Somlyo AV: Effects and subcellular distribution of magnesium in smooth and striated muscle. Fed Proc (40):2667-2671, 1981.

5. Somlyo AP, Somlyo AV, Shuman H, Endo M: Calcium and monovalent ions in smooth muscle. Fed Proc (41);2883-2890, 1982.

6. Somlyo AP, Devine CE, Somlyo AV, Rice RV: Filament organization in vertebrate smooth muscle. Phil Trans Roy Soc B (265):223-229, 1973.

7. Butler TM, Siegman M: Chemical energy usage and myosin light chain phosphorylation in mammalian smooth muscle. Fed Proc (43):57-61, 1983.

8. Adelstein RS, Eisenberg RE: Regulation and kinetics of the actin-myosin ATP interaction. Ann Rev Biochem (49):921-956.

9. Somlyo AV, Butler TM, Bond M, Somlyo AP: Myosin filaments have nonphosphorylated light chains in relaxed smooth muscle. Nature (294): 567-570, 1981.

10. Miller JR, Silver PJ, Stull JT: The role of myosin light chain kinase phosphorylation in Beta-adrenergic relaxation of tracheal smooth muscle. Molec Pharmacol (24):235-242, 1983.

11. Ashton FT, Somlyo AV, Somlyo AP: The contractile apparatus of vascular smooth muscle: Intermediate high voltage stereo electron microscopy. J Mol Biol (98):17-29, 1975.

12. Bond M, Somlyo AV: Dense bodies and actin polarity in vertebrate smooth muscle. J Cell Biol (95):403-413, 1982.

13. Berner PF, Frank E, Holtzer H, Somlyo AP: The intermediate filament proteins of rabbit vascular smooth muscle: Immunofluorescent studies of desmin and vimentin. J Musc Res Cell Motil (2):439-452, 1981.

14. Berner PF, Somlyo AV, Somlyo AP: Hypertrophy-induced increase of intermediate filaments in vascular smooth muscle. J Cell Biol (88): 96-101, 1981.

15. Jones A: Content and fluxes of electrolytes. In: Bohr DF, Somlyo AP, Sparks HV (eds) The handbook of physiology. Vascular smooth muscle. Williams and Wilkins Co., Baltimore, MD, 1980, pp 253-299.

16. Van Breeman C, Lesser P: The absence of increased membrane calcium permeability during norepinephrine stimulation of arterial smooth muscle. Microvasc Res (3):113-114, 1971.

17. Somlyo AP, Somlyo AV: Electrophysiological correlates of the inequality of maximal vascular smooth muscle contraction elicited by drugs. In: Bevan JA, Furchgott RF, Maxwell RA, Somlyo AP (eds) Vascular neuro-effector systems. S. Karger, Basel, Switzerland, 1971, pp 216-226.

18. Brading AF: Ionic distribution and mechanisms of transmembrane ion movements in smooth muscles. In: Bulbring E, Brading AF, Jones AW, Tomita T (eds) Smooth muscle: an assessment of current knowledge. Edward Arnold, Ltd, London, England, 1981, pp 65-92.

19. Casteels R: Electro- and pharmacomechanical coupling in vascular smooth muscle. Chest (78):150-156, 1980.

20. Blaustein M: Sodium ions, calcium ions, blood pressure regulation, and hypertension: a reassessment and a hypothesis. Am J Physiol (232):C165-C173, 1977.

21. Bozler E: Role of calcium in initiation of activity of smooth muscle. Amer J Physiol (216):671, 1969.

22. Somlyo AP, Devine CE, Somlyo AV, North SR: Sarcoplasmic reticulum and the temperature-dependent contraction of smooth muscle in calcium-free solutions. J Cell Biol (51):722-741, 1971.

23. Devine CE, Somlyo AV, Somlyo AP: Sarcoplasmic reticulum and excitation-contraction coupling in mammalian smooth muscle. J Cell Biol (52): 690-718, 1972.

24. Mangel AW, Nelson DO, Connor JA, Prosser CL: Contractions of cat small intestinal smooth muscle in calcium-free solution. Nature (281):582-583, 1979.

25. Somlyo AV, Somlyo AP: Strontium accumulation by sarcoplasmic reticulum and mitochondria in vascular smooth muscle. Science (174):955-958, 1971.

26. Somlyo AP, Somlyo AV, Shuman H: Electron probe analysis of vascular smooth muscle: Composition of mitochondria, nuclei and cytoplasm. J Cell Biol (81):316-335, 1979.

27. Raeymaekers L, Hasselbach W: CA^{2+} uptake, Ca^{2+}-ATPase activity, phosphoprotein formation and phosphate turnover in a microsomal fraction of smooth muscle. Eur J Biochem (116):373, 378, 1981.

28. Vallieres J, Scarpa A, Somlyo AP: Subcellular fractions of smooth muscle: Isolation, substrate utilization and Ca^{++} transport by main pulmonary artery and mesenteric vein mitochondria. Arch Biochem Biophys (170):659-669, 1975.

29. Wikstrom M, Ahonen P, Luukkainen T: The role of mitochondria in uterine contractions. FEBS Lett (56):77-88, 1975.

30. Somlyo AP, Somlyo AV, Shuman H, Sloane B, Scarpa A: Electron probe analysis of calcium compartments in cryosections of smooth and striated muscles. Ann NY Acad Sci (307):523-544, 1978.

31. Somlyo AP, Somlyo AV, Kitazawa T, Bond M, Shuman H, Kowarski D: Ultrastructure, function and composition of smooth muscle. Ann Biomed Engr (BMES) in press.

32. Somlyo AP, Devine CE, Somlyo AV, North SR: Sarcoplasmic reticulum and the temperature-dependent contraction of smooth muscle in calcium-free solutions. J Cell Biol (51):722-741, 1971.

33. Somlyo AP, Shuman H: Electron probe and electron energy loss analysis in biology. Ultramicroscopy (8):219-234, 1982.

34. Somlyo AV, Somlyo AP: Electromechanical and pharmacomechanical coupling in vascular smooth muscle. J Pharmacol Exp Ther (159):129-145, 1968.

35. Morgan JP, Morgan KG: Vascular smooth muscle: The first recorded Ca^{2+} transients. Pfluegers Arch (395):75-77, 1982.

36. Fay FS, Shlevin HH, Granger WC Jr, Taylor SR: Aequorin luminescence during activation of single isolated smooth muscle cells. Nature (280):506-508, 1979.

37. Grand RJA, Perry SV: Calmodulin-binding proteins from brain and other tissues. Biochem J (183):285-295, 1979.

38. Chacko S, Rosenfeld A: Regulation of actin-activated ATP hydrolysis by arterial myosin. Proc Natl Acad Sci USA (79):292-296, 1982.

39. Somlyo AV, Gonzalez H, Shuman H, McClellan G, Somlyo AP: Calcium release and ionic changes in the sarcoplasmic reticulum of tetanized muscle: An electron probe study. J Cell Biol (90):577-594, 1981.

40. Johansson B: Structural and functional changes in rat portal veins after experimental portal hypertension. Acta Physiol Scand (98): 381-383, 1976.

41. Junker JL, Wasserman AJ, Berner PF, Somlyo AP: Electron probe analysis of sodium and other elements in hypertrophied and sodium-loaded smooth muscle. Cir Res (54):in press.

42. Jones AW, Somlyo AP, Somlyo AV: Potassium accumulation in smooth muscle and associated ultrastructural changes. J Physiol (London)

(232):247-273, 1976.
43. Garfield RE, Daniel EE: Light and dark smooth muscle cells in estrogen-stimulated rat myometrium. Can J Physiol Pharmacol (54): 8220833, 1976.

7

ROLE OF THE NA[+] PUMP IN VASCULAR SMOOTH MUSCLE CONTRACTILITY

JULIUS C. ALLEN, RICHARD D. BUKOSKI, STEPHEN S. NAVRAN & CHARLES L. SEIDEL

INTRODUCTION

Although it is well-known that calcium is required for contraction in vascular smooth muscle, little is known about the mechanisms which regulate its free cytoplasmic concentration. There are a number of areas within the cell which may participate in this process but a unified hypothesis has yet to be proposed regarding selective roles of these various specific membrane areas. While studies with intact tissue have clearly identified compartmentation of Ca^{++} levels in vascular smooth muscle, successful identification of any compartment with a specific organelle, remains to be accomplished (1).

The two major areas which have been considered as being involved in regulation of cytoplasmic calcium are the sarcolemma and sarcoplasmic reticulum. The suggestion that mitochondria may also be involved has been made by a number of workers. The current thinking, however, is that membrane areas play a more direct role in vascular smooth muscle, and that mitochondria may serve as a reserve source for Ca^{++}, although this is still disputed.

One of the major problems in delineating the role of these two distinct membrane areas is the fact that it has been extremely difficult to isolate and separate the two, and therefore, to characterize their separate calcium sequestering capabilities. Daniel and his co-workers (2), have reported significant purification of the cell membrane area using as markers 5'-nucleotidase and ouabain inhibitable K^+ stimulated paranitrophenyl phosphatase (K^+-phosphatase) activities. Their conclusions are that cell membrane is the major area for regulation of cytoplasmic calcium for both arterial and venous smooth muscle. Allen et al. (3) essentially agree with this conclusion based on the presence of latent Na^+,K^+-ATPase activities and Ca^{++} sequestering capacities in heterogeneous fractions of canine aorta.

Ca^{++} sequestering capacities of both cardiac and skeletal muscle tissue (based on yield of sarcoplasmic reticulum per gram tissue x Ca^{++} sequestering capacity of the SR, in umoles Ca^{++}/g SR protein) suggests that the organelle in the intact tissue can sequester enough Ca^{++} to decrease cytoplasmic Ca^{++} levels to a low enough value to effect relaxation. Such calculations for vascular smooth muscle using similar criteria, suggest that the membranes being assessed, either SL or SR alone, or together cannot sequester enough Ca^{++} to effect relaxation.

Because it has been difficult to assign specific roles regarding Ca^{++} sites to a specific membrane area and because of the apparent inability of cellular membranes to sequester sufficient Ca^{++} to effect relaxation, we wish to suggest that Na^+,K^+-ATPase may play an important modulating role in vascular smooth muscle contraction and relaxation, and contribute to the heterogeneity of contractile responses. Such a role has been postulated by others for the Na^+-pump in the mechanism of K^+-induced relaxation of vascular smooth muscle. In such cases it has been suggested that pump stimulation can effect a decrease in cytoplasmic Ca^{++} by either a Na–Ca^{++} exchange mechanism, or membrane hyperpolarization.

For these reasons we have recently been studying the Na^+-pump in vascular smooth muscle both indirectly and directly. Indirect studies have involved mechanical studies, and have assumed that K^+-induced relaxation of NE-contracted arteries is a manifestation of Na^+-pump function.

Kinetic models of the Na^+ pump based on both isolated cell-free systems (7) and intact tissue (8) suggest that external Na^+ can compete with external K^+ for the K^+-activation site of the Na^+ pump. Our working hypothesis was that if the Na^+ pump is the rate-limiting step of K^+-induced relaxation, then alterations in external Na^+ should produce predictable affects on the K^+-induced relaxation event.

Direct studies have involved both whole tissue measurement of ouabain-sensitive ^{86}Rb uptake, as well as Na^+,K^+-ATPase and ^3H-ouabain binding to isolated cell free systems from various sources of vascular smooth muscle. The data from both of these directions strongly suggest that the Na^+-pump is directly involved in regulation of vascular smooth muscle contractile state.

INDIRECT STUDIES

In 1977 Webb and Bohr (4) suggested that when an isolated strip of vascular smooth muscle was contracted by norepinephrine in a K^+-free medium that the relaxation occurring when K+ was added back to the bathing solution was a measure of the Na+-pump. Recently, we have published a number of experiments using this "K^+-relaxation" protocol, which have suggested that this may not be universally true, because of selected effects of the agonist in question on the Na+-pump (5,6). We have performed extensive contractile characterizations of the renal and femoral arteries of the dog. These studies compared the responsiveness of the renal and femoral arteries of the dog, and Figure 1 shows a schematic diagram of the "K^+-relaxation" protocol.

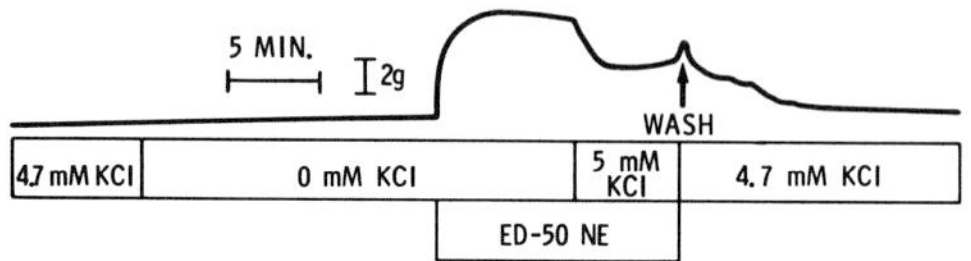

FIGURE 1: Drawing of a typical K^+-induced relaxation procedure. See text for description (reproduced by permission from reference 5)

The tissue is bathed in a normal equilibrating Krebs solution, which is then replaced by a K^+-free Krebs. This solution effects an inhibition of the Na^+-pump, because of the absence of K^+ to activate the external K^+-activation site. Norepinephrine is then added in an appropriate amount to cause a contraction. After equilibrium is reached, K^+ is returned to the bath, inducing a relaxation. Both the rate of this K^+-induced relaxation, and the total amount of relaxation may be used as indicators of pump activity.

Regardless of which specific parameters of relaxation we measured, either the rate or amount of relaxation, the renal artery always relaxed to a greater extent or at a faster rate than the femoral artery, as can be seen in Figure 2. If K^+-induced relaxation was indeed a measure of the quantity or capacity of the Na^+-pump, then this would suggest that the Na^+-pump of these two arteries are significantly different.

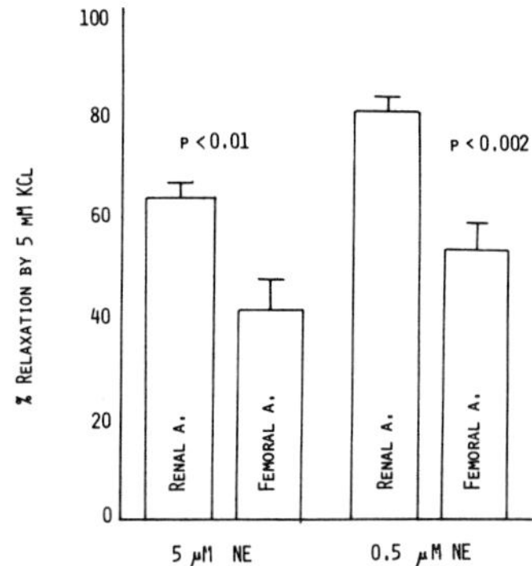

FIGURE 2: K^+-induced relaxation in canine renal and femoral arteries. See Figure 1 for protocol. Tissues were contracted by either 0.5 uM or 5 uM norepinephrine in K^+-free Krebs. After equilibrium was reached, K^+ was added to effect relaxation. % relaxation was calculated based on the contractile response to norepinephrine representing 100%, or the maximum amount that the tissue could relax.

We further studied this hypothesis using a model of Na^+-pump that was developed both for isolated cell-free (7) systems and intact gastrointestinal smooth muscle (8). Both models suggested that if the external Na^+ levels were decreased then the external K^+ would be more effective in stimulating the Na^+-pump. This was based on the fact that there seems to be competition for Na^+ at the external K^+ site of the pump. Therefore, it was our contention that in both of these tissues if the external Na+ level were lowered then K^+-relaxation ought to be enhanced. The femoral artery did indeed respond in this manner (Fig. 3). When the external Na^+ was lowered, K^+ became more effective in inducing femoral relaxation. However, the renal artery did not respond in the same manner, even though the sensitivity of K^+-relaxation of the renal artery to K^+ was higher than that of the femoral artery. When external Na+ was lowered there was no increase in the K-sensitivity in the renal artery.

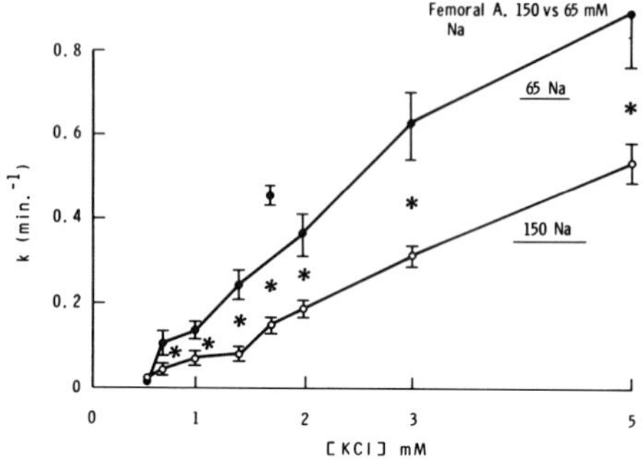

FIGURE 3: Effect of different external Na concentrations (●——●, 65 mM Na; o——o 150 mM Na$^+$) on initial rate of K$^+$-induced relaxation as a function of external K$^+$ concentration in femoral arteries (reproduced by permission from reference 5).

Our conclusions from those experiments were that in the renal artery the Na+-pump was not simply reflected by K+-induced relaxation, since the pump did not respond in a manner predicted by Na$^+$ pump kinetics, whereas in the femoral artery the response was consistent with the hypothesis that external Na+ could modulate the K+ effect on the external membrane. This lead us to suggest that either the pumps of the two arteries are not the same or that K+-relaxation does not universally "measure" the Na+-pump.

<u>DIRECT STUDIES</u>

1. Na$^+$,K$^+$-ATPase

Since K$^+$-relaxation is only an indirect way of measuring the Na$^+$ pump, and assessing its involvement in contractile regulation, we went to more direct measures: 1) Na$^+$,K$^+$-ATPase isolation and ^{3}H-ouabain binding, 2) ouabain sensitive ^{86}Rb-uptake. Na$^+$,K$^+$-ATPase and ^{3}H-ouabain binding fractions were isolated using the standard procedures developed in this laborataory. It should be noted that this enzyme activity has been difficult to isolate and study in vascular smooth muscle, mainly because of the very large Mg$^+$-ATPase component that is

not appear to be consistent with our hypothesis, i.e. that there was a difference between the Na^+-pumps of the two arteries. It rather supported the contention that the pumps of the arteries are identical.

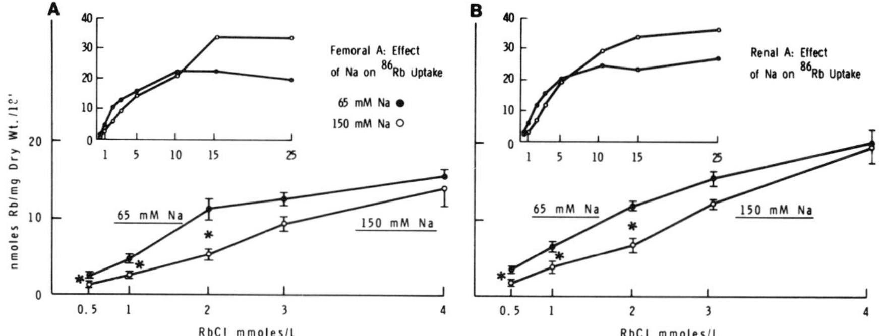

FIGURE 4:   A comparison of effects of lowered external Na^+ on ^{86}Rb uptake by femoral and renal arteries (●——● 65 mM Na^+, o——o, 150 mM Na^+).

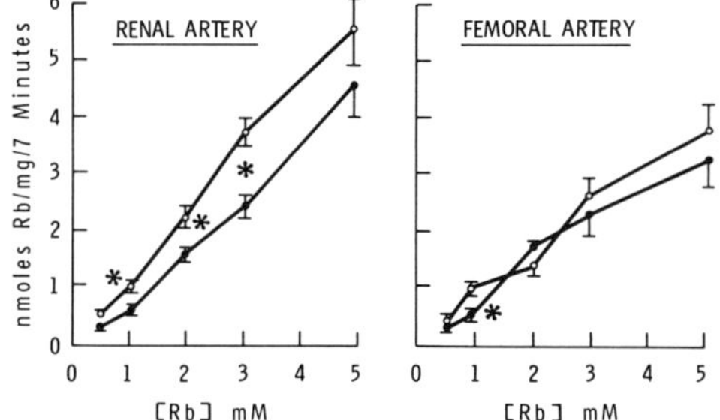

FIGURE 5:   Effect of 3.5 uM Norepinephrine (o——o) on ^{86}Rb uptake of renal and femoral arteries (reproduced by permission from reference 6).

There was, however, a major difference between the procedures of measuring ^{86}Rb-uptake and K^+-relaxation, since the latter required the presence of the contractile agonist, norepinephrine. Consenquently, we studied the effect of an ED_{50} dose of norepinephrine, on ^{86}Rb uptake. The use of 3.5 uM norepinephrine consistently stimulated ^{86}Rb-uptake (Figure 5) in the renal artery but not in the femoral artery. If the Na+,K+-ATPase enzymes were studied in cell free systems from both arteries no affects were seen so it is difficult to identify the

generally found with any measurable Na^+,K^+-ATPase activity. Isolation of the Na^+,K^+-ATPase, measurement of its enzyme activity, quantitation of the number of ouabain-binding sites and the qualitative aspects of ouabain-binding indicated that there was no difference in the cell free enzyme systems of the two arteries. Therefore, it seems highly unlikely that the pumps have inherent differences, yet they seem to respond differently when assessing their role in K^+-relaxation as indicated earlier. It can be concluded, therefore, that the Na^+,K^+-ATPase, as manifested in a cell-free system, is not exactly reflective of the pump working _in situ_ in a vascular smooth muscle cell membrane. Data to be discussed below, using antibodies from purified canine renal medullary Na^+,K^+-ATPase enhance this concept.

2. ^{86}Rb uptake

Since the Na^+,K^+-ATPase activity and ouabain-binding parameters were identical in the renal and femoral artery, it was important to study the functioning pump _in situ_, using ouabain sensitive ^{86}Rb to assess kinetic behavior and Na^+-pump capacity. Initial work by a number of workers, suggested that ^{86}Rb-uptake is a direct manifestation of the Na^+-pump (9). Using the same kinetic criteria that we used to relate Na^+-pump function to contractility (i.e. modulation of the external K^+ (or Rb) site by alterations in external Na^+) we were able to show that in both renal and femoral arteries, lowering external Na^+ significantly increased ouabain sensitive ^{86}Rb-uptake (Fig. 4) Therefore, both the arterial pump systems were responding to lowered external Na^+ with increased affinity for ^{86}Rb, as predicted. However, it should be recalled that with K^+-relaxation, only the femoral artery responded to a decrease in external Na^+ levels. Thus the ^{86}Rb data did

mechanism of norepinephrine's affect *in situ*. We have not yet been
able to demonstrate norepinephrine effects on vascular smooth muscle
Na+,K+-ATPase in studies done in a manner similar to Scheid et al. who
have actually shown norepinephrine stimulation of the enzyme in frog
stomach muscle (10). However, Limas and Cohn (11) did show a
stimulation of canine mesenteric artery Na^+,K^+-ATPase by a number of
agents. It was our hypothesis therefore that the "native" Na^+-pumps
were similar but that the nature of the *in situ* phospholipid: Na^+,K^+-
ATPase complex and the effect of ionic and electrical gradients on its
function may be different between the two arteries.

In order to further identity Na^+-pump similarity, we studied the
effect of antibodies raised in the rabbit to purified Na^+,K^+-ATPase
isolated from canine renal medulla. Our hypothesis was that if all
Na^+,K^+-ATPases from the same species are similar then there should be a
response of the Na^+,K^+-ATPase isolated from various tissues in the same
animal to this antibody. The observed data supported this hypothesis.
We were able to show that all of the canine Na^+,K^+-ATPase preparations
studied interacted with the Anti-Na^+,K^+-ATPase antibody. Sources of
canine Na^+,K^+-ATPase studied were aorta, renal artery, femoral artery,
heart and kidney. In each case the Na^+,K^+-ATPase enzyme was inhibited
by interaction with the antibody as predicted, and also demonstrated
positive reaction with both at least two antibody specific tests,
Ouchterlouney gels and western transfer. The antibody had no affect on
various non-Na^+,K^+-ATPase, activities from dog (i.e. Mg ATPase). In
addition, there was no interaction with the antibody with rat heart or
kidney Na^+,K^+-ATPase (Figure 6).

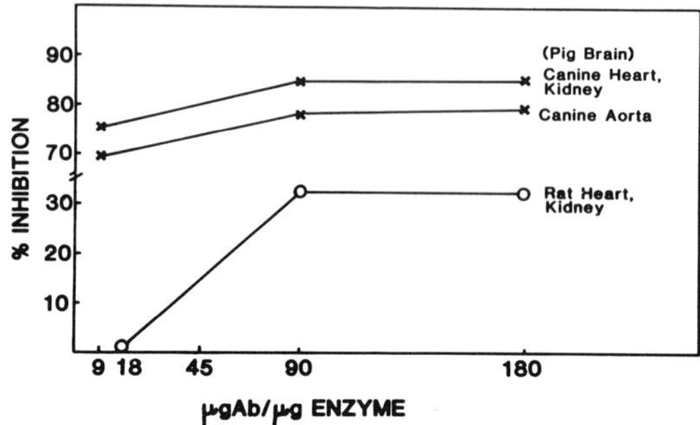

FIGURE 6:   Effects of antibodies to canine kidney medullary Na$^+$,K$^+$-ATPase on Na$^+$,K$^+$-ATPase activities of various canine preparations.

All these data have lead us to suggest that the basic unit of the Na$^+$-pump from different tissues is similar in a given species. However, when that protein complex is placed in a membrane its function can be altered by specific membrane components and electrochemical forces.   Thus, the Na$^+$,K$^+$-ATPase molecule as placed in the renal artery may be juxtaposed to lipids or proteins which could respond to norepinephrine and hence stimulate the pump, whereas its placement in the femoral artery membrane may be too distant from these components for it to respond to norepinephrine or they may be dissimilar in the two arteries.   In short, this is to say that the cell-free system of Na$^+$,K$^+$-ATPase does not exactly reflect the functional aspects of the pump as it exists in the cell membrane.   The enzyme protein may be the fundamental pump but and in different tissues it can be modulated differently by the microenvironment.

PRIMARY AND SECONDARY MODULATION OF THE Na$^+$ PUMP

The concept of such pump modulation allows much speculation regarding the role of the pump in regulation of contractility.   There are essentially two ways the pump can be regulated.   One is directly

(Primary) by altering the amount of Na^+ or K^+ present to interact with the pump. The other is indirectly (Secondary) by alterations of the protein itself by modulators which may alter pump sensitivity to cations.

Such differences in regulatory characteristics can be shown by ^{86}Rb experiments. Pump function can be studied in both Na^+ loaded and normal Na^+ tissues. The purpose of using Na^+ loaded tissues is to assess maximum pump rate. This maximal ^{86}Rb uptake rate is generally achieved by incubating the tissue in K^+-free solutions, which inhibits the pump, allowing the tissue to become loaded with Na^+. Subsequent administration of ^{86}Rb (tor K^+) maximally stimulates the pump.

The other condition for study of the pump is at low (or normal) internal Na^+ levels. This can be accomplished by preincubation for a period of time (such as 2-3 hrs) in regular Krebs medium, which allows the pump to reach equilibrium as it returns ionic conditions to their resting levels after tissue dissection and manipulation. If ouabain-sensitive ^{86}Rb-uptake is measured at this time, i.e. in the presence of low (normal) intracellular Na^+, it is significantly less than in Na^+ loaded conditions. If, however, the Na^+ ionophore, monensin is added to the medium, the ^{86}Rb-uptake is stimulated to the same level as that which occurs in Na^+-loaded tissue (Table 1). Presumably the reason for this is that the monensin increases the $[Na^+]$ on the inside of the cell.

TABLE 1:

^{86}Rb Uptake in Canine Renal Arteries

(nmoles/mg dry wt/20')

Na$^+$ loaded		Low Na$^+$	
C	Monensin	C	Monensin
16.6	15.7	5.2	12.7

There are a number of agonists which have been found to modulate the pump under normal Na$^+$ conditions. In these situations the Na$^+$-pump is presumably being regulated by the Na$^+$ gating effect of these agonists (12). However, we have recently shown that a number of agonists can actually stimulate the pump when monensin has no further effect suggesting that their mechanism of action cannot involve a gating effect of Na$^+$. Our hypothesis is that these compounds may alter the membrane environment adjacent to the pump or even the pump protein itself to alter sensitivity to either external K$^+$ or internal Na$^+$ (secondary modulating affects).

Recently we have used the compound forskolin (a direct activator of adenylate cyclase) to try to stimulate the Na$^+$-pump in renal and femoral arteries. Indeed, in all cases, ouabain sensitive ^{86}Rb uptake in the renal artery was stimulated by forskolin (Fig. 7), whereas the femoral artery was not (13) (data not shown). These data are similar to those of Figure 4, with norepinephrine. Since forskolin can stimulate ^{86}Rb uptake when monensin cannot forskolin may exert its affect other than by increasing intracellular Na$^+$ content. Indeed, it may be altering the pump by affecting the membrane environment, which can then alter pump function.

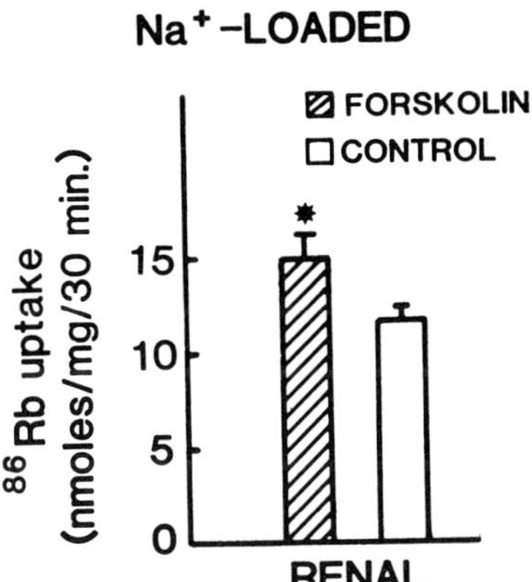

FIGURE 7: Effect of forskolin on ^{86}Rb uptake of canine renal artery.

The concept that the pump may be stimulated in a manner in addition to increasing internal Na$^+$ to a maximum, leads one to suggest that there may be many modulators of pump activity in these tissues. This we may call pump reserve. What this essentially says is that in a certain "activated" state the pump can be stimulated more by a given concentration of cation (in this particular case Na$^+$. The pump is stimulated by forskolin, for example, at both normal (resting) cellular Na$^+$ levels as well as high Na$^+$ levels. The absolute quantity of stimulation appears to be equal at both these high and low levels of internal Na$^+$ although the percent stimulation of basal pump rate is more at the lower levels of Na$^+$. This would provide a cell many areas of control resulting from altered pump function. For example, at low levels of internal Na+ (that is normal levels of cellular Na+) the pump could be modulated, effecting an altered membrane state (hyperpolarization?) which could then lead to altered effects, such as relaxation. The altered pump becomes   more responsive to a resting level of Na^+, so that the pump can be stimulated even though internal Na^+ has not been changed. While this does <u>not</u> provide any further evidence regarding the mechanism of Ca^{++} withdrawal from contractile proteins it does implicate the Na^+ pump as a possible control point. There is an increased affinity of the pump for Na^+, that is caused by forskolin.

<u>SUMMARY</u>

We have presented data which implicates Na^+,K^+-ATPase and the Na^+-pump in regulation of vascular smooth muscle contractility. We have shown that the pump can be stimulated in two ways, directly by altering internal Na^+ and indirectly, whereby the pump itself or adjacent proteins and/or lipids residing in the membrane are altered such that the pump sensitivity to ionic control is altered. Such mechanisms could involve phosphorylation of the enzyme or a subunit, altered membrane fluidity or allosteric regulation, altering K_M or V_{max}. Thus at both normal and high Na^+ levels the possibility exists that the pump could be modulated to play a role in vascular smooth muscle contractile regulation. If any differences exist between membrane micro-environments of differing arteries it is easy to postulate how alterations in pump function could play a role in vascular smooth muscle contractile heterogeneity.

<u>ACKNOWLEDGEMENTS</u>

Original work in this manuscript was supported by HL 07282 and HL 24585. We thank Elaine Hughes for her expert secretarial assistance.

1. Allen, J.C. and Bukoski, R.A.: Current status of vascular smooth muscle subcellular calcium regulation. In Vascular Smooth Muscle: Metabolic, Ionic and Contractile Mechanisms. Crass, M.F. and Barnes, C.D. (eds.), Academic Press, New York, 1982, pp. 99-134.

2. Daniel, E.E., Grover, A.K., and Kwan, Y.: Calcium. In Biochemistry of Smooth Muscle, Vol. III. Stephens, N.L. (ed), CRC Press, Boca Raton, Florida, 1983, pp. 1-88.

3. Allen, J.C., Smith, D.J., and Gerthoffer, W.T.: Ca-accumulation and latent Na-K-ATPase activity of heterogenous membrane fractions of vascular smooth muscle. Life Sci. 28:945-950 1981.

4. Webb, R.C. and Bohr, D.F.: Potassium-induced relaxation as an indicator of Na^+,K^+-ATPase activity in vascular smooth muscle. Blood Vessels 15:198-207, 1978.

5. Bukoski, R.D., Seidel, C.L., and Allen, J.C.: Differences in K^+-induced relaxation of canine femoral and renal arteries. Am. J. Physiol. 245:H598-H603, 1983.

6. Bukoski, R.D., Seidel, C.L., and Allen, J.C.: Ouabain binding, Na^+, K^+-ATPase activity, and ^{86}Rb uptake of canine arteries. Am. J. Physiol. 245:H604-H609, 1983.

7. Lindenmayer, G.E., Schwartz, A., and Thompson, H.: A kinetic description for sodium and potassium effects on $(Na^+ + K^+)$-adenosine triphosphatase: a model for a two nonequivalent site potassium activation and an analysis of multiequivalent site models for sodium activation. J. Physiol. London 236:1-28, 1974.

8. Widdicombe, J.H.: Ouabain-sensitive ion fluxes in the smooth muscle of the guinea pig's taenia coli. J. Physiol. London 266:235-254, 1977.

9. Overbeck, H.W., Pamnani, M.B., Akera, T., Brody, T.M., and Haddy, F.J.: Depressed function of a ouabain-sensitive sodium-potassium pump in blood vessels from renal hypertensive dogs. Circ. Res. 38 (Suppl. II):48-52, 1976.

10. Scheid, C.R., Honeyman, T.W., and Fay, F.S.: Mechanism of β-adrenergic relaxation of smooth muscle. Nature 277:32-36, 1979.

11. Limas, C.J. and Cohn, J.N.: Stimulation of vascular smooth muscle sodium, potassium-adenosine triphosphatase by vasodilators. Circ. Res. 35:601-607, 1974.

12. Akera, T., Yamamoto, S., Temma, K., Kim, D-H, and Brody, T.M.: Is ouabain-sensitive rubidium or potassium uptake a measure of sodium pump activity in isolated cardiac muscle? Biochim. Biophys. Acta 640:779-790, 1981.

13. Allen, J.C., Navran, S.S., Seidel, C.L., and Strong, R.: Correlation of vascular smooth muscle relaxation and Na^+ pump stimulation by forskolin. The Physiologist 26:A-12, 1983.

8

REGULATION OF MYOSIN PHOSPHORYLATION IN SMOOTH MUSCLE

J.T. STULL, J.R. MILLER AND P.J. SILVER

1. INTRODUCTION

Contraction of smooth muscle is thought to be dependent upon an increase in the concentration of sarcoplasmic free Ca^{2+} which activates the contractile elements. The source of activator Ca^{2+} may be extracellular or intracellular, and varies with the physiological or pharmacological agent producing the contraction (1-3). For example, K^+ depolarization stimulates influx of extracellular Ca^{2+} through potential-dependent Ca^{2+} channels in the sarcolemma. On the other hand, cholinergic stimulation is thought to stimulate extracellular Ca^{2+} influx through potential-independent as well as potential-dependent sarcolemmal channels and, in addition, stimulates release of Ca^{2+} from intracellular sites (4,5).

Calcium regulates several intracellular processes mainly by binding to the ubiquitous Ca^{2+} receptor protein, calmodulin (6). Among these processes are activation of myosin light chain kinase and phosphorylase kinase which may result in an increase in the extent of phosphorylation of the respective protein substrates, the phosphorylatable myosin light chain (P-light chain) and phosphorylase. There is substantial biochemical evidence which implicates myosin P-light chain phosphorylation in the Ca^{2+}-dependent regulation of smooth muscle actin-myosin interactions (7-9). However, alternative hypotheses, suggesting that Ca^{2+}-dependent regulation resides in other contractile elements, also exist (10-12). In intact smooth muscle, the relationship between the extent of isometric force development and extent of P-light chain phosphorylation is not straightforward. As originally reported by Dillon et al. (13) for arterial smooth muscle and later by Silver and Stull (14) and Gerthoffer and Murphy (15) for tracheal smooth muscle, the phosphate content of the P-light chain increases during the initial development of isometric force and then declines during the subsequent maintenance of isometric force.

It has been suggested that myosin P-light chain phosphorylation is not required for steady-state force maintenance in response to a contractile stimulus due to the formation of latched myosin cross bridges (13,15,16). Phosphorylation of P-light chain stimulates the rate of myosin cross-bridge cycling and hence has been correlated to shortening velocity in intact arterial smooth muscle. No unique relationship has been found between developed isometric force and the extent of P-light chain phosphorylation. Based on measurements at steady state, it has been proposed that a higher sarcoplasmic Ca^{2+} concentration appears to be necessary for P-light chain phosphorylation than for force maintenance (17). Thus, two Ca^{2+}-dependent mechanisms have been proposed to regulate the mechanical performance of smooth muscles: (1) myosin phosphorylation and shortening velocity and (2) a second unidentified site that allows force maintenance with low cross-bridge cycling rates (latch).

We have analyzed changes in phosphorylation of myosin P-light chain in tracheal smooth muscle following contractions elicited by two distinct methods, K^+ depolarization and stimulation of cholinergic muscarinic receptors, which presumably increase the intracellular concentration of calcium. The primary focus of this study was to determine if isometric force generation was independent of myosin P-light chain phosphorylation, i.e., could isometric force be generated without P-light chain phosphorylation if a second Ca^{2+} regulatory site is more sensitive to activation by Ca^{2+} than myosin light chain kinase?

It is known that beta-adrenergic stimulation of many types of smooth muscle results in relaxation. Some previously advanced hypotheses relate beta-adrenergic stimulation to a reduction in intracellular Ca^{2+} concentration (18-20). Alternatively, it is possible that the sensitivity of the contractile proteins to activation by Ca^{2+} is decreased. Consistent with the latter hypothesis, myosin light chain kinase purified from turkey gizzard smooth muscle has recently been shown to be phosphorylated by cyclic AMP-dependent protein kinase (21). When phosphorylation occurred in the absence of calmodulin, myosin light chain kinase exhibited a reduced sensitivity to activation by the $Ca^{2+} \cdot$calmodulin complex, i.e., the calmodulin concentration necessary for half-maximal activation increased from 1.2 nM to 25 nM (21). Similar results have been obtained with myosin light chain kinase purified from bovine aortic and stomach smooth muscle (22,23). Additional evidence for this hypothesis has been provided from studies of smooth muscle native actomyosin (11) and chemically skinned smooth muscle fiber systems (25,26). In these studies large amounts of cyclic AMP-dependent protein kinase were added. Beta-adrenergic stimulation does inhibit myosin light chain phosphorylation concomitant with inhibition of isometric force development in intact tracheal smooth muscle (14). However, these results by themselves do not assess the contributions of multiple mechanisms, such as phosphorylation of myosin light chain kinase and reduction of cytoplasmic Ca^{2+} concentrations, for inhibition of contraction. Both types of mechanisms would decrease P-light chain phosphorylation. To date, evidence that phosphorylation of myosin light chain kinase occurs in intact smooth muscle, and is a component of the regulation of smooth muscle contraction, is lacking. Since purified proteins phosphorylated by protein kinases are not necessarily phosphorylated in vivo (9), it is essential that phosphorylation of myosin light chain kinase as well as the anticipated change in the activation properties of the enzyme be demonstrated in living smooth muscle. We have developed an activity ratio assay for smooth muscle myosin light chain kinase that determines whether there is any change in the calmodulin activation properties, which might accompany phosphorylation by cyclic AMP-dependent protein kinase. This procedure is analogous to activity ratio measurements used to assess phosphorylation states of phosphorylase, phosphorylase kinase, glycogen synthase, hormone-sensitive lipase, etc., and has been used to determine whether beta-adrenergic stimulation in intact tracheal smooth muscle leads to a decrease in the affinity of myosin light chain kinase for calmodulin.

2. PROCEDURE

2.1. Material and methods

2.1.1. <u>Intact tracheal smooth muscle strip preparation</u>. Trachealis smooth muscle strips were prepared as previously described (14). Briefly, muscles were removed from fresh bovine trachea, dissected free of the intimal and adventitial layers, and cut into transverse strips. The strips were mounted vertically in a jacketed muscle bath (36° ± 1°C) with a passive force of 1.5 g applied to the strips. The muscle strips were exposed to the pharmacological agents and quick-frozen at the indicated times by rapidly lowering the muscle bath and immersing the strips in dichlorodifluoromethane cooled in liquid nitrogen (14). Following freezing, the clipped ends of the muscle strips were chipped away and discarded; the remaining portions were stored in airtight containers at -65°C prior to biochemical analysis.

2.1.2. _Biochemical analyses_. Frozen portions of each muscle strip were divided into approximately equal halves weighing 5-7 mg (frozen wet weight). Each portion was assayed for either P-light chain phosphate content, extent of phosphorylase _a_ formation or myosin light chain kinase activity ratio.

The phosphate content of the P-light chain was quantitated by a combination of two electrophoretic procedures as detailed previously (27). Briefly, frozen portions of muscle strips were homogenized in 15-20 vols (w/v) of an extraction buffer containing 100 mM sodium pyrophosphate pH 8.8, 5 mM ethyleneglycol-bis(β-aminoethyl ether),N,N'-tetraacetic acid, 50 mM sodium fluoride, 10% glycerol, 15 mM 2-mercaptoethanol, 1 mM phenyl-methylsulfonyl fluoride, 0.1 mM leupeptin, 100 units/ml aprotinin (Trasy-lol) and centrifuged at 7,000 x g for 20 min. The supernatant fraction was mixed with 20 μL of a saturated sucrose solution and an aliquot of this mixture (30-40 μL) was subjected to pyrophosphate-polyacrylamide gel electrophoresis to isolate native myosin from other cellular proteins. Following brief staining with Coomassie Blue R-250, the protein band representing myosin and a portion of the top of the pyrophosphate gel were excised, homogenized in an isoelectric focusing denaturant buffer containing 8 M urea, and subjected to isoelectric focusing on polyacrylamide gels to separate the phosphorylated from the non-phosphorylated form of the myosin P-light chain. Following staining by an ammonial-silver staining procedure, the phosphate content of the P-light chain was quantitated by measuring the relative amounts of the phosphorylated and non-phosphorylated forms of the P-light chain by densitometry.

To determine phosphorylase _a_ content, frozen muscle portions were homogenized in 15 vols (w/v) of an extraction buffer containing 20 mM β-glycerolphosphate, pH 6.8, 20 mM sodium fluoride, 2 mM ethylenediamine-tetraacetic acid, 0.01% bovine serum albumin, and 15 mM 2-mercaptoethanol. Following homogenization, acid washed Norite (10 mg/ml final concentration) was added and the extracts were centrifuged at 3,000 x g for 10 min. Phosphorylase _a_ activity in the supernatant fraction was determined using an enzyme coupled fluorometric procedure (14). The phosphorylase _a_ activity ratio was expressed as the ratio of activity measured in the absence and presence of 5'-AMP.

The activation of myosin light chain kinase involves two sequential reactions:

$$\text{calcium} + \text{calmodulin} \rightleftharpoons \text{calcium} \cdot \text{calmodulin}$$

$$\text{calcium} \cdot \text{calmodulin} + \text{myosin light chain kinase} \rightleftharpoons$$
$$\text{calcium} \cdot \text{calmodulin} \cdot \text{myosin light chain kinase}$$

The calcium·calmodulin·myosin light chain kinase complex is the active form of the enzyme. It has been proposed that the Ca_4^{2+}·calmodulin complex is the form of calmodulin that activates myosin light chain kinase (28).

The two-step reaction mechanism for activation of myosin light chain kinase indicates that an increase in the K_{CM} value will result in an increase in the calcium concentration required for activation although there are no changes in the affinity of calmodulin for calcium. The myosin light chain kinase activity ratio assesses the degree of activation of myosin light chain kinase at a submaximal concentration of the activating complex, Ca_4^{2+}·calmodulin. Myosin light chain kinase activity was determined as previously described (28), except that the reaction mixtures contained 1 μM calmodulin and either 4 or 100 μM free calcium. The lower concentration of calcium was controlled by the use of a calcium/EGTA buffer system. The myosin light chain kinase activity ratio is the ratio of kinase activities measured at 4 μM and 100 μM free calcium, respectively. The quantitative model for the activation of myosin light chain kinase (28) predicts that this ratio will decrease in response to a modification of the enzyme, e.g., phosphorylation, which increases K_{CM}, the concentration of Ca_4^{2+}·calmodulin necessary for half-maximal activation. For example, when $K_{Ca}2+ = 12$ μM (intrinsic activation constant, the product of the K_D values for the 4 divalent metal binding sites on calmodulin) and K_{CM}, the concentration of Ca_4^{2+}· calmodulin necessary for half-maximal activation, is increased from 1 nM to 20 nM, the activity ratio decreases from 0.80 to 0.16. These changes in K_{CM} values are similar to those reported for myosin light chain kinase after phosphorylation by the catalytic subunit of cyclic AMP-dependent protein kinase (21). Thus, measurement of the myosin light chain kinase activity ratio could be used to evaluate changes in calmodulin activation (i.e., in K_{CM}) expected with phosphorylation of myosin light chain kinase by cyclic AMP-dependent protein kinase (29). This ratio is easily determined in a dilute tissue extract obtained in the presence of inhibitors of protein kinases and phosphoprotein phosphatases. Free Ca^{2+} concentrations are controlled in the assay system by the use of a Ca^{2+}/EGTA buffer system, and the content of endogenous calmodulin in the diluted extract (1 to 10 nM) is much less than the amount added to the assay mixture (1 μM).

3. RESULTS

3.1. Isometric force and P-light chain phosphorylation

3.1.1. _Temporal comparisons of isometric force and P-light chain phosphorylation_. Differences in the temporal responses in both P-light chain and phosphorylase phosphorylation were apparent during the development and maintenance of isometric force in the presence of 1 μM carbachol or 60 mM KCl (30).

Table 1. Comparison of temporal responses to carbachol and KCl

Agent	Time (min)	Force (g)	P-Light Chain (mol P/mol LC)
Carbachol, 1 μM	0	0.0	0.14
	0.5	7.0	0.33
	1	8.8	0.79
	3	10.9	0.49
	30	10.9	0.26
	120	12	0.11
KCl, 60 mM	0	0.0	0.11
	0.5	4.8	0.41
	1	6.0	0.59
	3	6.0	0.40
	120	6.3	0.38

All values, with the exception of P-light chain phosphate content at 120 min with carbachol, were significantly ($p < 0.05$) different from control values at 0 min. Each value represents the mean for 3-8 samples from a total of 12 trachea. Statistical comparisons were made by the Student's t-test.

These concentrations of carbachol (1 µM) and KCl (60 mM) produced near maximal contractile responses, respectively; contractions with KCl were elicited in the presence of 0.1 µM atropine to minimize possible effects due to K^+ depolarization and release of acetylcholine from cholinergic nerve terminals. As shown in Table 1, the maximum extent of isometric force developed in the presence of KCl was approximately 55% of that obtained with carbachol; likewise, the maximum extent of P-light chain phosphorylation was appreciably greater with carbachol (0.79 mol phosphate per mol P-light chain) than with KCl (0.59 mol phosphate per mol P-light chain). These maximum levels of P-light chain phosphorylation occurred 1 min after the addition of either carbachol or KCl while maximum force development occurred after 3 min for carbachol and 1 min for KCl. The maximum isometric force developed in the presence of either agent was maintained for up to 120 min, yet the phosphate content of the P-light chain declined during this interval. The rate and magnitude of this decline was dependent upon the contractile agent. Muscles stimulated in the presence of KCl showed decreases in phosphate content from 0.59 to 0.40 mol phosphate per mol P-light chain after 3 min; this value was unchanged after 120 min. In contrast, muscles contracted in the presence of carbachol showed a continued decrease from the maximal value obtained at 1 min (0.79) and reached basal levels (0.11 mol/mol) after 120 min. When compared with the marked differences in steady-state isometric force at 120 min (12 g with carbachol; 6.3 g with KCl), these findings further emphasize the lack of correlation between the maintained isometric force and steady-state phosphate content of the P-light chain in smooth muscle.

3.1.2. <u>Concentration-response relationships between isometric force and P-light chain phosphorylation</u>. The relationships between concentration of either contractile agent and isometric force development and P-light chain phosphate content were also examined (Table 2). Concentration-dependent increases in isometric force development were paralleled by concomitant concentration-dependent increases in P-light chain phosphate content during stimulation with either contractile agent. This similarity is reflected in the estimations of concentrations required for half-maximal responses for each agent. The concentrations of carbachol required for half-maximal responses for force and P-light chain phosphorylation were 45 nM and 44 nM, respectively. The concentrations of KCl required for half-maximal

Table 2. Comparison of concentration-response relationship to carbachol
and KCl measured at 1 min.

Agent	Concentration	Force (g)	P-Light Chain (mol P/mol LC)
Carbachol	0.00 μM	0.0	0.10
	0.01	1.0	0.21
	0.03	3.7	0.42
	0.10	4.8	0.59
	0.25	5.6	0.62
	0.50	7.7	0.75
	1.0	7.5	0.79
	5.0	8.6	0.64
KCl	0 mM	0.00	0.10
	20	1.9	0.24
	30	3.0	0.36
	45	5.0	0.39
	60	6.9	0.59
	90	7.1	0.55

All values were significantly ($p < 0.05$) different from control values.
Each value represents the mean for 3-8 samples from a total of 12 trachea.
Statistical comparisons were made by the Student's t-test.

responses were 28 mM and 23 mM, respectively, for force and P-light chain
phosphorylation.

3.2. <u>Phosphorylation of myosin light chain kinase</u>

3.2.1. <u>Phosphorylation of purified myosin light chain kinase.</u> Purified
myosin light chain kinase from bovine tracheal smooth muscle had a
molecular weight of 150,000 on polyacrylamide gels electrophoresed in the
presence of SDS. The enzyme was phosphorylated by incubation at 30°C with
the catalytic subunit of cyclic AMP-dependent protein kinase and 1 mM [γ-
^{32}P]ATP. Radiolabelled phosphate was incorporated into myosin light chain
kinase to the extent of 2.02 ± 0.2 mol ^{32}P per mol enzyme within 30 minutes

(n=4). Measurements of the myosin light chain kinase activity ratio were performed on the enzyme before and after phosphorylation. Phosphorylation of the kinase was accompanied by a decrease in the activity ratio from a control value of 0.79 to 0.24, corresponding to a 12-fold increase in the Ca_4^{2+}·calmodulin concentration necessary for half-maximal activity.

To determine whether the decrease in the activity ratio would be maintained during tissue extraction procedures, aliquots of the phosphorylated kinase were diluted 5-fold in 1:400 (w/v) homogenates of bovine tracheal smooth muscle containing EDTA and buffered with potassium phosphate or MOPS. After a 10-min incubation, protein-bound ^{32}P in this mixture was 99% of that measured with the purified enzyme before addition to the homogenate. The activity ratio of myosin light chain kinase following incubation in the homogenate was 0.27. Thus, in the presence of inhibitors of protein kinase and phosphoprotein phosphatase activities, the ratio appears to be stable enough to permit measurement in an extract of intact smooth muscle. Qualitatively similar data were obtained with phosphorylation of purified myosin light chain kinase from aortic smooth muscle. Phosphorylation decreased the activity ratio from 0.79 to 0.21. Addition of the phosphorylated enzyme to homogenates of tracheal smooth muscle did not result in reversal of the activity ratio.

Table 3. Recovery of phosphorylated myosin myosin light chain kinase added to homogenates of tracheal smooth muscle.

Treatment	Extent of phosphorylation[a]	Activity ratio	cpm[b]
Control	--	0.79	--
^{32}P-MLCK + buffer	2.36	0.24	5950
^{32}P-MLCK + homogenate	2.34	0.27	5904

[a] Mol ^{32}P incorporated per mol myosin light chain kinase.

[b] Protein-bound ^{32}P measured in aliquots of buffer or homogenate removed 20 min after addition of phosphorylated myosin light chain kinase.

3.2.2. <u>Phosphorylation of myosin light chain kinase in intact smooth muscle</u>. Initial studies using intact tracheal smooth muscle tested the ability of isoproterenol to relax isolated strips precontracted by exposure to carbachol. At 0.1 µM carbachol, isometric force was approximately 75% of that elicited by maximal concentrations of carbachol. Isoproterenol was added to the bath in increasing cumulative concentrations from 1 nM to 10 µM for 3 min at each concentration. At 10 µM isoproterenol, active force was abolished. The average force decreased to 26% of control values, at 0.3 µM isoproterenol, and this concentration was chosen for further studies.

The effect of beta-adrenergic stimulation of intact smooth muscle was studied by the addition of 0.3 µM isoproterenol to a muscle bath containing trachealis muscle strips which had not been precontracted. The strips were quick-frozen after incubation periods from 0 to 5 minutes. Measurements of the myosin light chain kinase and phosphorylase activity ratios were performed on homogenates of the frozen strips. The results (Table 4) indicate that phosphorylase <u>b</u> to <u>a</u> conversion was elevated significantly from control values at times between 1 and 5 minutes, while the myosin light chain kinase activity ratio did not differ from the control value of 0.80 at any time studied. Treatment with isoproterenol also did not affect the total amount of myosin light chain kinase activity extracted from the tissue, i.e., that activity measured at 100 µM calcium.

Table 4. Time course of changes in myosin light chain kinase and phosphorylase activity ratios following exposure to 0.3 µM isoproterenol.

Time	Myosin Light Chain Kinase	Phosphorylase
min	activity ratios	
0	0.80	0.08
1	0.82	0.18
2	0.80	0.23
5	0.79	0.28

In further experiments, the extent of phosphorylation of the myosin light chain during isoproterenol-mediated relaxation of carbachol contracted trachealis muscles was determined. As previously reported by Silver and Stull (14), the phosphate content of the myosin light chain initially increases then decreases, while maximal isometric force is maintained, in trachealis muscles contracted with 1 μM carbachol. From the rate of decline in these previous data, it was estimated that the extent of phosphorylation would return to basal values (approximately 0.10 mol phosphate/mol myosin light chain) after 2 hours of sustained contraction with carbachol. This estimate was close to actual values (0.11 ± 0.05 mol phosphate/mol myosin light chain) determined after 2 hours. Addition of 5 μM isoproterenol at this time produced immediate, near maximal relaxation (88%) without decreasing the phosphate content of the light chain (0.13 ± 0.05 mol phosphate/mol myosin light chain). Further evidence of activation of the cyclic AMP system was obtained with phosphorylase _a_ activity ratio measurements. Ratios measured after 2 hours of carbachol-stimulated contraction (0.28 ± 0.03) more than doubled during this interval of incubation with isoproterenol (0.63 ± 0.02). These data show that relaxation of maximally contracted trachealis smooth muscle by the beta-adrenergic agonist may occur with no change (decrease) in the phosphate content of the myosin light chain, and further suggest that beta-adrenergic relaxation of intact smooth muscle does not necessarily involve phosphorylation of myosin light chain kinase.

4. DISCUSSION

4.1. Isometric force and P-light chain phosphorylation

This study shows that the development of isometric force in intact bovine tracheal smooth muscle is directly correlated to the extent of phosphorylation of the myosin P-light chain. This correlation occurs over the range of concentrations of both carbachol and KCl for isometric force development. Thus, myosin P-light chain phosphorylation may play an important role in determining the extent of development of isometric force in tracheal smooth muscle regardless of the conditions producing the contraction.

In previous studies on smooth muscle, the dissociation between steady-state force and phosphorylation of P-light chain has been emphasized (13-17). Based on responses to changes in Ca^{2+} concentrations in physiological saline solution, it was proposed that isometric force was maintained at lower Ca^{2+} concentrations than P-light chain phosphorylation (17). If force generation and P-light chain phosphorylation are independent events, low Ca^{2+} concentrations should lead to force generation without P-light chain phosphorylation. At low concentrations of KCl and carbachol, the amount of Ca^{2+} released into the sarcoplasm for activation of the contractile elements would be expected to be low. In these experiments on bovine trachealis smooth muscle, development of isometric force was proportional to the extent of phosphorylation of P-light chain measured at 1 min, even with low concentrations of KCl and carbachol. Thus, force generation in intact bovine tracheal smooth muscle was not dissociated from P-light chain phosphorylation. These results also indicate that it is important to establish temporal responses rather than measuring P-light chain phosphorylation at a single time after the maximal response. It is apparent that one could obtain significant steady-state force with little or no phosphorylation of P-light chain at extended periods of time.

P-light chain phosphorylation may act as a switch for smooth muscle contraction. Ca^{2+}-dependent P-light chain phosphorylation may stimulate cross-bridge cycling and initiate shortening or development of isometric force. The number of cross bridges that may be transformed to the attached, noncycling latch state will be proportional to the number of cross bridges that are initially phosphorylated and hence cycling. If P-light chain is not first phosphorylated, myosin may not be able to form the latch state. This hypothesis is consistent with the recent observation that myosin phosphorylation may be a prerequisite for the latch state in detergent-treated carotid arteries (31). There was no difference in the Ca^{2+} concentrations required for the initial stimulation of P-light chain phosphorylation and stress. However, the subsequent reduction in Ca^{2+} concentrations led to stress maintenance without proportional phosphorylation. Thus, the maintenance of isometric force with the decrease in myosin P-light chain phosphorylation may depend upon Ca^{2+} binding to another myofibrillar site that regulates the latch state.

Different temporal responses were apparent in bovine tracheal smooth muscle with the two agents producing contraction. Contractions by both KCl and carbachol were associated with transient increases in P-light chain phosphorylation; however, the rate and magnitude of the decline in extent of P-light chain phosphorylation was much less in KCl-contracted muscles than in carbachol-stimulated muscles. In carbachol-contracted muscles, the maximal extent of isometric force was maintained even though the phosphate content of the P-light chain had declined to basal levels. A similar difference in the temporal response was seen for phosphorylase _a_ formation; a decrease from maximal levels was observed with carbachol stimulation, yet no decline was observed with KCl (30). Since the regulation of the extent of phosphorylation of both the P-light chain and phosphorylase is Ca^{2+}-dependent, it is reasonable to assume that the decrease in the extent of phosphorylation of these two proteins may be due to a decrease in the levels of sarcoplasmic free Ca^{2+} during maintained isometric contractions. This decrease in Ca^{2+} concentration may be greater with carbachol, and thus a greater decrease in extent of phosphorylation of P-light chain and phos-phorylase would be expected. This hypothesis is supported by the recent findings of Morgan and Morgan (32). Calcium-dependent aequorin luminescence declined during maintained isometric force in smooth muscle, and the extent of the decrease was greater with a pharmacological agonist than with K^{+} depolarization. This hypothesis is also supported by studies with carotid arterial smooth muscle (17) in which the decrease in P-light chain phos-phorylation during K^{+}-depolarized contractions could be attenuated by increasing the concentration of extracellular Ca^{2+}.

In summary, there appears to be a good correlation between the extent of P-light chain phosphorylation and development of isometric force. Although these results are consistent with the hypothesis that P-light chain phos-phorylation may play an important role in regulating smooth muscle contraction, it is obvious that there are also other factors that affect regulation. Force maintenance does not require steady-state phosphoryla-tion of P-light chain. The role of P-light chain phosphorylation and its relationship to these other potentially important secondary mechanisms in smooth muscle contraction will require additional investigations.

4.2. Phosphorylation of smooth muscle myosin light chain kinase

We have found that, similar to the turkey gizzard smooth muscle kinase, purified bovine tracheal smooth muscle myosin light chain kinase is a sub-strate for cyclic AMP-dependent protein kinase. The results obtained from activity ratio measurements performed on the purified kinase demonstrate that bovine tracheal smooth muscle myosin light chain kinase is altered in its sensitivity to activation by Ca_{4}^{2+}·calmodulin, similar to the turkey gizzard kinase. Although the activity ratio measurement itself does not permit determination of the absolute value of K_{CM}, the values of the ratios v/V_{max} and $(v/V_{max})'$ obtained before and after phosphorylation, respectively, may be used to estimate a fold-change from K_{CM} to K_{CM}'.

$$\frac{(V_{max}/v)' - 1}{(V_{max}/v) - 1} = \frac{K_{CM}'}{K_{CM}}$$

Thus, a decrease in the activity ratio of purified myosin light chain kinase from 0.79 to 0.24 represents a 12-fold increase in the value of K_{CM} produced by phosphorylation, in close agreement with the findings of Conti and Adelstein (21).

To determine the sensitivity of myosin light chain kinase to calmodulin activation in intact tracheal smooth muscle tissue following beta-adrenergic stimulation, we studied trachealis muscle strips exposed to isoproterenol in the relaxed state, since Conti and Adelstein (21) suggest that phosphorylation resulting in a change in the activation properties of the kinase would be inhibited when the enzyme was activated, i.e., bound to calmodulin. If beta-adrenergic induced relaxation of tracheal smooth muscle were mediated by phosphorylation of myosin light chain kinase, then an effect on the myosin light chain kinase activity ratio should be manifest upon preincubation with 0.3 µM isoproterenol. Previous findings indicate that preincubation with isoproterenol will inhibit the force developed and P-light chain phosphorylation in tracheal smooth muscle (14). However, 0.3 µM isoproterenol produced marked relaxation and stimulation of the glycogenolytic cascade, but it did not alter the myosin light chain kinase activity ratio.

The relaxation effects of beta-adrenergic receptor stimulation on tracheal smooth muscle are not necessarily dependent upon decreased myosin light chain phosphorylation. Preincubation of tracheal smooth muscle with isoproterenol inhibited myosin light chain phosphorylation and isometric force development in response to carbachol (14). These observations alone do not explain whether a decrease in the availability of activating Ca^{2+}, phosphorylation of myosin light chain kinase, or both account for the apparent decrease in myosin light chain kinase activity. However, the extent of phosphorylation of myosin light chain in bovine tracheal smooth muscle is not maintained during prolonged isometric tension. Since beta-adrenergic stimulation produces marked relaxation even when the phosphate content of P-light chain has returned to control values, biochemical mechanisms other than phosphorylation of myosin light chain kinase are probably primary determinants of the relaxation response.

In summary, we have proposed measurement of the myosin light chain kinase activity ratio to measure changes in the calmodulin activation properties of myosin light chain kinase hypothesized to accompany phosphorylation of the enzyme. This technique has yielded evidence to suggest that myosin light chain kinase in purified form or in a smooth muscle homogenate may be phosphorylated in the presence of a sufficiently high concentration of cyclic AMP-dependent protein kinase catalytic subunit. Phosphorylation of smooth muscle kinase produces a decreased sensitivity to activation by Ca_4^{2+}·calmodulin. However, significant phosphorylation of the kinase in intact smooth muscle would depend upon several factors, including the cyclic AMP-dependent protein kinase content in the tissue, the degree of its activation by cyclic AMP following beta-adrenergic stimulation, and the catalytic rate of phosphorylation of myosin light chain kinase by cyclic AMP-dependent protein kinase. In fact, no changes in the activation properties of myosin light chain kinase were observed when intact tracheal smooth muscle strips were exposed to concentrations of isoproterenol sufficient to produce marked relaxation. These results suggest that beta-adrenergic stimulation did not result in phosphorylation of the enzyme. Among the possible explanations for this finding are 1) that calmodulin, with its calcium-binding sites partially occupied by Ca^{2+}, remains bound to myosin light chain kinase in resting smooth muscle (16), blocking the site of phosphorylation, 2) that the kinase is associated, in vivo, with myofibrillar proteins in a way which prevents its phosphorylation, and 3) that phosphorylation of the kinase in vivo occurs much too slowly to be an intermediate step in the response to beta-adrenergic stimulation. These possibilities may be resolved by additional studies on the properties of phosphorylation of purified smooth muscle myosin light chain kinase by cyclic AMP-dependent protein kinase.

5. ACKNOWLEDGMENTS

The authors wish to acknowledge the excellent, dedicated assistance of Ms. Nancy Bryant in the preparation of this manuscript and support from the National Institutes of Health (GM07062, HL06359, and HL26043).

6. REFERENCES

1. Bolton TB: Mechanisms of action of transmitters and other substances on smooth muscle. Physiol Rev (59): 606-718, 1979.
2. Weiss GB: Calcium release and accumulation at cellular sites and compartments in vascular smooth muscle. In: Flaim SF, Zelis R (eds) Calcium-blockers--mechanisms of action and clinical applications. Urban and Schwarzenberg, Baltimore, 1982, pp 65-76.
3. van Breemen C, Aaronson P, Cauvin C, Loutzenhiser R, Mangel A, Saida K: Plasmalemmal calcium movements and the calcium cycle in arterial smooth muscle. In: Flaim SF, Zelis R (eds) Calcium blockers-- mechanisms of action and clinical applications. Urban and Schwarzenberg, Baltimore, 1982, pp 53-63.
4. Farley JM, Miles PR: The sources of calcium for acetylcholine-induced contractions of dog tracheal smooth muscle. J Pharmacol Exp Ther (207): 340-346, 1978.
5. Brading AF, Sneddon P: Evidence for multiple sources of calcium for activation of the contractile mechanism of guinea pig taenia coli on stimulation with carbachol. Br J Pharmacol (70): 229-240, 1980.
6. Brostrom CO, Wolff DJ: Properties and functions of calmodulin. Biochem Pharmacol (30): 1395-1405, 1981.
7. Adelstein RS, Eisenberg E: Regulation and kinetics of the actin-myosin-ATP interaction. Ann Rev Biochem (49): 921-933, 1980.
8. Hartshorne DJ, Gorecka A: Biochemistry of the contractile proteins of smooth muscle. In: Bohr DF, Somlyo A, Sparks HV Jr (eds) Handbook of physiology, the cardiovascular system, Vol. II. American Physiological Society, Bethesda, 1980, pp 93-120.
9. Stull JT: Phosphorylation of contractile proteins in relation to muscle function. Adv Cyclic Nucleotide Res (13): 39-93, 1980.
10. Nonomura Y, Ebashi S: Calcium regulatory mechanism in vertebrate smooth muscle. Biomedical Res (1): 1-14, 1980.
11. Walters M, Marston SB: Phosphorylation of the calcium ion-regulated thin filaments from vascular smooth muscle. Biochem J (197): 127-139, 1981.
12. Chacko S, Rosenfeld A: Regulation of actin-activated ATP hydrolysis by arterial myosin. Proc Natl Acad Sci USA (79): 292-296, 1982.
13. Dillon PF, Aksoy MO, Driska SP, Murphy RA: Myosin phosphorylation and the cross-bridge cycle in arterial smooth muscle. Science (211): 495-497, 1981.
14. Silver PJ, Stull JT: Regulation of myosin light chain and phosphorylase phosphorylation in tracheal smooth muscle. J Biol Chem (257): 6145-6150, 1982.
15. Gerthoffer WT, Murphy RA: Myosin phosphorylation and regulation of cross-bridge cycle in tracheal smooth muscle. Am J Physiol (244): C182-C187, 1983.
16. Aksoy MO, Murphy RA, Kamm KE: Role of Ca^{2+} and myosin light chain phosphorylation in regulation of smooth muscle. Am J Physiol (242): C109-C116, 1982.
17. Aksoy MO, Mras S, Kamm KE, Murphy RA: Ca^{++}, cAMP, and changes in myosin phosphorylation during contraction of smooth muscle. Amer J Physiol (245): C255-C270, 1983.
18. Bhalla RC, Webb RC, Singh D, Brock T: Role of cyclic AMP in rat aortic microsomal phosphorylation and calcium uptake. Am J Physiol (234): H508-H514, 1978.

19. Webb RC, Bohr DF: Relaxation of vascular smooth muscle by isoproterenol, dibutyryl-cyclic AMP and theophylline. J Pharmacol Exp Ther (217): 26-35, 1981.
20. Scheid C, Honeyman T, Fay F: Mechanism of β-adrenergic relaxation of smooth muscle. Nature (Lond) (277): 32-36, 1979.
21. Conti MA, Adelstein RS: The relationship between calmodulin binding and phosphorylation of smooth muscle myosin kinase by the catalytic subunit of 3':5'cAMP-dependent protein kinase. J Biol Chem (256): 3178-3181, 1981.
22. Vallet B, Molla A, DeMaille JG: Cyclic adenosine 3',5'-monophosphate-dependent regulation of purified bovine aortic calcium/calmodulin-dependent myosin light chain kinase. Biochim Biophys Acta (674): 256-264, 1981.
23. Walsh MP, Hinkins S, Flink IL, Hartshorne DJ: Bovine stomach myosin light chain kinase: purification, characterization and comparison with the turkey gizzard enzyme. Biochemistry 21:6890-6896, 1982.
24. Silver PJ, DiSalvo J: Adenosine 3':5'-monophosphate mediated inhibition of myosin light chain phosphorylation in bovine aortic actomyosin. J Biol Chem (254): 9951-9954, 1979.
25. Kerrick WGL, Hoar PE: Inhibition of smooth muscle tension by cyclic AMP-dependent protein kinase. Nature (292): 253-255, 1981.
26. Ruegg JC, Paul RJ. Vascular smooth muscle: calmodulin and cyclic AMP-dependent protein kinase alter calcium sensitivity in porcine carotid skinned fibers. Circ Res (50): 394-399, 1982.
27. Silver PJ, Stull JT: Quantitation of myosin light chain phosphorylation in small tissue samples. J Biol Chem (257): 6137-6144, 1982.
28. Blumenthal DK, Stull JT. Activation of skeletal muscle myosin light chain kinase by calcium (2+) and calmodulin. Biochemistry (19): 5608-5614, 1980.
29. Miller JR, Silver PJ, Stull JT: The role of myosin light chain kinase phosphorylation in beta-adrenergic relaxation of tracheal smooth muscle. Mol Pharmacol (24): 235-242, 1983.
30. Silver PJ, Stull JT: Phosphorylation of myosin light chain and phosphorylase in tracheal smooth muscle. Mol Pharmacol (in press).
31. Chatterjee M, Murphy RA: Calcium-dependent stress maintenance without myosin phosphorylation in skinned smooth muscle. Science (221): 464-466, 1983.
32. Morgan JP, Morgan KP: Differential effects of vasoconstrictors on intracellular Ca^{++} levels in mammalian vascular smooth muscle as detected with aequorin. Fed Proc (42): 571, 1983.

9

AUTONOMIC NERVES, AGGREGATING PLATELETS AND CONTRACTION OF CORONARY
ARTERIAL SMOOTH MUSCLE

P.M. VANHOUTTE

The exact physiological role of the vascular smooth muscle cells of
large coronary arteries is uncertain. However, it is now generally
admitted that exaggerated contraction of these cells ("coronary vasospasm")
can endanger myocardial perfusion to the point of causing angina pectoris,
or even myocardial infarction. This paper summarizes work on isolated
canine epicardial coronary arteries which may be relevant to the
understanding of the etiology of vasospastic episodes, with special
emphasis on the potential involvement of the substances released from
autonomic nerves and aggregating platelets.

1. AUTONOMIC NERVES

1.1. _Adrenergic nerves_. Experiments in the intact animal, treated with
beta-adrenergic blocking agents, suggest that activation of the sympathetic
nerves can cause coronary vasoconstriction, indicating a continual opposing
action of metabolically induced vasodilatation by the adrenergic transmitter
(1-6). The beta-adrenergic blockade required to demonstrate alpha-
adrenergically mediated constriction may mask a dominant, beta-adrenergic
inhibitory effect of released norepinephrine on the coronary smooth muscle
cells. This conclusion is supported by a variety of observations on
isolated coronary arteries. Thus, in the absence of beta-adrenergic
blockade, exogenous norepinephrine causes relaxation of coronary smooth
muscle in vitro (7-9). If endogenous norepinephrine is released from the
adrenergic nerve endings in large canine coronary arteries, either by
electrical impulses or indirect sympathomimetic amines, only relaxation
ensues under normal conditions; contractions are observed only after
beta-adrenergic blockade (Fig. 1; 10). These contractions are inhibited
by alpha-adrenergic blocking drugs (10). Thus, released norepinephrine
can activate both alpha- and beta-adrenoceptors of coronary arterial
smooth muscle. The lack of contraction to sympathetic nerve stimulation,

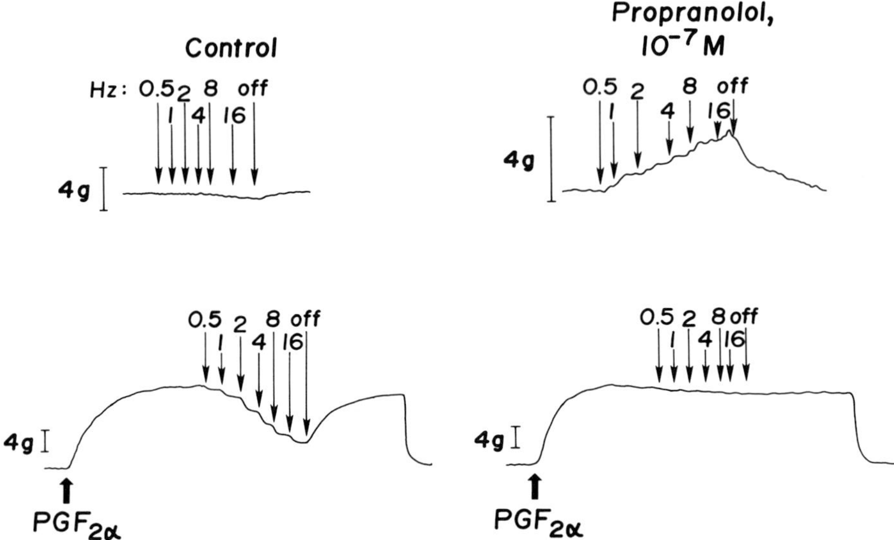

FIGURE 1. Response of canine left circumflex coronary artery to transmural electrical stimulation (10V, 0.25 msec) in control solution (left) and in the presence of propranolol (right). In the presence, but not in the absence of propranolol, electrical stimulation causes contraction under basal conditions (top). When tension is induced with prostaglandin $F_{2\alpha}$ (2 x 10^{-6}M, bottom), relaxations occur which are blocked by propranolol (data from ref. 10).

in the absence of beta-adrenergic blocking agents, indicates that the beta-adrenergic effect of released norepinephrine predominates. Alpha-adrenergically mediated contractions are observed in main coronary arteries, but not in the ventricular branches; the transition in alpha-adrenergic responsiveness is abrupt at the branching point (Fig. 2; 10). The available pharmacological evidence suggests that, at least in the dog, the postjunctional alpha-adrenoceptors belong to the $alpha_1$-adrenoceptor subtype (Fig. 3; 11); the contractions evoked by alpha-adrenergic activation are mediated exclusively by the entry of Ca^{2+} from the extra-cellular space (11,12).

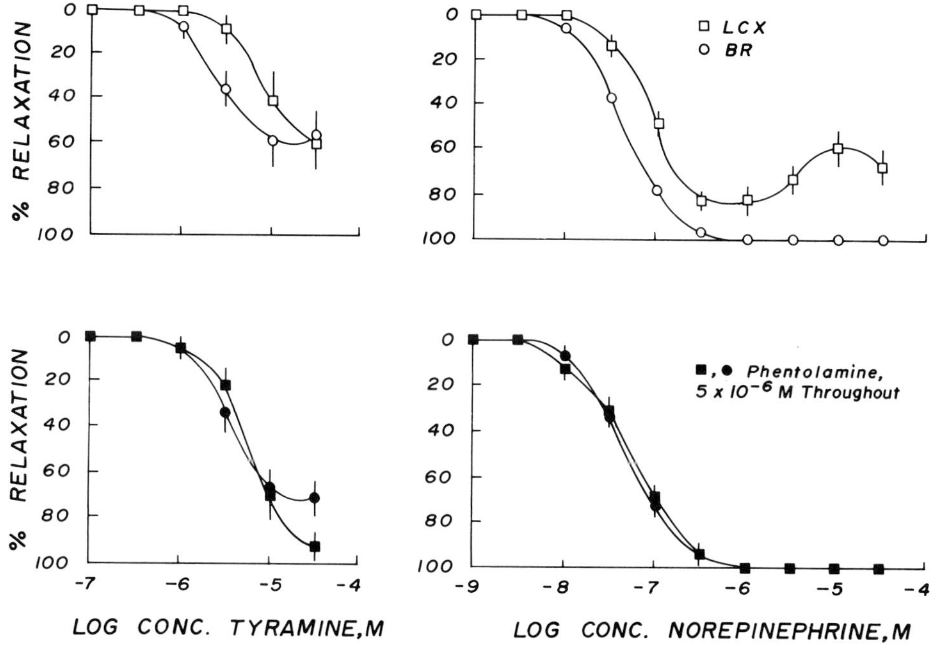

FIGURE 2. Effect of phentolamine on response of canine left circumflex and branch coronary arteries to tyramine and norepinephrine. In the absence of the alpha-adrenergic antagonist, left circumflex artery (LCS) rings are less sensitive to tyramine and norepinephrine than are branch artery rings (BR). In the presence of phentolamine, there is no difference in the sensitivity of the left circumflex and branch artery to either agonist; the sensitivity of the branch artery is unchanged from that obtained in control solution. Data shown as means $\pm$ S.E. of rings of each vessel from six dogs and expressed as percent relaxation of contraction evoked by prostaglandin $F_{2\alpha}$ (2 x 10^{-6}M) (data from ref. 10).

The assessment of the effects of adrenergic blocking drugs during activation of the sympathetic nerves are complicated by the prejunctional effects they have. The sympathetic nerve endings possess both alpha- and beta-adrenergic receptors; the former exert a negative feedback on the release of norepinephrine, the latter facilitate it (13-15). In the coronary wall, alpha-adrenergic blockers which inhibit prejunctional alpha$_2$-adrenoceptors, but not those selective for postjunctional alpha$_1$-adrenoceptors (e.g. prazosin) augment the release of norepinephrine, and thus exaggerate the relaxations induced by stimulation of the adrenergic

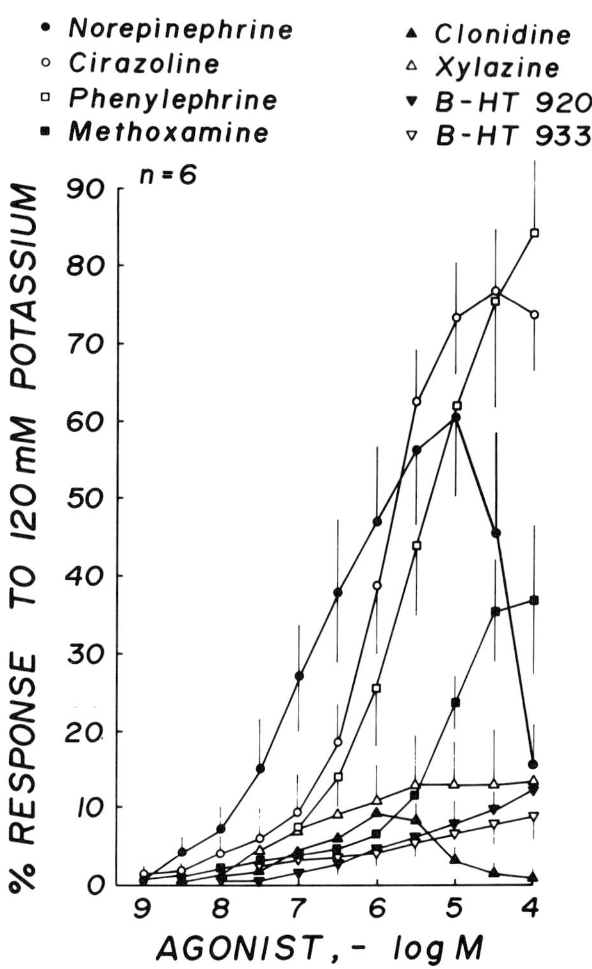

FIGURE 3. Response of canine left circumflex arteries to alpha-adrenergic agonists with varying degrees of selectivity for postjunctional alpha$_1$- and alpha$_2$-adrenoceptors. Significant contractions occur only in response to alpha$_1$-selective agonists (cirazoline, phenylephrine, methoxamine). The experiments were performed in the presence of propranolol (to block beta-adrenoceptors) and inhibitors of neuronal and extraneuronal uptake (from ref. 11, by permission).

nerves (Fig. 4; 10). Conversely, it can be predicted, that in conditions where levels of epinephrine are augmented, beta-adrenergic blockers would prevent the augmented release of norepinephrine caused by the catecholamine (14,16,17).

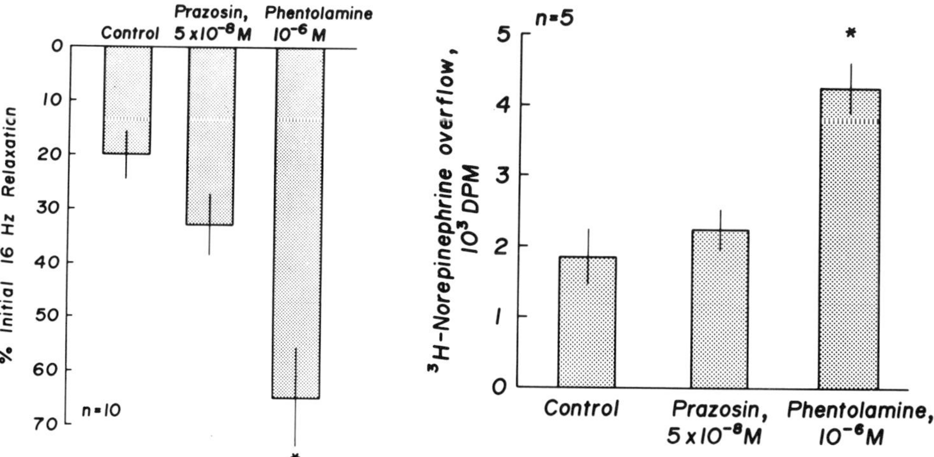

FIGURE 4. Left: Effects of prazosin and phentolamine on response of left circumflex artery to 2 Hz electrical stimulation. Data are means $\pm$ S.E. of the relaxation during prostaglandin $F_{2\alpha}$-induced (2 x 10⁻⁶M) contractions. Phentolamine, but not prazosin, significantly augmented the relaxation caused by 2 Hz stimulation (11). Right: Effect of prazosin and phentolamine on the release of ^{3}H-norepinephrine evoked in canine left circumflex artery by 2 Hz electrical stimulation. Data are means $\pm$ S.E. Phentolamine, but not prazosin significantly augmented the evoked release of adrenergic transmitter (from ref. 11, by permission of the American Heart Association).

It is still uncertain how norepinephrine released from sympathetic nerves, and epinephrine secreted by the adrenal medulla regulate coronary blood flow in normal and pathological situations. Alpha-adrenergic stimulation would tend to cause vasoconstriction by direct activation of the smooth muscle cells of larger coronary arteries, as well as by inhibiting the release of endogenous transmitter; non-selective alpha-adrenergic blockers would cause dilatation by opposing both the pre- and postjunctional effects of the catecholamines (Fig. 5). Beta-adrenergic activation and blockade would have the opposite effects, thus greatly favoring coronary vasoconstriction upon stimulation of the sympathetic nerves. These effects may explain the clinical finding that attacks of epicardial coronary artery spasms become more severe during treatment with beta-adrenergic antagonists; under these conditions an augmented sympathetic nerve activity causes unopposed alpha-adrenergic activation. Alpha-adrenoceptor antagonists can alleviate such spastic episodes (18-20).

1.2. <u>Cholinergic nerves</u>. Exogenous acetylcholine, by acting on muscarinic receptors of the adrenergic nerve endings, inhibits the release of norepinephrine in a variety of systemic blood vessels from different species, including man (14,21,22). Endogenously released acetylcholine has a similar effect in the heart and the gastric circulation (22). Preliminary evidence in the canine coronary artery suggests that acetylcholine, whether exogenously added or endogenously released curtails the release of norepinephrine during activation of the sympathetic nerves and hence reduces the relaxation induced by sympathetic nerve stimulation (Cohen, Shepherd and Vanhoutte, unpublished observations). In addition, in isolated coronary arteries of several species, including man, acetylcholine causes direct activation of the smooth muscle cells (23-28). If this were to occur in the intact organism coronary vasoconstrictor responses could result (e.g. 29,30), which could be greatly reinforced by prejunctional inhibition of adrenergic neurotransmission, resulting in less beta-adrenergically mediated relaxation of the coronary smooth muscle (Fig. 6).

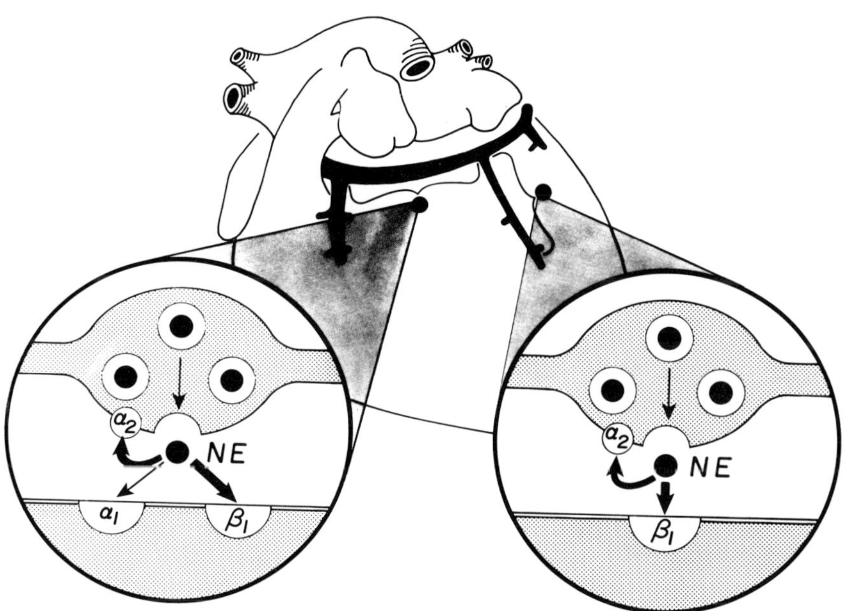

FIGURE 5. Sympathetic neuroeffector junction in canine epicardial coronary arteries. The predominant response to norepinephrine released from adrenergic nerve terminals is relaxation mediated at beta$_1$-adrenoceptors in proximal left circumflex artery, as well as in the smaller branch artery. Postjunctional alpha$_1$-adrenoceptors can moderate the relaxation in the larger vessel only. In both vessels, prejunctional alpha$_2$-adrenoceptors limit the relaxation response by inhibiting norepinephrine release.

As in a variety of systemic arteries and veins (e.g. 31,32), exogenous acetylcholine causes endothelium-dependent relaxations of the canine coronary artery (31-36). However, preliminary evidence suggests that acetylcholine released from cholinergic nerves does not (Cohen, Shepherd and Vanhoutte, unpublished observations). In view of the lack of evidence demonstrating cholinergic innervation of the endothelial cells, endothelium-dependent dilatation probably does not contribute to the response to activation of cholinergic nerves (Fig. 6; 16).

2. AGGREGATING PLATELETS

When quiescent isolated canine coronary arteries are exposed to aggregating platelets, they contract. The contractions are larger and

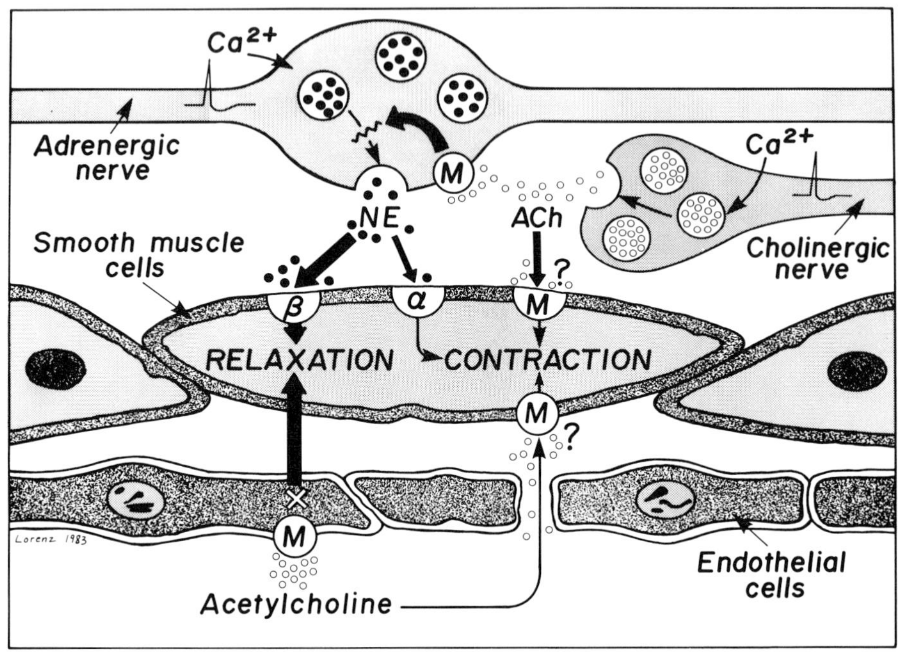

FIGURE 6. Possible interaction of endogenous and exogenous acetylcholine with adrenergic nerve endings, vascular smooth muscle cells and endothelial cells in the coronary arterial wall. ACh; o = acetylcholine; NE; ● = norepinephrine; α = alpha-adrenoceptor; β = beta-adrenoceptor; M = muscarinic receptor; x = unknown mediator; Μ = inhibitory effect.

sustained in preparations denuded of the endothelium, while in arteries with intact endothelium they are attenuated and transient (36). These contractions are attenuated by several serotonergic antagonists (36), indicating that they are due in part to the release of serotonin. When the arteries are contracted first, aggregating platelets cause further contractions in the absence of endothelium, but marked relaxations in its presence (Fig. 7; 36). These experiments suggest that the endothelial cells mediate an inhibitory response of the vascular smooth muscle to products released by the aggregating platelets, and as a consequence, prevent, or at least reduce, the vasoconstriction due to the release of vasoactive substances such as serotonin and thromboxane A_2. Similar findings were obtained with exogenous serotonin; certain serotonergic inhibitors inhibit the endothelium-mediated relaxations caused by

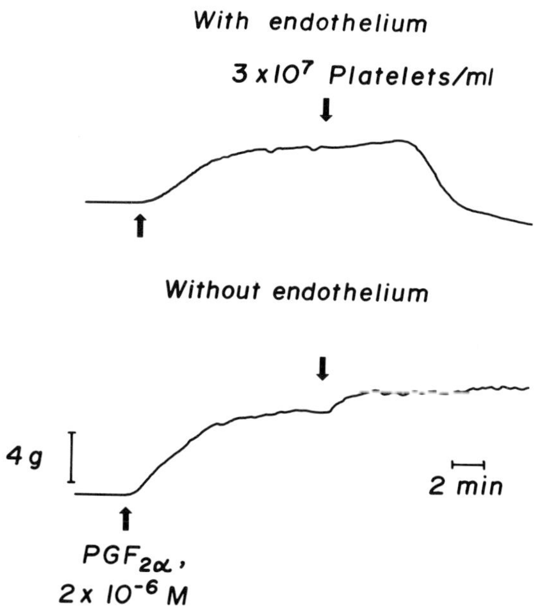

FIGURE 7. Response of isolated canine left circumflex artery rings to
aggregating platelets. Tracings are of isometric tension of two rings
suspended in physiological salt solution; in one ring (lower), the
endothelium had been removed by gentle rubbing. Both rings were con-
tracted by adding prostaglandin $F_{2\alpha}$ (PGF$_{2\alpha}$, 2 x 10^{-6}M). A concentrated
suspension of autologous platelets in calcium-free citrate buffer was
then added to the salt solution. The platelets, which aggregated upon
addition to the salt solution caused a transient contraction, followed
by a prolonged relaxation of the ring with endothelium. Only further
contraction resulted in the ring denuded of endothelium (from ref. 36,
copyright 1983 by the American Association for the Advancement of
Science).

aggregating platelets and exogenous serotonin (36,37). Thus, serotonin

released by aggregating platelets must also contribute to the endothelium-

dependent relaxation they cause. It is possible that other substances

released by platelets contribute to the inhibitory response mediated by

the endothelium. Thus, adenosine diphosphate, which is also stored and released by the platelets, causes endothelium-dependent relaxations in systemic and coronary arteries (31,38,39).

The interactions between aggregating platelets and the blood vessel wall may be particularly relevant in the etiology of coronary vasospasm. The endothelial cells may help prevent vasospastic episodes in coronary arteries (40). These cells form a barrier which because of surface characteristics and secretion of prostacyclin, prevents platelet aggregation (41,42). The access of serotonin, released by the aggregating platelets, to the vascular smooth muscle cells will be reduced considerably by enzymatic destruction in the endothelial cells (43). Thus, endothelial lesions would predispose to platelet aggregation and vasospasm in response to serotonin and other vasoconstrictor substances released by the aggregating platelets. Thrombosis and vasospasm probably contribute to myocardial infarction (44,45). The fact that aggregating platelets may induce coronary vasodilatation by the action of released serotonin, adenosine diphosphate, and possibly other substances, on the endothelial cells should help prevent spasm. Platelet aggregation, induced by blood coagulation and the production of thrombin, should also trigger endothelium-dependent inhibition of coronary smooth muscle (35,39,46). The end result might be an increase in flow which would favor removal of the forming thrombosis (Fig. 8; 47,48).

3. SUMMARY

In the canine epicardial coronary artery, the inhibitory beta-adrenergic action of endogenously released norepinephrine predominates over its alpha-adrenergic vasoconstrictor effect, and norepinephrine-induced constrictions are seen only in the presence of beta-adrenergic blocking drugs. Non-selective alpha-adrenergic blockers favor coronary relaxation by their actions both at pre- and postjunctional sites. Exogenous acetylcholine causes endothelium-dependent relaxation, as well as prejunctional inhibition of norepinephrine release. The latter also occurs upon activation of cholinergic nerves, which will result in vasoconstriction when the main action of norepinephrine is to cause beta-adrenergically mediated relaxations. Aggregating platelets release vasoactive substances, including serotonin, which cause relaxation of coronary smooth muscle in the presence of endothelial cells, but contraction in their absence.

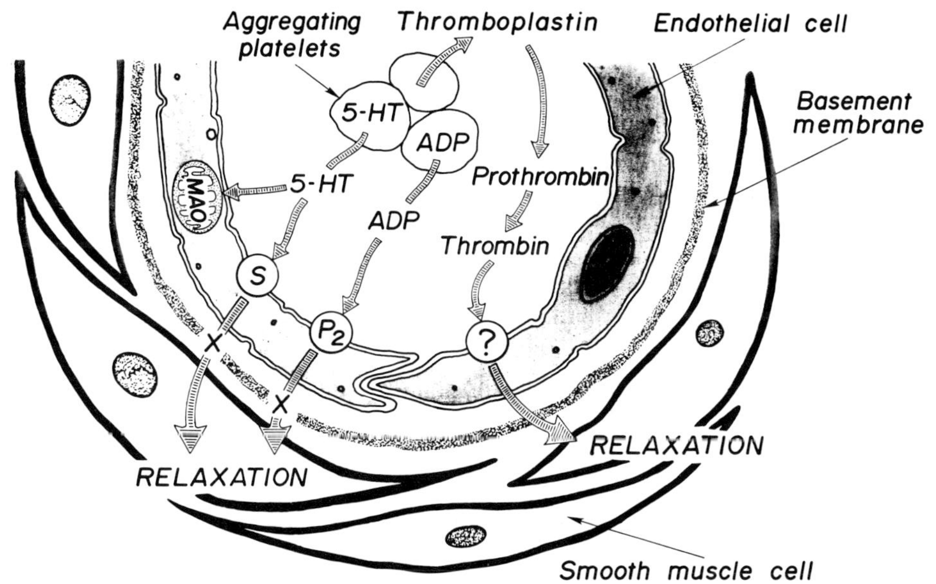

FIGURE 8. Role of the endothelium in preventing vasoconstriction. The protective role of the endothelium depends not only on enzymatic destruction of serotonin (5-HT) by endothelial monoamine oxidase (MAO) but also on the fact that adenosine diphosphate (ADP) and serotonin, released from aggregating platelets, and thrombin can trigger endothelium-mediated relaxations of the smooth muscle cells of the arterial media. S = serotonergic receptor; P_2 = P_2-purinergic receptors; ?,X = unknown mechanism (from ref. 47, by permission).

ACKNOWLEDGEMENTS

The material presented has been collected during two years of a most enjoyable collaboration with Drs. Richard A. Cohen and John T. Shepherd. The author thanks Mrs. Janet Beckman for typing the manuscript and Mr. Robert Lorenz for preparing the figures.

REFERENCES

1. Berne RM, Rubio R: Coronary circulation. In: Geiger SR (ed) Handbook of Physiology, The Cardiac System, sec. 2, vol. 1. American Physiological Society, Washington, D.C., 1979, pp. 873-952.
2. Feigl EO: Coronary physiology. Physiol Rev (63): 1-205, 1982.
3. Feigl EO: Sympathetic control of coronary circulation. Circ Res (20): 262-271, 1967.

4. Kelley KO, Feigl EO: Segmental α-receptor-mediated vasoconstriction in the canine coronary circulation. Circ Res (43): 908-917, 1978.

5. Powell JR, Feigl EO: Carotid sinus reflex coronary vasoconstriction during controlled myocardial oxygen metabolism in the dog. Circ Res (44): 44-51, 1979.

6. Stone HL: Control of the coronary circulation during exercise. Ann Rev Physiol (45): 213-227, 1983.

7. Brine F, Cornish EJ, Miller RC: Effects of uptake inhibitors on responses of sheep coronary arteries to catecholamines and sympathetic nerve stimulation. Br J Pharmacol (67): 553-561, 1979.

8. Toda N: Response of isolated monkey coronary arteries to catecholamines and to transmural electrical stimulation. Circ Res (49): 1228-1236, 1981.

9. Zuberbuhler RC, Bohr DF: Responses of coronary smooth muscle to catecholamines. Circ Res (16): 431-440, 1965.

10. Cohen RA, Shepherd JT, Vanhoutte PM: Prejunctional and postjunctional actions of endogenous norepinephrine at the sympathetic neuroeffector junction in canine coronary arteries. Circ Res (52): 16-25, 1983.

11. Rimele TJ, Rooke TW, Aarhus LL, Vanhoutte PM: Alpha$_1$-adrenoceptors and calcium in isolated canine coronary arteries. J Pharmacol Exp Ther (226): 668-672, 1983.

12. Vanhoutte PM, Rimele TJ: same symposium.

13. Starke K, Docherty JR: Recent developments in α-adrenoceptor research. J Cardiovasc Res (2, suppl 3): S269-S286, 1980.

14. Vanhoutte PM, Verbeuren TJ, Webb RC: Local modulation of adrenergic neuroeffector interaction in the blood vessel wall. Physiol Rev (61): 151-247, 1981.

15. Vanhoutte PM: Beta-adrenergic blocking drugs, adrenergic neuro-effector interaction and systemic vascular resistance. In: Zanchetti A (ed) Advances in Beta-Blocker Therapy II, Proceedings of the 2nd Internationa Symposium. Excerpta Medica, Amsterdam, 1982, pp 279-289.

16. Vanhoutte PM: Why is acetylcholine a vasodilator? In: Vanhoutte PM, Leusen I (ed) Vasodilatation. Raven Press, New York, 1981, pp 67-72.

17. Verbeuren TJ, Lorenz RR, Aarhus LL, Shepherd JT, Vanhoutte PM: Prejunctional beta-adrenoceptors in human and canine saphenous veins. J Autonomic Nervous System (8): 261-271, 1983.

18. Levene DL, Freeman MR: α-Adrenoceptor-mediated coronary artery spasm. JAMA (236): 1018-1022, 1976.

19. Yasue H, Omote S, Takizawa A, Nagao M, Miwa K, Tamaka S: Exertional angina pectoris caused by coronary arterial spasm: effects of various drugs. Am J Cardiol (43): 647-652, 1979.

20. Yasue H, Touyama M, Kato H, Tanaka S, Akiyama F: Prinzmetal's variant form of angina as a manifestation of alpha-adrenergic receptor-mediated coronary artery spasm: documentation by coronary arteriography. Am Heart J (91): 148-155, 1976.

21. Vanhoutte PM: Cholinergic inhibition of adrenergic transmission. Fed Proc (36): 2444-2449, 1977.

22. Vanhoutte PM, Levy MN: Prejunctional cholinergic modulation on adrenerg neurotransmission and the cardiovascular system. In: Levy MN, Vassalle M (ed) Excitation and Neural Control of the Heart. The American Physio-logical Society, Washington, D.C., 1982, pp 243-255.

23. Sakai K: Coronary vasoconstriction by locally administered acetylcholin carbachol and bethanechol in isolated, donor-perfused, rat hearts. Br J Pharmacol (68): 625-632, 1980.

24. Turlapaty PDMV, Altura BM: Magnesium deficiency produces spasm of coronary arteries: relationship to etiology of sudden death ischemic heart disease. Science (208) 198-200, 1980.
25. Ginsburg R, Bristow MR, Stinson EB, Harrison DC: Studies with isolated coronary arteries. Chest (78): 180S, 1980.
26. Kalsner S: The effects of periarterial nerve activation on coronary vessel tone in an isolated and perfused slab of beef ventricle. Can J Physiol Pharmacol (57): 291-297, 1979.
27. Kalsner S: Vasoconstrictors, spasm and acute myocardial events. In: Kalsner S (ed) The Coronary Artery. Croom Helm, London, 1982, pp 551-595.
28. Garland CJ, Keatinge WR: Constrictor actions of acetylcholine, 5-hydroxytryptamine and histamine on bovine coronary artery inner and outer muscle. J Physiol (327): 363-376, 1982.
29. Brachfeld N, Monroe RG, Gorlin R: Effect of pericoronary denervation on coronary hemodynamics. Am J Physiol (199): 174-178, 1960.
30. Guzman SV, Swenson E, Jones M: Intercoronary reflex. Demonstration by coronary angiography. Circ Res (10): 739-745, 1962.
31. Furchgott RF, Zawadzki JV, Cherry PD: Role of the endothelium in the vasodilator response to acetylcholine. In: Vanhoutte PM, Leusen I (ed) Vasodilatation. Raven Press, New York, 1981, pp 49-66.
32. Vanhoutte PM, Rimele TJ: Role of the endothelium in the control of vascular smooth muscle function. J de Physiol (78): 681-686, 1983.
33. Furchgott RF, Zawadzki JV: The obligatory role of endothelial cells in the relaxation of arterial smooth muscle by acetylcholine. Nature (288): 373-376, 1980.
34. Cherry PD, Furchgott RF, Zawadzki JV, Jothianandan D: Role of endothelial cells in relaxation of isolated arteries by bradykinin. Proc Natl Acad Sci USA (79): 2106-2110, 1982.
35. Ku DD: Coronary vascular reactivity after acute myocardial ischemia. Science (218): 576-578, 1982.
36. Cohen RA, Shepherd JT, Vanhoutte PM: Inhibitory role of the endothelium in the response of isolated coronary arteries to platelets. Science (221): 273-274, 1983.
37. Cohen RA, Shepherd JT, Vanhoutte PM: Involvement of the endothelium in response of vascular smooth muscle to intra- versus extraluminal applications of vasoactive substances. Fed Proc (42): 1263, 1983.
38. De Mey JG, Vanhoutte PM: Role of the intima in cholinergic and purinergic relaxation of isolated canine femoral arteries. J Physiol (316): 347-355, 1981.
39. Cohen RA, Shepherd JT, Vanhoutte PM: 5-Hydroxytryptamine can mediate endothelium-dependent relaxation of coronary arteries. Am J Physiol (245): H1077-H1080, 1983.
40. Luchi RJ, Chahine RA, Raizner AE: Coronary artery spasm. Ann Int Med (91): 441-449, 1979.
41. Sherry S, Scriabine A: Platelets and Thrombosis. University Park Press, Baltimore, 1974.
42. Moncada S: Biological importance of prostacyclin. Br J Pharmacol (76): 3-31, 1982.
43. Gillis C: Metabolism of vasoactive hormones by pulmonary vascular endothelium: possible functional significance. In: Bevan, et al (ed), Vascular Neuroeffector Mechanisms. Raven Press, New York, 1980, pp. 304-314.

44.   Oliva PB, Breckinridge JC: Arteriographic evidence of coronary
      arterial spasm in acute myocardial infarction.   Circulation (56):
      366-374, 1977.
45.   Maseri A, L'Abbate A, Baroldi G, Chiercha S, Marzilli M, Ballestra
      AM, Sereri S, Parodi O, Biagini A, Distante A, Pesola A: Coronary
      vasospasm as a possible cause of myocardial infarction.   N Engl J
      Med (299): 1271-1277, 1978.
46.   De Mey JG, Claeys M, Vanhoutte PM: Endothelium-dependent inhibitory
      effects of acetylcholine, adenosine triphosphate, thrombin and
      arachidonic acid in the canine femoral artery.   J Pharmacol Exp
      Ther (222): 166-173, 1982.
47.   Vanhoutte PM, Cohen RA: The elusory role of serotonin in vascular
      function and disease.   Biochem Pharmacol (32): 3671-3674, 1983.
48.   Cohen RA, Shepherd JT, Vanhoutte PM: Vasodilatation mediated by the
      coronary endothelium in response to aggregating platelets.   In:
      Vanhoutte PM, Vatner SF (ed) Vasodilator Mechanisms.   Karger, Basel,
      1984, in press.

III
FUNCTIONAL ABNORMALITIES OF THE HYPERTROPHIED AND FAILING HEART

Section III of this volume presents reviews and original research papers dealing with abnormalities of myocardial function which accompany cardiac hypertrophy and failure. Initially there is a series of chapters which review important fields of interest such as molecular changes within the hypertrophied and failing myocyte, changes in autonomic neural control which accompany heart failure, the altered inotropic responsiveness of the hypertrophied and failing heart to drugs, hormones and neurotransmitters and, finally, a very concise and informative review of the host of new inotropic agents that are now under development. Original research papers follow this series. One study shows that with age the spontaneously hypertensive rat predictably develops congestive heart failure. This finding should open the way for understanding the transition of hypertrophy into failure and allow studies of interventions into this transition. Another study in intact dogs deals with the effect of exercise on cardiac contractile state in normal hearts and hearts hypertrophied by pressure overload. The next chapter by Dr. Schwartz and co-workers introduces a series of chapters dealing with molecular changes which accompany hypertrophy. She reports experiments dealing with the interesting idea, put forth by others, that cardiac hypertrophy is accompanied by a shift in myosin ATPase activity from a "fast" to "slow" isoenzyme. Finally, there is a series of chapters dealing with that all important divalent ion, calcium, and abnormalities of its metabolism in hypertrophy. Taken collectively, the chapters that comprise the third part of this book present a timely overview of research in the area of cardiac hypertrophy and failure.

10

SUBCELLULAR CHANGES IN COMPENSATED AND FAILING HYPERTROPHIED
HEARTS

CONSTANTINOS J. LIMAS

It is difficult to overestimate the importance of
cardiac hypertrophy as an adaptation to chronic overload.
Since the capacity of the myocardial cell to proliferate is
retained for only a short time after birth (1), the task of
maintaining pump performance in adulthood depends heavily on
an increase in muscle cell mass (hyertrophy). This requires
an extensive mobilization of structural and metabolic processes to achieve two often competing goals: (a) maintain
the steady-state energy balance of cardiac myocyte, and (b)
preserve adequate systolic and diastolic function of the
heart. To the extent that these goals are met, hypertrophy
is a truly compensatory adaptation to cardiac overload.
Unfortunately, varying degrees of contractile performance
decline frequently accompany the establishment of hypertrophy. A large number of studies over the last few years
have demonstrated the functional heterogeneity of hyprtrophy
and have begun to unravel the subcellular mechanisms responsible for this heterogeneity. It is becoming increasingly
apparent that several factors, including the severity of
hypertrophy, its rate of development and the nature of the
inciting stimulus, collectively define the functional consequences of hypertrophy. In addition, the structural
responses of nonmuscle cardiac tissues as well as the activation of neurohumoral systems determine the limits to the
effectiveness of hypertrophy as an adaptive process.

This chapter gives a brief, personal overview of some
issues related to the role of hypertrophy as a compensatory
adjustment to increased functional demands on the heart. It

focuses particularly on changes at the subcellular level which may affect the overall pump performance of the heart. It is obvious that we have only begun to explore the complex biochemical readjustments of the myocyte in the course of hypertrophy and that basic questions remain unanswered. It is hoped that even this succinct and selective review will stimulate further research into this important area of cardiovascular research.

(1) Is the hypertrophied cardiac myocyte simply a bigger cell?

In its simplest interpretation, the term "hypertrophy" refers to the most identifiable morphologic characteristic of this process, i.e. that the cell size has increased. It is advisable, therefore, to stress that extensive structural, biochemical and functional remodeling during hypertrophy results in a cell distinctly different from its normal, smaller-sized counterpart. In this sense, hypertrophy should perhaps be distiguished from the increase in cell size that occurs as part of normal growth during post-natal development and reflects cell differentiation under genetic programming.

Experimental studies on the nature and functional significance of cardiac hypertrophy have utilized a number of different methods to increase the pressure or volume work load of the heart. Concomitant changes in neurogenic and humoral influences also take place and may modify the impact of the initial stimulus to hypertrophy.

It is clear that a sustained increase in functional demands on the heart leads predictably to an increase in muscle mass; mobilization of inotropic reserve is utilized only as a transient adaptation. The importance of hypertrophy as an adaptive process is demonstrated by the rapid onset of heart failure when protein synthesis in response to acute overload is prevented (2). There is also suggestive evidence that in some instances, failure to maintain pump function on a chronic basis may be attributed to inadequate degrees of hypertrophy (3). It is not surprising, therefore, that considerable attention has been given to the pathways which regulate the initiation and maintenance of hypertrophy. Although, as implied in the introduction, cardiac hypertrophy involves the structural remodeling of a wide range of cell constituents, the following discussion will be restricted to aspects of protein synthesis control. The preponderance of evidence to date indicates that cardiac protein synthesis is mainly regulated at the transcriptional level (4). One can, therefore, rephase the question about initiation and maintenance of hypertrophy to refer to control mchanisms of RNA synthesis in the nucleus. Some of the pertinent aspects of these mechanisms have recently been reviewed (4).

It is fair to say that we are most ignorant about the earliest steps in the activation of cardiac protein synthesis which involve the transduction of the hypertrophic stimuli to the nucleus where gene transcription is initiated. Since the cell membrane is the first site of action of regulatory influences, it is logical to assume that the flow of information is from the cell membrane through the cytosol to the nucleus. Indeed, recent studies have reported the presence in hypertrophied heart extracts of substances which will stimulate RNA synthesis in normal hearts (5,6). Little is known about the nature of these substances except that they are not species-speciic. This is the most elementary type of study and, although encouraging, needs to be considerably refined before it adds to our knowledge of the signal(s) to hypertrophy and their regulation. Studies in other cell systems have identified in crude extracts a number of protein factors involved in the control of RNA polymerase activity or specific steps in the gene transcription process (7,8). The origin and control of these factors are currently unknown. In some forms of experimental cardiac hypertrophy, evidence has been presented for a requirement for polyamine synthesis (9-11). Since polyamines are thought to be involved in the regulation of cell growth (12), the demonstration of an early activation is not, however, adequate proof of polyamine involvement in the initiation of hypertrophy. Recent studies with specific inhibitors of ornithine decarboxylase, the rate-limiting enzyme, have supported the idea that polyamines are needed for isoproterenol-mediated (15), but not thyroxine-induced (15,16) hypertrophy. Similar studies have not been carried out with other models.

In regard to membrane events, the only speculation so far has focused on the possible role of adrenergic hormone-receptor interactions. There are still enthusiasts for unitary theories such as the postulated role of norepine-phrine as the mediator of hypertrophy (17). Although final judgement is not possible on the basis of existing evidence, it is probably unlikely that a single substance will control such a fundamental process as cell growth. Obviously, more work is urgently needed in this area.

Beyond the question of how the stimulus to hypertrophy is translated into RNA synthesis initiation, lies the matter of quantitative and qualitative controls. The former refer to mechanisms by which the magnitude of protein synthesis is controlled; the latter, to selective activation of a single, or only a few, genes. Both types of control have important functional impliations. As stated above, there is now evidence that, occasionally, the extent of cardiac hyper-trophy may be inappropriately small with consequent decrease in pump performance. This may, conceivably, be the result of a failure to sustain the intensity of the transcriptional and/or post transcriptional mechanisms which control the rate of protein synthesis. On the other hand, it is well known that qualitative changes of several important proteins involved in contractility also occur in hypertrophy. The best studied example is the shift in myosin isoenzymes in response to hormonal stimuli and hypertrophy (18-20). This subject is reviewed elsewhere (21). Briefly, the ratio of isoenzymes wth different enzymatic properties (V_1, corre-sponding to the $\alpha\alpha$ homodimer, V_2 or $\alpha\beta$ heterodimer, and V_3 or $\beta\beta$ homodimer) varies in rats and rabbits according to the physiological or pathological state of the cardiac muscle. For example, V_3 [which, in rats, is the predominant fetal myosin form (18)] reappears in hypothyroidism (22) and pressure-induced hypertrophy (19,23) and may explain the lower Ca^{2+}-activated myosin ATPase activities in these states. Thyroid hormones, on the other hand, mediate a shift to the V_1 isoenzyme (18,20). Four points are worth noting in this regard: (a) myosin isoenzyme redistribution in hypertrophy occurs quite rapidly; (b) it is reversible, therefore under cellular control; (c) the pattern of change is in the same direction as that of contractility, i.e., models with decreased contractility are associated with a V_1 to the V_3 shift and those with enhanced contractility with a V_3 to V_1 shift; and (d) the magnitude of the changes in Ca^{2+} ATPase activity and isomyosin distribution is related most closely to the severity of hypertrophy and there is little evidence so far that a V_1 to V_3 shift is a marker for the transition from a compensated to a decompensated state. Indeed, this transition regularly occurs at a time when pump performance is still preserved and the suggestion has been made that it may increase the metabolic efficiency of the myocardium (24,25). Finally, there is species variation in the isoenzymic distribution of myosin and the shits in response to functional overload. Recent studies (26,27) strongly suggest that isomyosin shifts, although possible in humans, are quantitatively small, do not influence ATPase activity and do not correlate with the severity of hypertrophy. Possibly, different control mechanisms for the regulation of ATP hydrolysis operate in humans. Those negative results do not negate the importance of isomyosin studies since it would be extremely helpful to understand the nature of the restraints on isomyosin redistribution in humans. Furthermore, the possibility still exists (28) that contractility could be manipulated upwards by pharmacologically effectuating a V_3 to V_1 shift in humans.

Although the changes in isomyosin distribution are the best known example of enzymatic adaptations in hypertrophy, they are not unique. At least two more examples can be cited: those of creatine phosphokinase and lactate dehydro-genase. Four CK isoenzymes have been identified (MM, BB, MB and the mitochrondial CK) with different electrophoretic migration and subcellular distribution (29). Recent experi-ments in the spontaneously hypertensive rat have shown (30) that, in hearts exhibiting impaired ventricular performance - from the 18-month old SHR - the total CK and MM-CK activities per unit mass are reduced by about 30% while the activity of the miotochondiral CK isoenzyme is reduced by 60%. These changes may have important implications for the energetic balance of the hypertrophied myocardium. Lactate dehydro-genase activity has been reported to increase in chronic hypertrophy and failure (31-33). In addition, there is an isoenzyme shift toward a more skeletal muscle type. An increase in the M subunits at the expense of the H subunits has been reported after pulmonary artery stenosis in dogs (31,32) and after aortic stenosis in quinea pigs (33) and rabbits (34). The significance of this redistribution is not clear but may make the heart muscle less susceptible to hypoxia.

Finally, the possibility of similar changes in the sarcoplasmic reticulum Ca^{2+} ATPase should be raised. There is considerable evidence that Ca^{2+} transport by cardiac sarcoplasmic reticulum is altered during the course of hypertrophy and this is associated with decreased Ca^{2+} ATPase function (35-38). The molecular basis for this dysfunction in hypertrophy and failure has not been eluci-dated. Heterogeneity of the Ca^{2+} ATPase has been demon-strated in skeletal muscle sarcoplasmic reticulum and has been ascribed to the presence of ATPase isoenzymes with distinct structural and kinetic properties (39,40). Whether such heterogeneity exists for cardiac muscle and the effects of hypertrophy on it have not been studied but represent a potentially important investigative area.

Beyond their potential importance for the understanding of contractility control, these enzymatic redistributions offer a unique opportunity to study the molecular mechanisms of single gene expression. Selective transcription of a single gene or restricted numbers of genes is currently incompletely understood. The mechanisms of RNA synthesis activation in the hypertrophied myocardium are only now being studied, and the general outlines begin to emerge (4).

In general, transcription requires the interaction of the responsible enzymes, RNA polymerases with their DNA template. In eukaryotic cells, however, mRNA production is not simply a question of transcribing the RNA since the transcription units are longer than the final product. Therefore, several processing steps occur to primary RNA transcripts, including methylation of the 5'-end, adenylation to create 3'-poly (A) segment, removal of specific intervening sequences (introns) and splicing of the remaining RNA pieces (exons) leading to the final product (41,46). Each of these steps represents a potential regularoty site but the most frequent type of control occurs at the initiation of transcription. Post-transcriptional events may also be important, especially changes in mRNA stability (43) and mRNA translation efficiency (44).

Although heterogeneity of the RNA polymerase affords one level of transcriptional selectivity, this is limited to the class of RNA snthesized (mRNA, tRNA, rRNA). Quantitative control over the amount of RNA transcribed is exerted by increasing the numbers of transcribing RNA polymerase molecules. At least during the initiation of cardiac hypertrophy, however, this increase is realized through shifts of the enzyme from the free to the engaged (functionally active) enzyme (45,46). These shifts imply changes in the nature of the interaction between the polymerase and its template.

A large body of evidence over the last few years has underscored the importance of changes in the structure and composition of chromatin in determining tanscriptional activity. The structure of the bulk chromatin is too compact to allow accessibility of the large RNA polymerase molecule to its template (41,17). Intuitively, therefore, there is a requirement for a generalized or localized relaxation of chromatin structure before transcription can be initiated. The basic unit of chromatin is the nucleosome which consists of 146-240 base pairs of DNA wrapped twice around a histone core made up of two molecules each of the four major histone classes. The first level of organization is the 100 A "beads-on-a-string" fiber generated by folding of the inter-nucleosomal linker DNA. This fiber is then coiled into a 300 A fiber to yield a structure with a packing ratio of 25:1, close to that of interphase chromatin. To make a mitotic chromosome from the 300 A fiber, a further two orders of magnitude of compaction are generated.

Thre is considerable experimental evidence that trans-cribed genes are in an altered configuration (41). The simplest probe of that conformational change is the altered susceptibility of transcriptionally active chromatin to digestion by nucleases. In particular, deoxyribonuclease I sensitivity is increased in the "active" fraction of chromatin (48-50) but this increase reflects the potential of the gene to be transcribed rather than the transcription process itself. In other words, the conformational change which is reflected in the enhanced nuclease sensitivity is a require-ment but not an adequate condition per se for the initiation of transcription.

The structural basis for the altered conformation of the active genes resides largely in the protein composition of the chromatin. Chromatin-associated proteins include histones and non-histone proteins (51-53). Both protein classes include a large number of structural components common to different cell types and invariant with gene activation. Considerable attention has, however, been focused on the possibility that some non-histone proteins act as positive regulators of transcription (54). Indirect support for such a role comes from a consideration of the properties of these chromosomal proteins: they are hetero-geneous, tissue-specific, bind to homologous DNA, undergo reversible postsynthetic modifications (including phosphory-lation, acetylation and poly (ADP) ribosylation), stimulate

<u>in</u> <u>vitro</u> RNA synthesis and change during the course of gene activation. Most studies on the role of non-histone proteins in gene transcription have been carried out with nonmuscle cells. Only recently have cardiac non-histone proteins been subjected to scrutiny and have been found to have properties similar to those in other cell types. Changes in the composition and properties of cardiac muscle non-histone protein have been described in relation to normal postnatal development (55,56), thyroxine-induced hypertrophy (57), spontaneous hypertension (58), and genetic cardiomyopathy (59-61). In addition, evidence has been presented that protein kinase activities associated with the non-histone protein fraction are intimately involved in the regulation of the "active" chromatin structure (55,57,62,63).

A more detailed study of the involvement of non-histone proteins in cardiac RNA synthesis was carried out in the hypertrophied myocardium of spontaneously hypertensive rats (58). The enhanced DNase I sensitivity of cardiac nuclei from hypertensive rats (SHRs) compared to age-matched normotensive (WKY) rats was abolished by 0.35 M NaCl extraction and was restored by reconstitution with salt extract. The active ingredient was identified as the high-mobility-group (HMG) non-histone proteins (64). Interestingly, reconstitution of salt-extracted nuclei with HMG did not abolish the differences in DNase I susceptibility between SHRs and WKYs suggesting that additional factors contribute to these differences. Experiments in other cell systems have shown that HMGs 14 and 17 induce DNase I sensitivity and that there is direct correspondence between chromatin regions which are capable of interacting with HMGs and regions which are highly sensitive to DNase I (65,66). However, the specificity of HMG binding seems to be dictated by factors residing in the residual salt-depleted chromatin (67). A tentative scheme for the initiation of gene transcription would involve, as a first step, the relaxation of the higher order of chromatin which would then allow the RNA polymerase access to specific DNA regions with consequent initiation of

transcription. The intensity of the transcriptional response
may be dictated initially by the extensiveness of chromatin
unfolding and the rate of the "read-out" by the RNA polymerase.
It is not known at this point whether the numbers of RNA
polymerase molecules ever become rate limiting.

Some consideration should be also be given to the
mechanism by which selective synthesis of key proteins or
functionally important isoenzyme shifts take place. Different
controls probably determine "en masse" activation of RNA
synthesis and selective transcription of only a limited
number of genes. In analogy with the model suggested above,
selective transcription may be regulated by very localized
"unwinding" of DNA regions (such as are thought to be mediated
by DNA-binding proteins or topoisomerases) (68) or even
modification of the DNA itself (e.g. methylation, conversion
to Z-DNA) (69,70). On the other hand, isoenzyme shifts may
depend on selective repression of one or more of the isoenzymes in addition to general stimulation of RNA synthesis.
One mechanism through which such selective repression could
occur is localized methylation of the DNA regions containing
the "down" regulated gene. Our knowledge about the control
of selective transcription will be greatly expanded when the
powerful tools of molecular biology are applied to specific
genes; the myosin gene is a logical candidate and some
progress has already been made in its isolation and characterization (71).

(2) Is heart failure exclusively a cardiac disease?

Although it sounds selfevident, it is frequently over-
looked that processes outside the cardiac myocyte have a
profound influence on its performance. These processes
include structural, neurogenic and hormonal influences.
Structural considerations pertain to: (a) the degree of
synthesis of collagen (72) and other macromolecular substances which affect the diastolic properties of the heart,
and (b) the adequacy of coronary vascular supply (73).
There are important considerations since the diastolic
properties of the heart have a direct impact on systolic

function and, in addition, may influence the completeness of hypertrophy regression after removal of the stimulus to hypertrophy. Similarly, adequacy of blood flow at rest and during exercise defines the limits of metabolic adaptation at the level of the cardiac myocyte.

Neurogenic and humoral influences are also important. It is well-known that cardiac hypertrophy and failure are associated with changes in tissue stores of catecholamines secondary to altered synthesis and release of norepinephrine (74,75). The syndrome of heart failure is associated with marked increases in circulating catecholamines (76,77) which have two important consequences: (a) they increase the afterload on the heart through peripheral vasoconstriction, and (b) they mediate a "loss" of cardiac beta-adrenoreceptors (78) perhaps through a process of "desensitization". The physiological consequences of the latter change is loss of the adrenergic support of the heart crucial for the maintenance of adequate pump function.

It should be stressed that other humoral responses are activated during hypertrophy and failure, including renin-angiotensin (79), and vasopressin (76). The consequences of this activation are, as yet, unclear but may have direct pertinence to the subcellular adaptations to hypertrophy. The importance of cnsidering extracardiac contributions to cardiac function has been clearly demonstrated by the beneficial effect of interfering with these contributions in clinical heart failure (80).

(3) <u>Is there an "energy crisis" in the hypertrophied cardiac cell</u>?

The possibility that the energy supply of the myocardial cell lags behind its demands and mediates cell dysfunction has attracted considerable attention. Oxygen consumption of the hypertrophied heart in increased significantly during the acute phase and returns to normal in the chronic compensated stage (81,82). This transition may reflect changes in ventricular wall stress during the evolution of hypertrophy (83). Experimental support, however, for this concept has not been forthcoming. Early studies have failed to confirm a deficiency of high-energy phosphate stores in the hypertrophied hearts (84, 85), and studies of oxidative phosphorylation with isolated mitochondira have yielded variable results (86). There are several reasons for the discrepancies: (a) different experimental models, including stimuli to hypertrophy, severity and duration of hypertrophy; (b) _in vitro_ experiments with isolated mitochondria under optimal conditions may not stimulate the _in vivo_ situation; (c) there is heterogeneity in mitochondrial populations (87) which further complicates the results.

It should be pointed out that myocardial cells operate under steady-state conditions so that energy demands and supply are balanced. An imbalance between the two can only occur transiently before it induces cell injury and necrosis. Energetic imbalance in the hypertrophied cell, therefore, really refers to the fact that energy demands have declined (e.g., by slowing down ATP-consuming pumps) rather than pointing to a mismatch between supply and demand. Of course, an imbalance could occur during stress or acute increases in work load but this has not been conclusively shown.

(4) <u>What determines the transition from compensated hypertrophy to cardiac failure</u>?

Several stages have been described in the spontaneous evolution of cardiac hypertrophy. In the scheme popularized by Meerson and his colleagues (88), an initial phase of hyperfunction is followed by a period of compensation during which pump function is normal, succeeded by decompensation and the clinical syndrome of congestive heart failure. Considerable effort has been spent to decipher the factors which determine the transition from one stage to the next but with limited success. In general, the evidence for a sequential evolution through the three stages has been decidely less than compelling. Outside the Meerson group there has been little support for the existence of an initial "hyperfunction" stage. Indeed, the degree of preservation of pump function appears to be related more to the severity of hypertrophy and adequacy of circulatory and systemic adaptations than to timing in relation to the Meerson three stages. One considerable difficulty with Meerson's concept is the assumption that progression occurs spontaneously, i.e., without any change in the imposed load on the heart. This assumption is difficult to support since the intensity of the stimulus to hypertrophy may change, the neurohumoral response may vary, loss of myocytes through ischemic or other damage will alter the load on the remaining cells and altered diastolic properties will secondarily affect systolic function.

It is logical to assume that there are lmits to the extent to which the heart can compensate for increased functional demands and that heart failure will occur whenever these limits are exceeded on either an acute or chronic basis. Within these limits there is a wide spectrum of compensation at the level of pump performance. Several studies have indicated that biochemical abnormalities precede the appearance of hemodynamic decompensation leading to the suggestion that these abnormalities are somehow responsible for the transition to heart failure. However, there has been to date no example of a biochemical change unique for this transition. Changes in Ca^{2+} transport or myosin ATPase activities may be quantitatively more severe in failing hearts but the difference is not of the degree that would be consistent with a cause-and-effect relationship. For example, in the study by Sordahl et al. (35), utilizing banding of the ascending aorta in rabbits, Ca^{2+} binding by the sarco-plasmic reticulum was decreased by 23% in animals without failure and by 30% in those with failure. Ito et al. (36), found a 41% decline in calcium transport in the presence of severe hypertrophy without overt failure and 56% in the presence of failure. In cardiomyopathic hamsters (89,90) during the failure stage, Ca^{2+} binding has been reported as 29-77% lower and in the absence of failure, normal or 32% lower. Mild degrees of hypertrophy are not associated with a decline in Ca^{2+} transport capacity (91). Conversely, correction of Ca^{2+} transport abnormalities in spontaneously hypertensive rats following pharmacologic normalization of blood pressure does not occur if hypertrophy does not regress (92). It should be pointed out that, although these Ca^{2+} transport abnormalities may contribute to decrease contractile performance and slower relaxation rates, to some extent they may be purposeful in that they promote the energetic efficiency of the myocardium in the same way as the myosin isoenzyme shifts. The functional significance of changes in Ca^{2+} transport mechanisms may, therefore, depend on their severity. Progression from compensation to failure may relate to a qunatitative decline to levels which affect performance adversely without affording further energetic protection. One hypertrophy model in which spontaneous transition to decompensation has been claimed to occur in the spontaneously hypertensive rat (93). Hemodynamic pump performance is maintained until age 18-24 months when the ejection fraction begins to decline. The degree of hypertrophy, however, continues to increase during this putative transition period. Therefore, the SHR does not really provide a steady-state model of a spontaneous shift from compensation to decompensation.

It is obvious that considerable additional work needs to be done before the molecular mechanisms by which cardiac failure is initiated are understood. It may be advisable to abandon the concept of spontaneous evolution through the three stages suggested by Meerson and, instead, think in terms of limitations to the adequacy of the adaptive mechanisms dependent on the severity of the load rather than its timing. A more fruitful approach would be to investigate the molecular mechanisms which define the limits to the compensatory adaptations and regulate the extent to which these adaptations are utilized.

REFERENCES

1. Klinge O: Proliferation und regeneration am myokard. Z Zellforsch 80: 488-517, 1967.
2. Morkin E, Garrett JC, Fischman AP: Effects of actinomycin D and hypophysectomy on development of myocardial hypertrophy in the rat. Am J Physiol 214: 6-9, 1968.
3. Gaasch WH: Left ventricular radius to wall thickness ratio. Am J Cardiol 43: 1189-1194, 1979.
4. Limas CJ: Control of RNA synthesis in the normal and hypertrophied myocardium. In: "Perspectives in Cardiovascular Research", RC Tarazi and JB Dunbar (eds), Vol 8, pp 93-109, 1983.
5. Hammond GL, Wieber E, Markert C: Molecular signals for initiating protein synthesis in organ hypertrophy. Proc Natl Acad Sci USA 76: 2455-2459, 1979.
6. Hammond GL, Lai YK, Markert CL: The molecules that initiate cardiac hypertrophy are not species-specific. Science 216: 529-531, 1982.
7. Natori S: Stimulatory proteins of RNA polymerase II from Ehrlich ascites tumor cells. Mol Cell Biochem 46: 173-187, 1982.
8. Tsai SY, Tsai MS, Kops LE, Minghetti PP, O'Mally BW: Transcription factors from oviduct and Hela cells are similar. J Biol Chem 256: 13055-13059, 1981.
9. Caldarera CM, Orlandini G, Casti A, Moruzzi G: Polyamine and nucleic acid metabolism in myocardial hypertrophy of overloaded heart. J Mol Cell Cardiol 6: 94-105, 1974.
10. Feldman MJ, Russell DH: Polyamine biogenesis in left ventricle of rat heart after aortic constriction. Am J Physiol 222: 1199-1203, 1971.
11. Chideckel EW, Rosovski SJ, Belur EB: Catecholamine-thyroid hormone interaction on myocardial ornithine decarboxylase. Am J Physiol 243: E305-E309, 1982.
12. Pegg AE, McCann PP: Polyamine metabolism and function. Am J Physiol 243: C212-C221, 1982.
13. Krelhaus W, Gibson K, Harris P: The effects of hypertrophy, hypobaric conditions and diet on myocardial ornithine decarboxylase activity. J Mol Cell Cardiol 7: 63-69, 1977.
14. Matsushita S, Sogani RK, Raben MS: Ornithine decarboxylase in cardiac hypertrophy in the rat. Circ Res 31: 699-709, 1972.
15. Bartolome J, Huguenard J, Slotkin TA: Role of ornithine decarboxylase in cardiac growth and hypertrophy.
16. Pegg AE: Effect of α-difluoromethylornithine on cardiac polyamine content and hypertrophy. J Mol Cell Cardiol 13: 881-888, 1981.
17. Ostman-Smith I: Cardiac sympathetic nerves as the final common pathway in the induction of adaptive cardiac hypertrophy. Clin Sci 61: 265-272, 1981.
18. Hoh JF, McGrath PA, Hale PT: Electrophoretic analysis of multiple forms of rat cardiac myosin: effect of hypophysectomy and thyroxine replacement. J Mol Cell Cardiol 10: 1053-1076, 1978.

19. Lompre AM, chwartz K, d'Albis A, Lacombe G, Thiem NV, Swynghedauw B: Myosin isoenzyme redistribution in chronic heart overload. Nature 282: 105-107, 1979.
20. Martin AF, Pagani ED, Solaro RJ: Thyroxine-induced redistribution of isoenzymes of rabbit ventricular myosin. Circ Res 50: 117-124, 1982.
21. Swynghedauw B, Delcayre C: Biology of cardiac overload. Pathobiol Ann 12: 137-183, 1982.
22. Schwartz K, Lompre AM, Bouveret P, Wisnewsky C, Whalen RG: Cardiac myosins at fetal stages, in young animals and in hypothyroid adults. J Biol Chem 257: 14412-14418, 1982.
23. Mercadier JJ, Lompre AM, Wisnewsky C, Samuel JL, Bercovici J, Swynghedauw B, Schwartz K: Myosin isoenzymic changes in several models of rat cardiac hypertrophy. Circ Res 49: 525-532, 1982.
24. Alpert NR, Mulieri LA: Increased myothermal economy of isometric force generation in compensated cardiac hypertrophy induced by pulmonary artery constriction in the rabbit. Circ Res 50: 491-500, 1982.
25. Kissling G, Rupp H, Malloy L, Jacob R: Alterations in cardiac oxygen consumption under chronic pressure overload. Significance of the isoenzyme pattern of myosin. Basic Res Cardiol 77: 255-270, 1982.
26. Schier JT, Adelstein RS: Structural and enzymatic comparison of human cardiac muscle myosins isolated from infants, adults and patients with hypertrophic cardiomyopathy. J Clin Invest 60: 816-825, 1982.
27. Mercadier JJ, Bouveret P, Gorza L, Schiaffino S, Clark WA, Zak R, Swynghedauw B, Schwartz K: Myosin isoenzymes in normal and hypertrophied human ventricular myocardium. Circ Res 53: 52-62, 1983.
28. Morkin E, Flink IL, Goldman S: Biochemical and physiologic effects of thyroid hormone on cardiac performance. Progr Cardiovasc Dis 25: 435-464, 1983.
29. Lang H: Introduction, in "Creatine Kinase Isoenzymes", H. Lang (ed) Springer-Verlag, New York, NY, 1981.
30. Ingwall JS: Changes in creatine kinase system during the transition from compensated to uncompensated hypertrophy in the spontaneously hypertensive rat. In: Perspectives in Cardiovascular Research, (Tarazi, RC and Dunbar, JB, eds), Vol. 8, pp 145-155, 1983.
31. Bishop SP, Altschuld RA: Increased glycolytic metabolism in cardiac hypertrophy and congestive failure. Am J Physiol 218: 153-159, 1970.
32. Fox AC, Reed GE: Changes in lactate dehydrogenase composition of hearts with right ventricular hypertrophy. Am J Physiol 216: 1026-1033, 1969.
33. Sobel BE, Henry PK, Ehrlich BJ, Bloor CM: Altered myocardial lactic dehydrogenase isoenzymes in experimental cardiac hypertrophy. Lab Invest 22: 23-27, 1970.
34. Revis NW, Cameron AJV: The relationship between fibrosis and lactate dehydrogenase isoenzymes in experimental hypertrophic heart of rabbits. Cardiovasc Res 12: 348-357, 1978.

35. Sordahl LA, McCollum WB, Wood WF, Schwartz A: Mitochondria and sarcoplasmic reticulum function in cardiac hypertrophy and failure. Am J Physiol 224: 497-502, 1973.
36. Ho Y, Suko J, Chidsey CA: Intracellular calcium and myocardial contractility. V. Calcium uptake of sarcoplasmic reticulum fractions in hypertrophied and failing hearts. J Mol Cell Cardiol 6: 237-247, 1974.
37. Lamers JMJ, Stinis JT: Defective calcium pump in the sarcoplasmic reticulum of the hypertrophied rabbit heart. Life Sci 24: 2313-2320, 1979.
38. Limas CJ: Calcium transport ATPase of cardiac sarcoplasmic reticulum in experimental hyperthyroidism. Am J Physiol 235: H745-H757, 1978.
39. Damiani E, Betto R, Salvatori S, Volpe P, Salviati G, Margreth A: Polymorphism of sarcoplasmic reticulum adenoine triphosphatase of rabbit skeletal muscle. Biochem J 197: 245-248, 1981.
40. Wang T, Grassi de Gende AO, Schwartz A: Kinetic properties of calcium adenosine triphosphatase of sarcoplasmic reticulum isolated from cat skeletal muscles. A comparison of caudofemoralis (fast), tibialis (mixed) and soleus (slow). J Biol Chem 254: 10675-10678, 1979.
41. Weisbrod S: Active chromatin. Nature 297: 289-295, 1982.
42. Darnell JE Jr: Variety in the level of gene control in eukaryotic cells. Nature 297: 365-371, 1982.
43. Guyette WA, Matuski RJ, Rosen JM: Prolactin-mediated transcriptional and post-transcriptional control of casein gene expression. Cell 17: 1013-1023, 1979.
44. Rosenthal E, Hunt T, Roderman JV: Selective translation of mRNA controls the pattern of protein synthesis during early development of the surf clam, spisula solidissima. Cell 20: 487-494, 1980.
45. Limas CJ: Enhanced myocardial RNA synthesis in hyperthyroid rats; role of endogenous RNA polymerases. Am J Physiol 236: H451-H456, 1979.
46. Cutilletta AF: Muscle and non-muscle cell RNA polymerase activities in early myocardial hypertrophy. Am J Physiol 240: H901-H907, 1981.
47. Igo-Kemenes T, Horz W, Zachau HG: Chromatin. Ann Rev Biochem 51: 89-121, 1982.
48. Gazit B, Cedar H: Nuclease sensitivity of active chromatin. Nuclei Acids Res 8: 5143-5155, 1980.
49. Garel A, Axel R: Selective digestion of transcriptionally active ovalbumin genes from oviduct nuclei. Proc Natl Acad Sci USA 73: 3966-3970, 1976.
50. Miller DM, Turner P, Nienhuis AW, Axelrod DG, Gopalakrishnan TV: Active conformation of the globin genes in uninduced and induced mouse erytholeukemia cells. Cell 14: 511-524, 1974.
51. Allfrey VG, Littau VC, Mirsky AE: On the role of histones in regulating ribonucleic acid synthesis in the cell nucleus. Proc Natl Acad Sci USA 49: 414-421, 1963.

52. Elgin SCR, Weitraub H: Chromosomal proteins and chromatin structure. Ann Rev Biochem 44: 725-774, 1975.
53. Stein GS, Stein JL, Thomason JA: Chromosomal proteins in transformed and neoplastic cells: a review. Cancer Res 38: 1187-1201, 1978.
54. Hnilica LS: Chromosomal non-histone proteins. CRC Press, Boca Raton, Fla, 1983.
55. Limas CJ: Myocardial nuclear protein kinases during postnatal development. 234: H338-H344, 1978.
56. Limas CJ, Chan-Stier C: Nuclear chromatin changes during postnatal myocardial development. Biochmi Biophys Acta 521: 387-396, 1978.
57. Limas CJ, Chan-Stier C: Myocardial chromatin activation in experimental hyperthyroidism. Role of the nuclear nonhistone proteins. Circ Res 42: 311-316, 1978.
58. Limas CJ: Enhanced myocardial RNA synthesis in spontaneously hypertensive rats. Possible role of high-mobility-group non-histone proteins. Biochim Biophys Acta 646: 37-43, 1982.
59. Liew CC, Sole MJ: Nuclear proteins in the heart of the cardiomyopathic Syrian hamster. Fractionation of phenol-soluble non-histone proteins by two-dimensional polyacrylamide gel electrophoresis. Circ Res 42: 628-636, 1978.
60. Limas CJ, Einzig S, Noren GR: Nucleoprotein changes in the hearts of cardiomyopathic turkeys. Cardiovasc Res 16: 225- 232, 1982.
61. Limas CJ, Einzig S, Noren GR: Contrasting effects of spontaneous and induced cardiomyopathy on the nucleoproteins of turkey hearts. Cardiovasc Res 16: 263-268, 1982.
62. Limas CJ, Chan-Steir C: Cyclic 3'-5'-monophosphate-dependent protein kinases of myocardial nuclear non-histone proteins. Biochim Biophys Acta 477: 404-413, 1977.
63. Akhtar RA, Itzhaki S: Studies in vitro of the effects of adenosine 3'-5'-cyclic monophosphate on the phosphorylation of nuclear proteins in isolated rat heart nuclei. Biochem J 161: 487-497, 1977.
64. Johns EW: The HMG chromosomal proteins. Acad Press Inc, New York, NY, 1983.
65. Weisbrod S, Weintraub H: Isolation of a subclass of nuclear proteins responsible for conferring a DNase I-sensitive structure on globin chromatin. Proc Natl Acad Sci USA 76: 630-634, 1979.
66. Weisbrod S, Weintraub H: Isolation of actively transcribed nucleosomes using immobilized HMG 14 and 17 and an analysis of α-globin chromatin. Cell 23: 391-400, 1981.
67. Weisbrod S, Groudine M, Weintraub H: Interaction of HMG 14 and 17 with actively transcribed genes. Cell 19: 289- 301, 1980.
68. Smith GR: DNA supercoiling: another level for regulating gene expression. Cell 24: 599-600, 1981.

69. Nordheim A, Pardue ML, Lafer EM, Moller A, Stollar BD, Rich A: Antibodies to left-handed Z-DNA bind to inter-band regions of Drosophila polytene chromosomes. Nature 294: 417-422, 1981.

70. Behe M, Felsenfeld G: Effects of methylation on a synthetic polynucleotide: the B-Z transition in poly (dG-M^{5}dC)·poly (dG-M^{5}dC). Proc Natl Acad Sci USA 78: 1619-1623, 1981.

71. Mahdavi V, Periasamy M, Nadal-Ginard B: Molecular characterization of two myosin heavy chain genes expressed in the adult heart. Nature 297: 659-665, 1982.

72. Buccino RA, Harris E, Spann JF Jr, Sonnenblick EH: Response of myocardial connective tissue to development of experimental hypertrophy. Am J Physiol 216: 425-430, 1969.

73. Bache RJ, Vrobel TR: Myocardial blood flow in experimental left ventricular hypertrophy In: Perspectives in Cardiovascular Research, Tarazi, CRC and Dunbar, JB, eds), Vol 8, pp 261-271, 1983.

74. Spann JF, Sonnenblick EH, Cooper T, Chidsey CA, Willman VL, Braunwald E: Cardiac norepinephrine stores and the contractile state of heart muscle. Circ Res 19: 317-325, 1966.

75. Pool PE, Covell JW, Levitt M, Gibb J, Braunwald E: Reduction of cardiac tyrosine hydroxylase activity in experimental congestive heart failure. Circ Res 20: 349-353, 1967.

76. Cohn JN, Levine TB, Francis GS, Goldsmith S: Neurohormal control mechanisms in congestive heart failure. Am Heart J 102: 509-514, 1981.

77. Bito K, Kubo S, Saimyoji H: Role of endocrine factors in congestive heart failue with emphasis on catechol-amines. Jap Circ J 44: 117-127, 1980.

78. Bristow MR, Ginsburg R, Minobe W, Cubicciotti RS, Sageman WS, Lurie K, Billingham ME, Harrison DC, Stinson EB: Decreased catecholamine sensitivity and β-adrenergic-receptor density in failing human hearts. N Engl J Med 307: 205-211, 1982.

79. Curtiss C, Cohn JN, Vrobel T, Franciosa JA: Role of the renin-angiotensin system in the systemic vasocon-striction of chronic congestive heart failure. Circulation 58: 763-767, 1978.

80. Cohn JN: Vasodilator therapy for heart failure: the influence of impedance on left ventricular performance. Circulation 97: 5-9, 1973.

81. Cooper G IV, Puga FJ, Zujko KL, Harrison CE, Coleman HN III: Normal myocardial function and energetics in volume-overload hypertrophy in the sat. Circ Res 32: 140-148, 1973.

82. Burns AH, Montini J: Myocardium in hypertrophy: oxygen consumption by isolated cardiac myocytes and working hearts from spontaneously hypertensive rats. Life Sci 30: 29-37, 1982.

83. Huber D, Grimm J, Koch R, Krayenbuehl HP: Determinants of ejection performance in aortic stenosis. Circulation 64: 126-134, 1981.
84. Feinstein BB: Effects of experimental congestive heart failure, ouabain and asphyxia on the high-energy phosphate and creatine content of guinea pig heart. Circ Res 10: 333-346, 1962.
85. Pool PE, Chandler BM, Sonnenblick EH, Braunwald E: Integrity of energy stores in cat papillary muscle. Effect of changes in temperature and frequency of contraction on high energy phosphate stores. Circ Res 22: 213219, 1968.
86. Sordahl LA: Role of mitochondria in heart cell function. Texas Rep Biol Med 39: 5-18, 1974.
87. Palmer JW, Tandler B, Hoppell CL: Biochemical properties of subsarcolemmal and interfibrillar mitochondria isolated from rat cardiac muscle. J Biol Chem 252: 8731-8739, 1977.
88. Meerson FZ: The myocardium in hyperfunction, hypertrophy and heart failure. AHA Monograph no. 26, 1969.
89. McCollum WB, Grow C, Harigaya S, Bajusz E, Schwartz A: Calcium binding by cardiac relaxing system isolated from myopathic Syrian hamsters (strains 14.6, 82.62 and 40.54). J Mol Cell Cardiol 1: 445-457, 1970.
90. Gertz EW, Stam AC Jr, Sonnenblick EH: A quantitative and qualitative defect in the sarcoplasmic reticulum in the hereditary cardiomyopathy of the Syrian hamster. Biochem Biophys Res Commun 40: 748-755, 1970.
91. Limas CJ, Spier SS, Kahlon J: Enhanced calcium transport by sarcoplasmic reticulum in mild cardiac hypertrophy. J Mol Cell Cardiol 12: 1103-1106, 1980.
92. Limas CJ, Spier SS: Effect of antihypertensive therapy on calcium transport by the sarcoplasmic reticulum of spontaneously hypertensive rats. Cardiovasc Res 14: 692-699, 1980.
93. Pfeffer JM, Pfeffer MA, Fishbein MC, Frolich ED: Cardiac function and morphology with aging in spontaneously hypertensive rats. Am J Physiol 273: H461-H468, 1979.

11

AUTONOMIC NEURAL CONTROL OF THE FAILING HEART

M. J. SOLE

Cardiac function is tightly regulated by the coordinated interaction of neural, humoral and mechanical factors. The sympathetic nervous system provides a particularly important control mechanism by which the electrophysiological, mechanical and metabolic properties of the heart may be rapidly and appropriately coupled to physiological demands. The myocardium readily responds to circulating catecholamines; however, under normal circumstances short-term alterations in cardiac output largely reflect changes in cardiac sympathetic (or parasympathetic) nerve traffic.

In the absence of a sympathetic stimulus cardiac output can be moderately increased by means of the Frank-Starling relationship (20). The dilated or noncompliant heart, however, cannot take advantage of the length-tension relationship and, thus, is dependent on sympathetic stimulation in order to increase or indeed, maintain cardiac output (26,71). Parodoxically, however, profound abnormalities develop in this neuroregulatory mechanism with the development of cardiac hypertrophy and failure.

1. THE SYMPATHETIC NERVOUS SYSTEM AND HEART FAILURE

Cardiac sympathetic efferent traffic is primarily integrated in cardiovascular centers in the medulla and hypothalamus; short spinal sympathetic reflex loops may bypass these centers under certain pathophysiological conditions (75). The cell bodies of sympathetic preganglionic neurons are localized in the interomedio-lateral cell columns of the spinal cord. The axons concerned with cardiac control leave the spinal cord by the anterior roots of the upper thoracic nerves, synapse in the stellate and caudal cervical ganglia and project to complex but relatively well demarcated areas of the myocardium (46). More than

80 percent of cardiac norepinephrine stores are synthesized within the noradrenergic sympathetic nerve terminals of the heart (66).

1.1. Circulating and Cardiac Norepinephrine

A depletion of cardiac norepinephrine stores in congestive heart failure was first reported twenty years ago by Chidsey et al (12), in the United States and Meerson et al (42), in the U.S.S.R. These findings were confirmed over the next few years in a variety of animal models such as left heart failure produced by aortic constriction in the guinea pig (64), or rat (25), and right heart failure produced by pulmonic constriction in the cat (65), or hypoxic pulmonary hypertension in the steer (72), or pulmonary stenosis or tricuspid avulsion in the dog (13). The profound loss of neurotransmitter cannot be explained by the hypertrophic process alone for the reduction is seen in both ventricles regardless of which one is subjected to the hemodynamic stimulus. Noncardiac tissues, however, do not usually appear to be affected (56,64).

The depletion of cardiac catecholamine stores appears to have physiological significance. The electrical stimulation of cardiac sympathetic nerves during canine congestive heart failure is not reflected by an appropriate inotropic or chronotropic response (16). Furthermore, in patients with heart failure there is a marked decrease in the heart rate response to exercise, upright tilt or hypotension, not affected by the administration of atropine(29); the baroreceptor reflex in the dog is similarly impaired (31). Isometric hand grip exercise in patients with myocardial dysfunction fails to induce a net release of norepinephrine into the coronary sinus (30).

The impairment of the intrinsic sympathetic support of the failing heart is partially compensated by an increase in circulating norepinephrine that parallels the degree of cardiac dysfuction (14,37,69). During exercise with moderate degrees of cardiac decompensation, and even at rest in severe forms of heart failure, plasma norepinephrine often exceeds 1,500–2,000 pg/ml (14,37). At these levels plasma norepinephrine not only reflects general sympathetic tone, but also acts as a circulating hormone (53), and thus can contribute to cardiac inotropic support, increase peripheral vascular resistance, stimulate the release of other vasoactive substances such as renin and alter metabolism. The significance of this "sympathetic hormonal activity" in congestive heart failure has been underlined by the marked depression of cardiac function that results following the administration of catecholamine depletors (12), or beta blockers (71), on the one hand and possibly by the clinical benefits of afterload reducers on the other (14).

1.2. Cardiac Adrenergic Receptors

The effectiveness of cardiac sympathetic nerves or circulating catecholamines in supporting the failing heart will be dependent on the response of cardiac adrenergic receptors. It has been reported that plasma lymphocytes from patients with severe myocardial dysfunction fail to generate normal amounts of cyclic AMP after beta-adrenergic receptor stimulation with isoproterenol (69). Although, this study suggests that the high levels of circulating catecholamines found in heart failure may be less than optimally effective because of beta-adrenergic receptor desensitization or down regulation, the relevance of this observation to cardiac beta-adrenergic receptor response is unclear. The failing myocardium does not appear to exhibit a depressed inotropic or chonotropic response to exogenous beta stimulation (29,65). Furthermore, Limas (40) has reported an actual increase in the number of cardiac beta-adrenergic receptors in the hypertrophied rat heart. Similarly, Karliner et al have reported increases in both cardiac alpha 1 and beta adrenergic receptors in guinea pigs suffering from congestive heart failure due to chronic pressure overload (32) and in cardiomyopathic Syrian hamsters (33). The adrenergic stimulation of cyclic AMP generation in cell preparations from hypertrophied and failing hearts has been reported as both unchanged (23,55,67) and depressed (55,67). Recently, Bristow et al (8) found that failing left ventricles obtained from recipients undergoing cardiac transplantation exhibited a 50 percent reduction in beta-adrenergic receptor density with parallel and comparable reductions in maximal isoproterenol-mediated adenylate cyclase stimulation and in maximal isoproterenol-stimulated muscle contraction as compared to normal left ventricular tissue from human donors who died of non-cardiac causes. Whether these conflicting reports pertaining to beta-adrenergic receptor response and density are manifestations of varying degrees of myocyte loss and fibrosis in the myocardial specimens examined or represent true differences secondary to the differing pathological states examined is not clear. A reduction in beta-adrenergic receptor density could contribute to the impairment in the sympathetic control of cardiac function seen in heart failure; however, the significance of these changes will have to await further study. Perhaps cardiac beta-adrenergic receptors although exposed to increased circulating levels of catecholamines may or may not see an actual overall increase in norepinephrine exposure (thus, are or are not down-regulated) depending on the amount of neurotransmitter released at the nerve terminal.

1.3. Mechanism of Cardiac Norepinephrine Depletion

In the last few years it has become clear that the mechanism of norepinephrine depletion is dependent on the type of heart disease examined. Spann et al (64), observed a reduced ability of cardiac sympathetic nerves to retain infused, tritiated norepinephrine in the guinea pig with supravalvular aortic constriction. Such a decrease in norepinephrine reuptake by the failing human heart *in vivo* may be reflected by a reduction in epinephrine extraction across the coronary circulation (48). Spann et al (64), found no alteration in norepinephrine distribution in the noradrenergic nerve terminal and norepinephrine turnover was unchanged; thus, the reduction appeared to reflect a decrease in the actual number of normal nerve endings rather than an alteration in the rate of norepinephrine turnover. An increase in cardiac norepinephrine turnover has been reported, however, by Fisher et al (25), and Filczewski (24), in rats with myocardial hypertrophy secondary to aortic constriction.

A reduction in the number of histofluorescent adrenergic nerve endings in proximity to myocardial cells was observed by Vogel et al (72) in the bovine hypoxic pulmonary hypertension model of right ventricular overload. There was little or no change in fluorescence in the connective tissue septa or perivascular areas. Recovery from heart failure in two steers was associated with normalization of the histofluorescent appearance of the heart. Borchard (7), used both histofluorescent and silver impregnation methods in an extensive microscopic study of human heart tissue and arrived at different conclusions. A complete disappearance of cardiac sympathetic nerves was observed in areas of scar tissue; the remaining nerves were widely spaced as they coursed through the hypertrophied myocardium. Axons that were identified as noradrenergic were found to contain depleted granular vesicles. This heterogeneity of sympathetic innervation may be particularly relevant to the increased risk of sudden death experienced by patients with heart failure. A study by Coulson et al (15), suggested that such changes may only be partially reversible. The investigators reported that relief of right ventricular pressure overload in cats with pulmonary artery constriction leads to an incomplete recovery of depleted norepinephrine stores even in the nonhypertrophied left ventricle.

The enzymes that participate in norepinephrine synthesis and metabolism have also been examined. Pool et al (45), found a marked decrease in the activity of tyrosine hydroxylase, the usual rate-limiting enzyme for norepinephrine biosynthesis, in the myocardium of dogs with experimental heart failure. This observation was verified by Sassa (50) and Yamazaki and Ogawa (76), in rabbits with aortic stenosis and by DeQuattro et al (19) in humans. Schmid et al (52), have reported a decrease in tyrosine hydroxylase and dopamine-beta-hydroxylase in hypertrophied right ventricles in guinea pigs with pulmonary artery constriction. No changes in the activities of these enzymes were detected in stellate ganglia, sinoatrial node, atrioventricular node or left ventricle. Monoamine oxidase has been reported as increased (18,50,76), decreased (34), or relatively unchanged (76). Protein synthesis in sympathetic neurons subserving the heart was reported by Meerson et al (43), to be increased immediately following the induction of cardiac hypertrophy by experimentally-induced aortic stenosis. Protein synthesis returned to normal during the stage of "stable hyperfunction", ultimately with the advent of heart failure, neuronal protein synthesis decreased dramatically. Cardiac norepinephrine stores were reduced at all stages.

All of these studies were performed in acquired forms of heart disease. The majority of models required surgical intervention with possible damage to post-ganglionic cardiac sympathetic nerve fibers. Angelakos et al (1), had reported that a marked decrease in cardiac norepinephrine stores is also present in a genetic paradigm of chronic congestive heart failure, the cardiomyopathic Syrian hamster. This cardiomyopathy is transmitted by an autosomal recessive gene that is

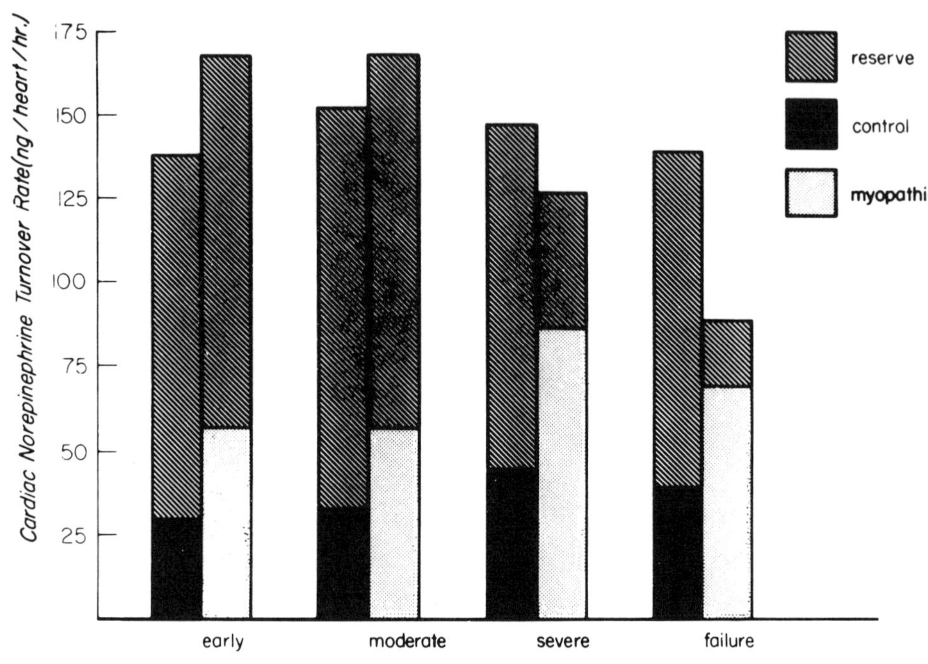

FIGURE 1. Calculated cardiac norepinephrine turnover rate per total
ventricular mass in control and cardiomyopathic hamsters at rest and
during immobilization stress. The hatched area represents the sympathetic
reserve — the amount by which resting norepinephrine turnover can be
increased during stress. (Reproduced from Sole MJ et al. Norepinephrine
turnover in heart and spleen of the cardiomyopathic Syrian hamster, Circ Res
(37):885-862, 1975. With permission of the American Heart Association, Inc.)

phenotypically expressed (cardiac dilatation, congestion) in 100 percent
of hamsters in affected lines (6). Our studies of the mechanism of
cardiac norepinephrine depletion in this natural model of heart failure
have revealed an entirely different set of biochemical abnormalities.

We observed that congestive heart failure in hamster cardiomyopathy is
associated with a marked increase in the rate constant for cardiac
norepinephrine turnover (56). The turnover rate in the resting failing
ventricle approaches the maximum values achievable under stress leaving
the failing hamster with little if any, cardiac sympathetic reserve
(Figure 1). This increase in sympathetic activity appears relatively

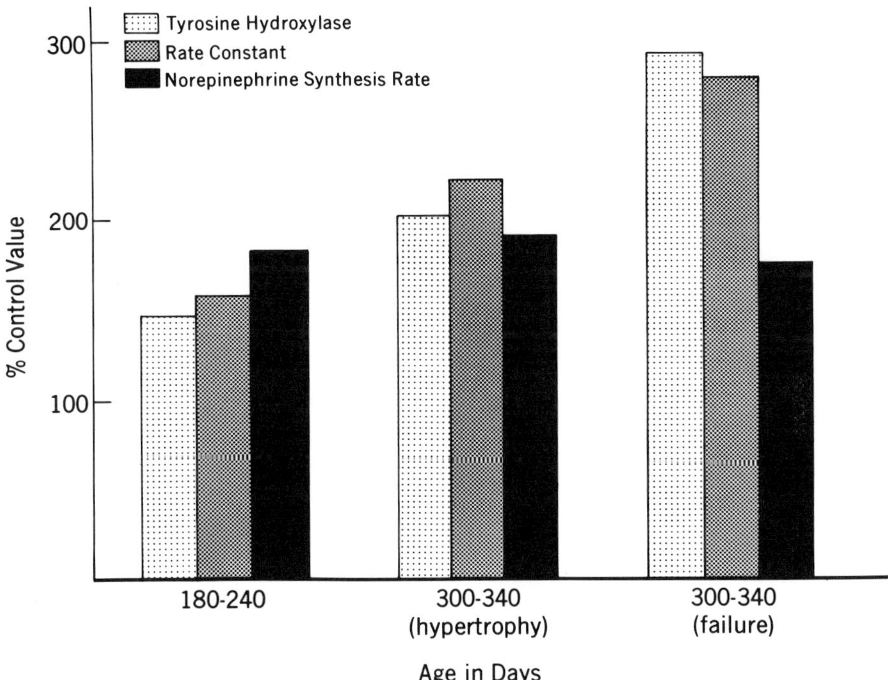

FIGURE 2. Relationship between tyrosine hydroxylase activity,
norepinephrine turnover rate constant, and norepinephrine synthesis
(turnover) rate and disease state in myopathic hamster hearts. Data are
calculated per heart to avoid the artifact of nerve terminal dilution by
the increased myocardial mass. Values are expressed as percentages of the
matched controls. (Reproduced from Sole MJ. Alterations in sympathetic
and parasympathetic neurotransmitter activity. In: Braunwald E, Mock MB,
Watson JT (eds) Congestive Heart Failure, Grune and Stratton, New York,
1982, pp 101-113. With the permission of Grune and Stratton).

specific for the heart as norepinephrine turnover is not increased in the
spleen (56), or skeletal muscle (57). Unlike other models of heart
failure, the hamster exhibits an increase (rather than a decrease) in
cardiac tyrosine hydroxylase activity with progression of the
cardiomyopathy (58). Schmid et al (51), have recently shown that this
increase also extends to the hamster's stellate ganglia. In spite of the
parallelism between norepinephrine turnover rate constant (a biochemical
index of sympathetic tone) and tyrosine hydroxylase activity (the putative
rate-limiting step), cardiac norepinephrine synthesis fails to increase
(Figure 2) and cardiac norepinephrine stores fall (56,57).

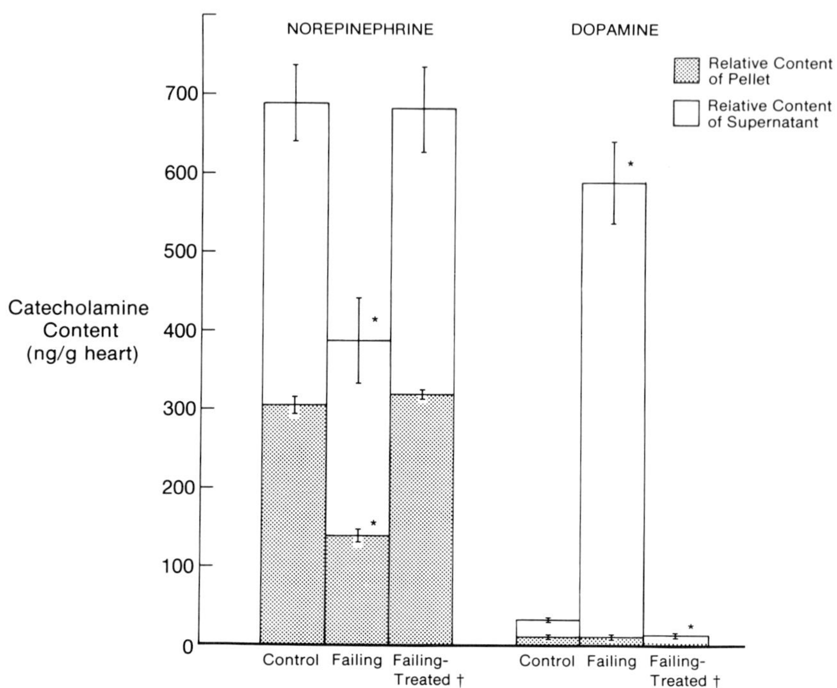

FIGURE 3. Content and distribution of dopamine and norepinephrine in control and failing hamster hearts. Chlorisondamine (10 mg/kg ip), a peripheral ganglionic blocker was given every 6 hours for 18 hours. The hamsters were sacrificed at 22 hours. Each value is the mean ± SE for at least 6 animals. *differs from control and treated p<0.001. (Reproduced from Sole MJ et al. Increased dopamine in the failing hamster heart: Transvesicular transport of dopamine limits the rate of norepinephrine synthesis, Am J Cardiol (49): 1682–1690, 1982. With permission of the American Journal of Cardiology).

These observations suggested to us that tyrosine hydroxylase may not be limiting norepinephrine synthesis in this model. In a subsequent study we observed that an increase in cardiac dopamine usually accompanies the fall in norepinephrine (57), supporting the hypothesis that the hydroxylation of dopamine is rate limiting. We found however that the activity of dopamine beta hydroxylase was increased during heart failure in this model and, thus, apparently is not the limitation to dopamine conversion (62). When we fractioned cardiac nerve terminals into soluble and particulate fractions, we found virtually all of the dopamine accumulated in the failing heart to be in the soluble fraction or extravesicular compartment (Figure 3), (62). Ganglionic blockade results in the complete restoration of both the content and distribution of norepinephrine and dopamine to that found in normal hearts (Figure 3). Conversely, a sustained increase in norepinephrine turnover in normal hearts, induced by immoblization stress, results in alterations of cardiac norepinephrine and dopamine content similar to that found in hamster heart failure (57). There is evidence to suggest that a deaminated metabolite(s) of dopamine in the extragranular space may inhibit dopamine transport across the membrane of the noradrenergic vesicle (62).

With the collaboration of Drs. C. J. Helke and D.M. Jacobowitz we performed histofluorescent studies during the terminal stages of hamster cardiomyopathy (62). These studies reveal two major alterations in the adrenergic nerves. First, the myopathic hearts show a marked reduction in the number of nerves in apposition to the myocardial muscle. Second, there is a sprouting of new fibers into connective tissue and lipofuscin pigment debris. There appears to be a normal number of nerve fibers around blood vessels.

We can conclude from these studies that cardiac norepinephrine depletion in hamster cardiomyopathy appears to be the result of a marked increase in cardiac sympathetic activity and tyrosine hydroxylase that eventually exceeds the rate at which the noradrenergic vesicle can take up dopamine – effectively shifting the rate-limiting step for norepinephrine synthesis from the hydroxylation of tyrosine to the tranvesicular transport of dopamine. There is evidence that this shift is a general manifestation of a marked increase in sympathetic nerve traffic rather than a peculiarity of hamster cardiomyopathy. Thus, the hamster model also supports a beginning literature which suggests that dopamine may have an independent role as a neurotransmitter in peripheral tissues (35,36).

Recently, alterations in the norepinephrine:dopamine ratio, similar to that described for the hamster have been discovered in human hearts taken from recipients suffering from idiopathic congestive cardiomyopathy during cardiac transplantation (G. Pierpont et al, Am. J. Cardiology, in press). Human correlates of hamster cardiomyopathy would be expected to show a net release of dopamine, its conjugate dopamine sulfate, or perhaps its deaminated metabolite, 3,4-dihydroxyphenylacetic acid (DOPAC) into the coronary sinus. The suggestion that such high catecholamine turnover states may exist in the failing heart is also particularly relevant in the light of recent Swedish studies (68), which report a beneficial affect of beta blockade in some cases of congestive cardiomyopathy

2. PARASYMPATHETIC NERVOUS SYSTEM AND HEART FAILURE

The parasympathetic nervous system also plays an important role in the regulation of cardiac function. The parasympathetic and sympathetic nerves of the human heart are anatomically separate; such a distinction is not found in many other mammalian species (47). Cardiac vagal afferent fibers enter the central nervous system and first terminate in the medulla in the nucleus tractus solitarii complex (44). Preganglionic cardiac vagal efferents also arise in the medulla, specifically originating in the nucleus ambiguus and in some species the dorsal motor nucleus of the vagus (27). There is evidence in the cat suggesting direct efferent links from the nucleus cuneatus and nucleus gigantocellularis as well (61). The preganglionic parasympathetic nerves synapse at cardiac ganglia which are particularly concentrated in the subepicardium of the posterior atrial walls. Both atria and ventricles exhibit evidence for a parasympathetic innervation; this innervation is relatively sparse in the ventricular myocardium save for around the proximal specialized conducting tissues.

Vagal stimulation causes a clear and significant inhibition of both chronotropic and inotropic responses to the activation of cardiac sympathetic efferent nerves (70). This adrenergic-cholinergic interaction has been described as "accentuated-antagonism" by Levy (38). The effect can be mimicked by the infusion of acetylcholine and blocked by the administration of atropine (39,70). Resting heart rate is under vagal control. A reflex increase in cardiac parasympathetic tone is evident during the onset and release phases of the Valsalva manoeuvre, during a simple faint, following infusion of drugs that increase blood pressure, or with carotid sinus stimulation (21,22). Conversely, the initial increase in heart rate during upright tilt or early in exercise reflects withdrawal of cardiac parasympathetic tone.

Under basal conditions there is a decrease in cardiac vagal tone in patients suffering from congestive heart disease (22). Furthermore these

patients exhibit a marked blunting of vagally–mediated cardiac slowing in
response to a pharmacologically induced elevation of arterial blood
pressure (22) or during the Valsalva manoeuvre. Studies designed to
characterize the origin of this abnormality in cardiac parasympathetic
control have been conflicting.

The sinus node has been shown to react normally to the stimulation of
vagal efferents in dogs with congestive heart failure (31). Meerson (41)
reported a normal content of cardiac acetycholine and a normal response to
efferent vagal stimulation in cardiac hypertrophy. Furthermore Roskoski
et al (49) examined choline acetyltransferase, the rate–limiting enzyme
for acetylcholine biosynthesis in several guinea pig models of hypertrophy
and failure. No absolute reduction in cardiac enzyme activity was found.
Dr. Jim Wells in collaboration with our laboratory has recently completed
an investigation of cardiac muscarinic receptors in hamster heart failure
by studying the binding, at equilibrium, of (–)-N-(3H)–methylscopolamine
(3H–NMS) in hamster cardiomyopathy (73). Inhibition of 1 nM 3H–NMS by
carbachol revealed three forms of the cardiac receptor, characterized by
high, medium and low affinity (–log Kd= 8.0–9.0, 6.5–7.0, 5.0–5.5) for the
agonist. The medium affinity state represented 45–60 percent of binding
in the atria and in both ventricles. The high affinity state was a minor
(12–17 percent) component in the atria, the right ventricle (less than 5
percent) and was absent from the left ventricle. In myopathic animals with
cardiac decompensation there was an increase in the fraction of the high
affinity form of the receptor. Receptors in all regions eventually lost
the modulatory effects of guanyl nucleotides. Ultimately there was an
actual disappearance of receptors from some of the regions studied.
Concomitant with these findings, we observed that 10nM carbacol arrests
the spontaneous beating of isolated atria from control hamsters but had
little effect on atria from failing animals. Thus heart failure, in the
cardiomyopathic hamster at least, is accompanied by profound changes in
cardiac muscarinic receptors.

3. STUDIES IN THE CENTRAL NERVOUS SYSTEM DURING HEART FAILURE

Recently, we have begun studies designed to identify and localize
brain neurotransmitters that participate in the integration of the neural
and humoral responses associated with heart failure. A decreased

sensitivity of cardiac receptors with vagal afferents for example could lead to impaired buffering of neurogenic drive in medullary cardiovascular centers and an increase in cardiovascular sympathetic efferent tone. A decreased sensitivity in left atrial receptors mediating a signal that inhibits both ADH release (at the hypothalamic level) and renal efferent sympathetic neural activity has been observed in dogs with heart failure (28). Nerve fibers containing the neurotransmitter serotonin have been demonstrated in brain regions believed to be important for cardiovascular control (11). Recent studies have supported a role for central serotonergic neurons in blood pressure regulation (2, 10, 11) and in the regulation of cardiac autonomic tone (2,60). Experimental evidence from our laboratory and those of others suggest that central serotonergic activity is inversely related to vagal and directly related to sympathetic cardiovascular efferent nerve traffic (11,60).

In order to determine whether changes in central serotonergic neural activity accompanies the development of heart failure, we examined serotonin metabolism in a variety of brain regions during the course of hamster cardiomyopathy. Congestive heart failure is associated with an increase in serotonergic activity in the pons-medulla and posterior hypothalamus (59). Using nuclear punch techniques (with the collaboration of Drs. R. deKloet and D. Versteeg) we were able to identify an increase in serotonergic activity in the ventromedial, periventricular and paraventricular nuclei of the hypothalamus and nucleus centralis superior in the raphe with the advent of hamster heart failure (5). Digitoxin restored the increase in the ventromedial nucleus and in the nucleus centralis superior to normal. At the same time, digitoxin partially restored cardiac catecholamines towards normal. (Sole et al, In preparation). There is little known regarding the cardiovascular functions of the nucleus centralis superior (interchangeably referred to as the nucleus medianis in the rat) and the ventromedial nucleus. Electrical stimulation of the nucleus centralis superior in the rat results in an increase in blood pressure; this response is abolished if brain serotonin is first depleted by p-chlorophenylalamine administration (54). We have shown, in other experiments (63), that serotonergic activity in the nucleus centralis superior is inhibited by the stimulation of cardiac vagal afferents. The serotonin concentration of the ventromedial nucleus has been shown to increase with immobilization stress (17). Electrical stimulation of (9), or the injection of serotonin into the posterior medial hypothalamus leads to an increase in blood pressure and sympathetic excitation (similar to the response to stimulation of the nucleus centralis superior). An injection of ouabain directly into the ventromedial hypothalamus is reported to produce a bradycardia which can be abolished by vagotomy (4). Stimulation of cardiac vagal afferents has no effect on serotonergic activity in the ventromedial nucleus, however (63).

The nucleus centralis superior projects axons throughout the central nervous system, particularly the forebrain; its fibers to the hypothalamus travel via the ventral part of the median forebrain bundle (3). It also appears to project to the pons medulla; indeed a lesion in the nucleus centralis superior can decrease serotonin in the pons-medulla by 25 percent. Thus, our observations suggest that at least two independent brain serotonin pathways are altered during hamster heart failure. Some or many of the changes we observed in brain serotonin probably underlie effects distinct from those which directly affect or modulate cardiovascular autonomic tone. However, our results suggest that one of these pathways perhaps a nucleus centralis superior-ventromedialis serotonergic pathway may participate in the modulation or integration of the increased cardiovascular sympathetic efferent response found in hamster heart failure.

4. CONCLUSIONS

The coupling of cardiac output to physiological demands in heart failure would appear to be dependent on appropriate cardiac regulation by the sympathetic nervous system. Paradoxically, however, profound abnormalities develop in this neural regulatory mechanism with the development of cardiac hypertrophy and failure. In some forms of heart failure, the sympathetic innervation of the heart exhibits reductions in norepinephrine content, norepinephrine reuptake, neuronal protein synthesis, the activity of tyrosine hydroxylase and dopamine beta hydroxylase, and perhaps the actual number of nerve terminals and adrenergic receptors. In congestive cardiomyopathy, at least as exhibited by the cardiomyopathic Syrian hamster, the abnormality in cardiac sympathetic innervation is primarily one of a marked increase in cardiac sympathetic tone and an ultimate inability of the noradrenergic vesicles to transport dopamine for hydroxylation to norepinephrine at a rate sufficient to meet demands. There is evidence to suggest that the defects in parasympathetic cardiovascular control may lie at vagal afferent, central nervous system and/or cardiac muscarinic receptor levels. Studies of the neurochemical integration of cardiac autonomic tone in the central nervous system during heart failure will be expected to contribute further to our knowledge of cardiac autonomic regulation in the coming decade.

REFERENCES
1. Angelakos ET, Carballo LC, Daniels JB, King MP, Bajusz E: Adrenergic neurohumours in the heart of hamsters with hereditary myopathy during cardiac hypertrophy and failure. In: Bajusz E and Ronna G (eds) Myocardiology: recent advances in studies of cardiac structure and metabolism. University Park Press, Baltimore, 1972, (1): 262–278.
2. Antonaccio MJ: Neuropharmacology of central mechanism governing the circulation. In: Antonaccio MJ(ed) Cardiovascular Pharmacology. Raven Press, New York, 1977, pp 131–165.
3. Azmitia EC: The serotonin-producing neurons of the midbrain median and dorsal raphe nuclei. In: Iversen LL, Iversen SD and Snyder SH (eds) Handbook of Psychopharmacology, Plenum, New York, 1978, (9): 233–314.
4. Basu Ray BN, Booker WM, Dutta SN, Pradhan SN: Effects of microinjection of ouabain into the hypothalamus in cats. Brit J. Pharmacol (45): 197–206, 1972.
5. Benedict CR, Sole MJ: Altered serotonin metabolism in specific brain nuclei during hamster heart failure; effects of digitoxin. Circ (66): II–307, 1982.
6. Bishop SP, Sole MJ, Tilley LP: Cardiomyopathies. In: Andrews CJ, Ward BC, Altman NH (eds) Spontaneous animal models of human disease. Academic Press, New York, 1979, pp 59–64.
7. Borchard F: The adrenergic nerves of normal and the hypertrophied heart. In: Bargmann W, Doer W (eds) Normal and pathological anatomy. George Thieme Publishers, Stuttgart, 1978, (33): 1–68
8. Bristow MR, Ginsberg R, Minobe W, Cubiciotti RS, Sageman WS, Lurie MSK, Billingham ME, Harrison DL, Stinson EB: Decreased catecholamine sensitivity and B-adrenergic-receptor density in failing human hearts. N. Engl. J. Med (307): 205–211, 1982.
9. Calaresu FR, Thomas MR: Electrophysiological connections in the brain stem involved in cardiovascular regulation. Brain Research (87): 335–338, 1975.
10. Chalmers JP: Brain amines and models of experimental hypertension. Circ Res (36): 469–480, 1975.
11. Chalmers JP, Wing LMH: Central serotonin and cardiovascular control. Clin Exp Pharmacol Physiol (2): 195–200, 1975.
12. Chidsey CA, Braunwald E, Morrow AG, Mason DT: Myocardial norepinephrine concentration in man. Effects of reserpine and of congestive heart failure. New Eng. J. Med (269): 653–659, 1963.

13. Chidsey CA, Kaiser GA, Sonnenblick EH, Spann JR Jr, Braunwald E: Cardiac norepinephrine stores in experimental heart failure in the dog. J. Clin Inves (43): 2386-2393, 1964.
14. Cody RJ, Franklin KW, Kluger J, Laragh JH: Sympathetic responsiveness and plasma norepinephrine during therapy of chronic congestive heart failure with captopril. Am J. Med (72): 791-797, 1982.
15. Coulson RL, Yazdanfar S, Rubio E, Bove AA, Lemole GM, Spann JR: Recuperative potential of cardiac muscle following relief of pressure overload hypertrophy and right ventricular failure in the cat. Circ Res (40): 41-49, 1977.
16. Covell JW, Chidsey CA, Braunwald E: Reduction of the cardiac response to postganglionic sympathetic nerve stimulation in experimental heart failure. Cir Res (19): 51-56, 1966.
17. Culman J, Kvetnansky R, Torda T, Murgas K: Serotonin concentration in individual hypothalamic nuclei of rats exposed to acute immobilization stress. Neuroscience (5): 1503-1506, 1980.
18. DeChamplain J, Krakoff LR, Axelrod J: Increased monoamine activity during the development of cardiac hypertrophy in the rat. Circ Res (23): 361-369, 1968.
19. DeQuattro V, Nagatsu T, Mendez A, Verska J: Determinants of cardiac noradrenaline depletion in human congestive failure. Cardiovasc Res (7): 344-350, 1973.
20. Donald DE, Ferguson DA, Milburn SE: Effect of beta-adrenergic receptor blockade on racing performance of greyhounds with normal and with denervated hearts. Circ Res (22): 127-134, 1968.
21. Eckberg DL: Parasympathetic cardiovascular control in human disease: a critical review of methods and results. Am J Physiol (239): H581-H593, 1980.
22. Eckberg DL, Drabinsky M, Braunwald E: Defective cardiac parasympathetic control in patients with heart disease. New Engl J Med (285): 877-883, 1971.
23. Epstein SE, Skelton GL, Levy GS, Entman M: Adenyl cyclase and myocardial contractility. Ann Intern Med (72): 561-578, 1970.
24. Filczewski M: Rate of catecholamine biosynthesis in the heart, brain and adrenals in experimental arterial hypertension and cardiomegaly. Acta Physiol Pol (26): 569-582, 1975.
25. Fisher JE, Horst WD, Kopin IJ: Norepinephrine metabolism in hypertrophied rat hearts. Nature, London, (207): 951-953, 1965.
26. Gaffney TE, Braunwald E: Importance of the adrenergic nervous system in the support of circulatory function in patients with congestive heart failure. A J. Med (34): 320-324, 1963.
27. Geis GS, Wurster RD: Horseradish peroxidase localization of cardiac vagal preganglionic somata. Brain Research (182): 19-30, 1980.
28. Gilmore JP, Zucker IH: Activity of atrial receptors under normal and pathological states. In: Hainsworth R, Kidd C, Linden FJ (eds) Cardiac Receptors. Cambridge University Press, Cambridge, 1979, pp 139-156 .
29. Goldstein RE, Beiser GD, Stampfer M, Epstein SE: Impairment of autonomically mediated heart rate control in patients with cardiac dysfunction. Circ Res (36): 571-578, 1975.
30. Haneda T, Miura Y, Arai T, Nakajima T, Miura T, Honna T, Kobayashi K, Sakuma, H, Adachi M, Miyazawa K, Yoshinsa K, Takishima T: Norepinephrine levels in the coronary sinus in patients with cardiovascular disease at rest and during isometric handgrip exercise. Am Heart J (100): 465-472, 1980.

31. Higgins CB, Vatner SF, Eckberg DL, Braunwald E: Alterations in the baroreceptor reflex in conscious dogs with heart failure. J. Clin Invest (51): 715-724, 1972.
32. Karliner JS, Barnes P, Brown M, Dollery C: Chronic heart failure in the guinea pig increases cardiac α_1-and B-adrenoreceptors. Eur J Pharmacol (67): 115-118, 1980.
33. Karliner JS, Alabaster C, Stephens H, Barnes P, Dollery C: Enhanced noradrenaline response in cardiomyopathic hamsters; possible relation to changes in adrenoreceptors studied by radioligand binding. Cardiovasc Res (15): 296-304, 1981.
34. Krakoff LR, Buccino RA, Spann JR, DeChamplain J: Cardiac catechol-O-methyltransferase and monoamine oxidase activity in congestive heart failure. Am J. Physiol (215): 549-552, 1968.
35. Lackovic Z, Relja M, Neff NH: Catabolism of endogenous dopamine in peripheral tissues: is there an independent role for dopamine in peripheral neurotransmission. J. Neurochem (38): 1453-1458, 1982.
36. Lackovic Z, Neff NH: Evidence that dopamine is a neurotransmitter in peripheral tissues. Life Sciences (32): 1665-1674, 1982.
37. Levine TB, Francis GS, Goldsmith SR, Simon AB, Cohn JN: Activity of the sympathetic nervous system and renin-angiotensin system assessed by plasma hormone levels and their relation to hemodynamic abnormalities in congestive heart failure. Am J. Cardiol. (49): 1659-1666, 1982.
38. Levy MN: Sympathetic-parasympathetic interactions in the heart. Circ Res (29): 437-445, 1971.
39. Levy NM, Blattberg B: Effect of vagal stimulation on the overflow of norepinephrine into the coronary sinus during cardiac sympathetic nerve stimulation in the dog. Circ Res (38): 81-85, 1976.
40. Limas CJ: Increased number of B-adrenergic receptors in the hypertrophied myocardium. Biochem Biophys Acta (588): 174-178, 1979.
41. Meerson FZ: The myocardium in hyperfunction, hypertrophy and heart failure. Circ Res, Suppl II, (25): II-143-II-145, 1969.
42. Meerson FZ, Manukhin BN, Pshennikova MG, Rosanova LS: On mediator exchange in compensatory hyperfunction and hypertrophy of the heart (in Russian). Patologischeskaya Fiziologiya: eksperimentalnaya terapia (1): 32-36, 1963.
43. Meerson FZ, Krokhina EM, Pshennikova MA, Saponicova VI: Dynamics of the rate of protein synthesis in sympathetic neurons as a factor determining the hyperfunction and hypertrophy of the heart. J. Molec Cell Cardiol (1): 411-423, 1970.
44. Palkovits M, Mezey E, Zaborsky L: Neuroanatomical evidences for direct neural connections between the brain stem baroreceptor centers and forebrain areas involved in the neural regulation of the blood pressure. In: Meyer P and Schmitt H (eds) Nervous system and hypertension. Wiley-Flammarion, Toronto, 1970, pp 18-30.
45. Pool PE, Covell JW, Levitt M, Gibb J, Braunwald E: Reduction of cardiac tyrosine hydroxylase activity in experimental congestive heart failure. Circ Res (20): 349-353, 1967.
46. Randall WC: Sympathetic control of the heart. In: Randall WC (ed) Neural Regulation of the Heart. Oxford University Press, New York, 1977, pp 43-92.
47. Randall WC, Armour JA: Gross and microscopic anatomy of the cardiac innervation. In: Neural Regulation of the Heart. Oxford University Press, New York, 1977, pp 15-39.

48. Rose CP, Burgess JH, Cousineau D: Reduced aortocoronary sinus extraction of epinephrine in patients with left ventricular failure secondary to long term pressure or volume overload. Circulation (68): 241-244, 1983.
49. Roskoski R Jr, Schmid PG, Mayer HE, Abboud FM: In vitro acetylcholine biosynthesis in normal and failing guinea pig hearts. Circ Res (36): 547-552, 1973.
50. Sassa H: Mechanism of myocardial catecholamine depletion in cardiac hypertrophy and failure in rabbits. Jap. Circ J. (35): 391-403, 1971.
51. Schmid PG, Lund DD, Roskoski R: Efferent autonomic dysfunction in heart failure. In: Abboud FM, Fozzard HA, Gilmore JP, Reis DJ (eds) Disturbances in neurogenic control of the circulation. American Physiological Society, Bethesda, 1981, pp 33-50.
52. Schmid PG, Lund DD, David JA, Whiteis CA, Bhatnager RK, Roskoski R: Selective sympathetic neural changes in hypertrophied right ventricle. Am J. Physiol (243): H175-H180, 1982.
53. Silverberg AB, Shah SD, Haymond MW, Cryer PE: Norepinephrine: hormone and neurotransmitter in man. J. Clin Invest (45): 228-236, 1978.
54. Smits JFM, Van Essen H, Struyker-Boudier HAJ: Serotonin mediated cardiovascular responses to electrical stimulation of the raphe nuclei in the rat. Life Sciences (23): 173-178, 1978.
55. Sobel BE, Henry PD, Robison A, Bloor C, Ross J Jr : Depressed adenyl cyclase activity in the failing guinea pig heart. Circ Res (24): 507-512, 1969.
56. Sole MJ, Lo C-M, Laird CW, Sonnenblick WH, Wurtman RJ: Norepinephrine turnover in the heart and spleen of the cardiomyopathic Syrian hamster. Circ Res (37): 855-862, 1975.
57. Sole MJ, Kamble AB, Hussain MN: A possible change in the rate-limiting step for cardiac norepinephrine synthesis in the cardiomyopathic Syrian hamster. Circ. Res (41): 814-817, 1977.
58. Sole MJ, Wurtman RJ, Lo C-M, Kumble AB, Sonnenblick EH: Tyrosine hydroxylase activity in the heart of the cardiomyopathic Syrian hamster. J. Mol Cell Cardiol (9): 225-233, 1977.
59. Sole MJ, Shum A, Van Loon GR: Alterations in brain serotonin during congestive heart failure in the cardiomyopathic Syrian hamster. Cardiovasc. Res (12): 373-375, 1978.
60. Sole MJ, Van Loon GR, Shum A, Lixfeld W, McGregor DC: Left ventricular receptors inhibit brain serotonin neurons during coronary artery occlusion. Science (201): 620-622, 1978.
61. Sole MJ, Hussain MN, Versteeg DHG, deKloet RE, Adams D, Lixfeld W: The identification of specific brain nuclei in which catecholamine turnover is increased by left ventricular receptors during acute myocardial infarction in the rat. Brain Res (235): 315-325, 1982.
62. Sole MJ, Helke CJ, Jacobowitz DM: Increased dopamine in the failing hamster heart: transvesicular transport of dopamine limits the rate of norepinephrine synthesis. Am. J. Cardiol (49): 1682-1690, 1982.
63. Sole MJ, Versteeg DHG, de Kloet ER, Hussain N, Lixfeld W: The identification of specific serotonergic nuclei inhibited by cardiac vagal afferents during acute myocardial ischemia, in the rat. Brain Res (265): 55-61, 1983.
64. Spann JF, Chidsey CA, Pool PE, Braunwald E: Mechanism of norepinephrine depletion in experimental heart failure produced by aortic constriction in the guinea pig. Circ Res (17): 312-321, 1965

65. Spann JF Jr, Buccio RA, Sonnenblick EH, Braunwald E : Contractile state of cardiac muscle obtained from cats with experimentally produced ventricular hypertrophy and heart failure. Circ Res (21): 341-35, 1967.
66. Spector S, Sjoerdsma A, Zaltzmann-Nirenberg P: Norepinephrine sythesis from tyrosine-C14 in isolated perfused guinea-pig heart. Science (139): 1299-1301, 1963.
67. Sulakhe PV, Dhalla NS: Adenyl cyclase activity in failing hearts of genetically myopathic hamsters. Biochem Med (6): 471-482, 1972.
68. Swedberg K, Hjalmarson A, Waagstein F, Wallentin I: Beneficial effects of long-term beta-blockade in congestive cardiomyopathy. Br Heart J. (44): 117-133, 1980.
69. Thomas JA, Marks BH: Plasma norepinephrine in congestive heart failure. Am J. Cardiol (41): 233-243, 1978.
70. Vanhoutte PM, Levy MN: Cholinergic inhibition of adrenergic neurotransmission in the cardiovascular system. In: Brooks McC C, Koizumi K, Sato A (eds) Integrative functions of the autonomic nervous system Elsevier/North Holland Biomedical Press, 1980, pp 159-176.
71. Vogel JHK, Chidsey CA: Cardiac adrenergic activity in experimental heart failure assessed with beta-receptor blockade. Am J. Cardiol (24): 198-208, 1969.
72. Vogel JHK, Jacobowitz D, Chidsey CA: Distribution of norepinephrine in the failing bovine heart: Correlation of chemical analysis and fluorescence microscopy. Circ Res (24): 71-84, 1969.
73. Wells JW, Wong H-M and Sole MJ: Muscarinic Receptors in Heart Failure. Proceedings of the Society of Neuroscience (7): 713, 1981 (Abstract).
74. Wing LMH, Chalmers JP : Participation of central serotonergic neurons on the control of the circulation ofthe unanesthesized rabbit. Circ Res (35): 504-513, 1974.
75. Wurster RD : Spinal sympathetic control of the heart. In Randall WC (ed) Neural regulation of the heart. Oxford University Press, New York, 1977, pp. 213-246.
76. Yamazaki N, Ogawa K : Cardiac catecholamine metabolism in heart failure. Jap Circ J. (35): 965-971, 1971.

12

THE INOTROPIC RESPONSIVENESS OF THE FAILING HEART

W.H. NEWMAN, M.B. FRANKIS, AND J.G. WEBB

1.   Introduction

A positive inotropic event is an increase in myocardial contractile state that is independent of an increase
in diastolic fiber length. The event represents the consequence of the interaction of some agent, usually a hormone,
a neurotransmitter or a drug, with the myocyte, which
ultimately causes an increase in the interaction of the
actin and myosin filaments. Increased interaction of the
filaments is measurable in the intact heart muscle as an
upward and rightward shift of the force-velocity curve and
an upward shift of the length-tension curve (1) (Figure 1).
Such shifts in both the strength and velocity of contraction
of the myocardium are an adaptive mechanism which permits
beat-to-beat adjustment of the cardiac contractile state in
order to match the changing hemodynamic load on the heart.
When this adaptive mechanism becomes compromised the heart
fails, and the classic signs of pump failure are manifest
as a decreased cardiac output, edema, and reduced renal
function. This compromised inotropic state of the myocardium - congestive heart failure - is classically treated
by the administration of drugs that have positive inotropic
action. The rationale behind such therapy is to elevate
the depressed contractile strength of the failing heart and
thereby improve pump function. The success of such a
rationale is evident in the fact that the positive inotropic
drug, digitalis, has been the mainstay in the therapeutic
regimen of heart failure for almost two hundred years.
Successful therapy with digitalis depends entirely on the

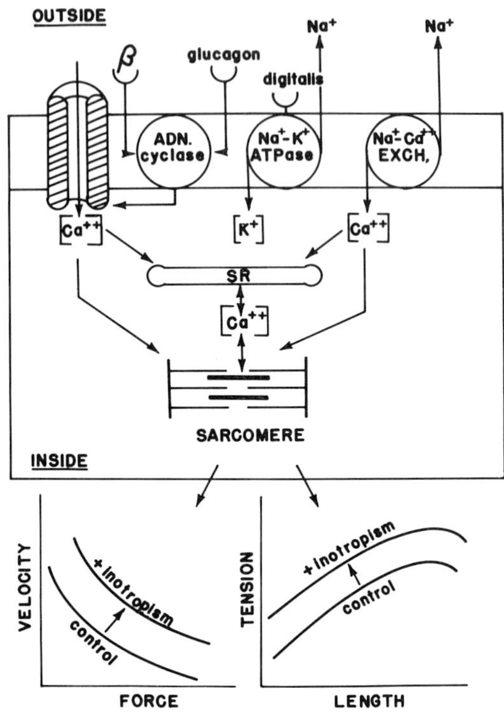

FIGURE 1.   A schematized illustration of a myocyte showing some known pathways to increased contractility.   From left-to-right: the slow calcium channel; the sarcolemmal adenylate cyclase system shown coupled to the receptors for β-adrenergic agonists and glucagon; sarcolemmal Na^+-K^+ ATPase system and the digitalis receptor; sarcolemmal Na^+-Ca^{2+} exchange.   A positive inotropic event involving any of these systems is believed to ultimately influence intracellular Ca^{2+} dynamics leading to increased interaction of actin with myosin in the sarcomere thus causing increased strength and velocity of contraction.

ability of the cardiac glycosides to increase the contractile state of the failing myocyte.   Similarly, the therapeutic usefulness of other newer positive inotropic agents such as the β-adrenergic receptor agonist prenalterol and the bipyridine derivatives, amrinone and milrinone - which to date act by an unknown mechanism (2) - will ultimately reside in the ability of these agents to cause a change in the inotropic state of failing heart muscle.   In failing heart muscle, many of the cellular systems which drugs influence to cause positive inotropism are abnormal (3). Therefore, it seems reasonable to suppose that the contractile response to some of agents would be altered in heart failure. In this chapter we will discuss the findings relative to this supposition.

2. <u>Responsiveness of the Failing Heart to the Sympathetic Nervous System</u>

One of the most important systems for beat-to-beat regulation of the contractile state is the sympathetic nervous system. Such regulation is brought about by release of norepinephrine from adrenergic nerve terminals, combination of the released transmitter with the β-adrenergic receptor on the myocyte sarcolemma, and consequent activation of the adenylate cyclase system. That heart failure is accompanied by an abnormality in this pathway was first discovered by Chidsey <u>et al</u>., (4) when they found that atrial tissue obtained from patients with heart failure contained about one-fourth the amount of norepinephrine per gram of tissue as was found in normal atria. This finding of reduced myocardial norepinephrine stores has since been confirmed in ventricular tissue from failing human hearts (5). Likewise reduced myocardial norepinephrine content has been measured in dog (6), guinea pig (7), cat (8) and bovine (9) models of acquired heart failure as well as in the failed heart of the Syrian hamster with genetic cardiomyopathy (10). Therefore, there is at least one alteration in this important inotropic regulatory pathway seen in heart failure of man and other animal species.

A functional derangement which accompanies the reduction of myocardial norepinephrine content is that activation of the sympathetic nervous system produces less of an increase in both heart rate and myocardial contractility in the failed heart versus the normal heart. This observation was made by Covell <u>et al</u>. (11) in dogs with heart failure from tricuspid insufficiency and pulmonic stenosis. When the cardioaccelerator nerve was stimulated in these dogs with failure, there was a reduced response of heart rate and of right ventricular contractile force (Figure 2) compared to normal dogs. Similarly, when papillary muscles from dogs (6) and from humans (12) with heart failure were exposed to increasing concentrations of tyramine, the response curves of contractile force were flattened and shifted to the right of dose-response curves obtained from normal papillary muscles. Since tyramine causes its inotropic effect by releasing norepinephrine from the sympathetic nerve endings, the loss of inotropic effect was compatible with the reduced myocardial norepinephrine levels found in these failed hearts. Reduced stores of neurotransmitters are also thought to play a primary

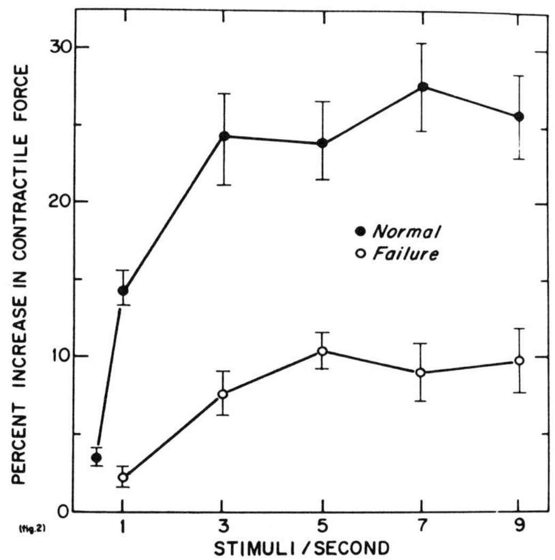

FIGURE 2. Response of right ventricular contractile force to cardiac accelerator nerve stimulation in normal dogs and dogs with heart failure. (From Covell, J.W. <u>et al</u>., Circ. Res. 19:51, 1966. Reproduced with permission of the American Heart Association, Inc.)

role in the impairment of autonomically mediated control of heart rate in patients with heart failure. Such patients have reduced chronotropic response to head up tilt and to the abrupt lowering of blood pressure by nitroglycerine (13).

Thus, heart failure is accompanied by loss of norepine-phrine from the myocardial adrenergic nerve endings, and the diminished release of transmitter may deprive the failing heart of reflex inotropic drive. The failing heart may then become increasingly dependent on extracardiac sources of catecholamines which are manifested as the increased plasma catecholamine levels seen in heart failure (14). Such a dependence is supported by the observed decline in cardiovascular status of patients with heart failure given propranolol, a β-adrenergic receptor blocking agent (15), or guanethidine (16), a drug which interferes with postganglionic synaptic transmission in the adrenergic nervous system. Clearly, high adrenergic tone is critical to some patients with heart failure, but, apparently, not to all patients with heart failure in light of recent studies reporting beneficial effects of β-adrenergic recep-tor blockade (17,18). If elevated circulating levels of catecholamines make an important contribution to the main-tenance of the cardiovascular status of some patients in heart failure, then knowledge of responsiveness of the failing heart to circulating and exogenous norepinephrine becomes important. Further, such knowledge could be important when considering the development and clinical testing of new inotropic agents.

3. Response of the Failing Heart to β-Adrenergic Agonists

The failing heart shows a blunted chronotropic and inotropic response to activation of the sympathetic nervous system, but the question of how the hypertrophied and failing heart responds to exogenously administered β-agon-ists or to postjunctional activation of the β-receptor-adenylate cyclase system by high circulating levels of catecholamines is more controversial. The initial studies regarding this question were done in isolated papillary muscles obtained from the failing right ventricle of dogs with tricuspid insufficiency and pulmonic stenosis (6). As mentioned above, in these muscles the response to tyramine was clearly reduced in that the dose-response curve of contractile force was shifted to the right and had a reduced maximum. This effect was in concert with the measured reduction of norepineprhine stores. Norepinephrine was added to the muscle bath in order to show that the muscles were capable of responding to β-adrenergic stimulation, but no detailed analysis of the dose response curves was reported. In 1966, similar studies evaluating tyramine responsiveness were done in papillary muscles obtained from failing human hearts (12). The tyramine response was found to be blunted in those muscles with reduced norepinephrine stores. Again, norepinephrine was used to show that the muscles were capable of responding to released catecholamine, but no evaluation of the contractile responsiveness of the failed muscles to exogenous catecholamine could be made since there was no normal group to serve as control. Covell et al. (11), in their study of dogs with right heart failure in which the response of right ventricular contractile force to cardioaccelerator nerve stimulation was found to be blunted, administered 3 μg/kg of norepinephrine and found no difference in the contractile response of the failing heart when compared to control dogs. Spann et al. (8) found that, in papillary muscle isolated from cats with right ventricular failure, introduction of 10^{-7} M norepinephrine to the muscle bath produced greater increments in force developed by failing muscles than by normal muscles. This result suggest a supersensitivity to exogenous norepinephrine in the failing heart. In contrast, Gold et al. (19), using the same model of heart failure in cats as Spann et al. (8), found that papillary muscles from failing hearts responded normally to increasing concentrations of norepinephrine (10^{-7} to 10^{-5} M) in the muscle bath. However, the positive inotropic action of glucagon was completely abolished in the failing isolated muscles (19).

We first studied this question of the responsiveness of the failing heart to β-adrenergic agonists in dogs with volume overload heart failure. The model, which is produced by creating a chronic arteriovenous fistula, is characterized by signs of heart failure that include: 1) ascites, 2) pulmonary and limb edema, 3) elevated left ventricular end diastolic pressure, 4) elevated plasma norepinephrine levels which averaged 240 pg/ml in the control state and rose to 860 pg/ml in failure, 5) elevated plasma renin activity which averaged 1.3 ng/ml/hr in the control state and 12.4 ng/ml/hr when heart failure was present, and 6) a depressed abbreviated left ventricular length-tension curve (20-24). A depressed length-tension curve with an abbreviated ascending limb is a hallmark of myocardial muscle failure. In these dogs, while under anesthesia, heart rate, arterial blood pressure and left ventricular contractile force were recorded. Graded doses of norepinephrine were administered by intravenous bolus injection or by continuous intravenous infusion, and the response of rate, pressure and contractile force was recorded. Figure 3 shows the mean dose-response curves to norepinephrine bolus injections that were obtained in one of our studies with this model (20). In the dogs with heart failure the inotropic response was blunted while the incremental response of heart rate and of blood pressure remained normal. When isoproterenol was given, a similar result was seen, i.e. there was a depressed inotropic response while rate and pressure responded normally (20). The depressed contractile response to catecholamines has also been observed using left ventricular dP/dt as the index of myocardial contractility in anesthetized dogs (25) and in conscious dogs (26) with heart failure from volume overload. Additionally, the depressed contractile response persists for up to twelve weeks after the AV fistula, which induced the heart failure, had been closed (21,26). Finally, Bristow _et al._ (27) have recently shown that papillary muscles obtained from failing human hearts exhibited depressed inotropic response to isoproterenol.

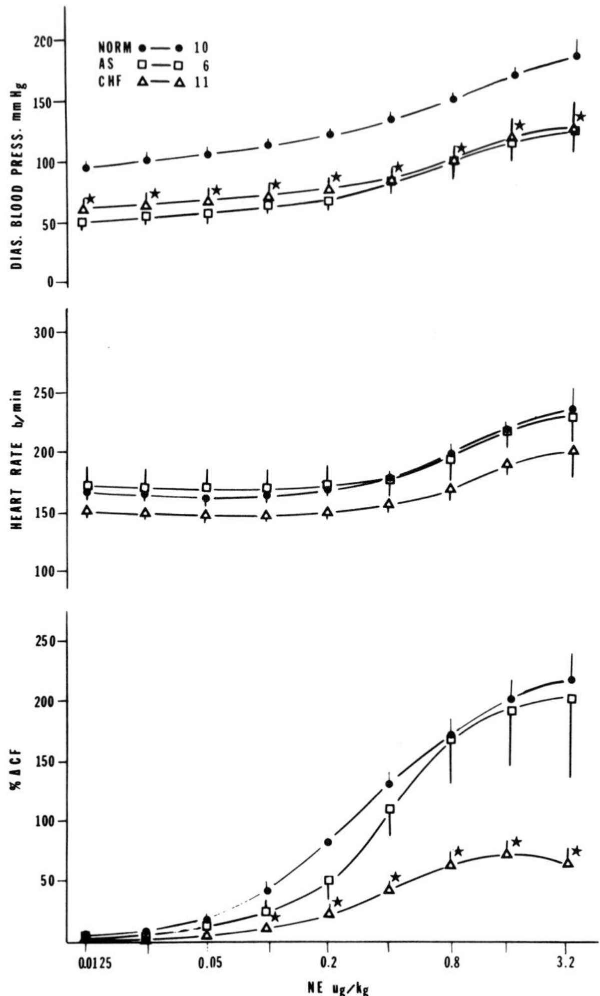

FIGURE 3. Dose-response curves of aortic blood pressure, heart rate, change in left ventricular contractile force (%ΔCF) to norepinephrine obtained from normal dogs, from dogs with heart failure (CHF) and from dogs with acute arteriovenous shunts (AS). (From Newman, W.H. Am J. Physiol. 235:H690, 1978 with permission of the American Physiological Association.)

Figure 4 shows the data for contractile force plotted in three different ways in order to illustrate the effect of a changing baseline contractile state that accompanies

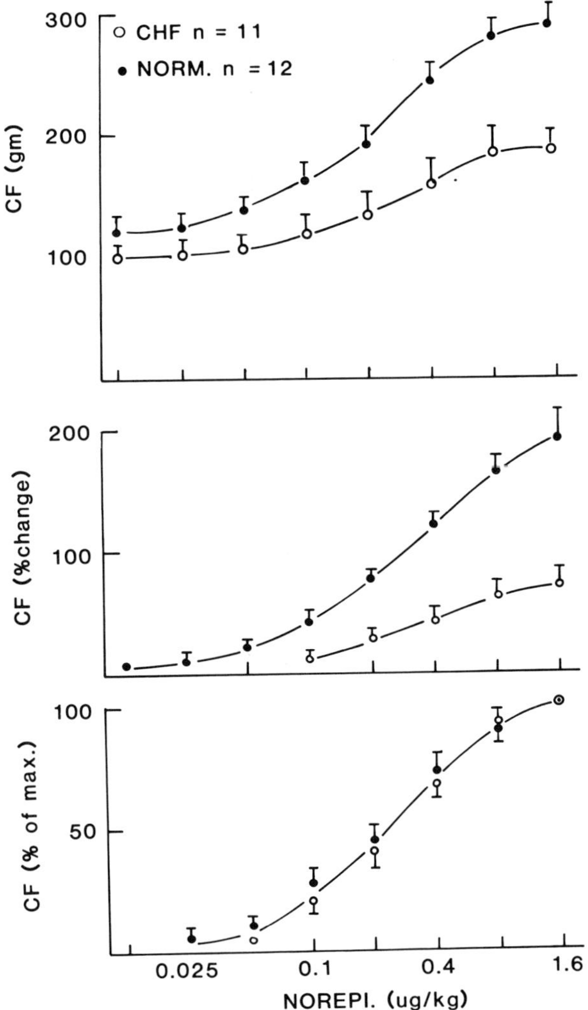

FIGURE 4. Contractile force data plotted in three different formats. See text for discussion.

heart failure on the dose-response relationships. The top panel compares the change in absolute grams of contractile force produced by norepinephrine injection in normal dogs and dogs with heart failure. The downward shift of the failure dose-response curve when compared to control does not necessarily represent a depressed inotropic responsiveness but could reflect only a depression of the basal contractile state seen in this heart failure model. Such would be the case if the downward displacement of the curve was in an entirely parallel manner. In the middle panel the response is expressed as percent change from the respective basal level of contractility in the normal and heart failure group. Expressed in such a manner the data clearly show that the shift in the contractile force curve was not in a parallel manner but that the increment of force produced by each dose of the drug was less in the failing heart than in the normal heart. For instance, in the normal heart the maximum effect of norepinephrine was a 200% increase in contractility while in heart failure this maximum effect was reduced to 75%. Plotted in this way the data indicate that the consequence of the combination of drug with receptor, i.e., a change in myocardial contractility, is depressed in the failing heart. The bottom panel shows the data from the top panel plotted as a percent of the respective maximum effect. The two curves are superimposable. If this were the only manner in which the data were examined, the conclusion might be that heart failure does not alter the contractile responsiveness to β-adrenergic agonists. The usefulness of such a plot as in the bottom panel is that it provides data concerning the affinity of the receptor for combination with agonists. In this case the plot is compatible with the idea that this model of heart failure is not associated with a change in the affinity of the cardiac β-adrenergic receptor since there was no change in ED_{50}. Indeed, estimates of β-receptor affinity obtained by radioligand binding methodology in membrane preparations obtained from failing heart muscle support the above contention (27). The point of Figure 4, then, is that dose-response curves obtained from failing hearts where the basal contractile state has changed must be carefully examined.

The response pattern of heart rate, blood pressure and contractile force in heart failure is interesting from another standpoint. Both the heart rate and contractile force responses are considered to result from activation of the cardiac β_1-adrenergic receptor. However, one response, contractile force, was depressed while the other, heart rate, remained normal in the failing state. Similarly, the increments in pressure produced by norepinephrine injection remained normal suggesting that the sympathetic α-adrenergic receptor was unchanged in heart failure. Therefore, it appears that the high circulating levels of plasma norepinephrine associated with this model did not bring about a systemic "down regulation" of the adrenergic receptors as might have been predicted. It appears, then, that heart failure may be accompanied by a reduction in the contractile response to β-adrenergic agonists while other adrenergic receptor mediated responses remain normal.

4. <u>Response of the Hypertrophied Compensated Heart to β-Adrenergic Agonists</u>.

The results presented above were obtained from animals and from man with end-stage congestive heart failure. When these experiments were done, the cardiac compensatory mechanisms were failing, and the signs of a decompensated pump were evident. The reduced contractile responsiveness to β-adrenergic stimulation could be limited to this decompensated state. Alternatively, the reduced responsiveness could occur earlier in the adaptation of the heart to chronic hemodynamic overload, i.e., when the heart is compensated and cardiac hypertrophy is present but there are no signs of cardiac pump failure. In our initial experiments we studied dogs with pressure overload cardiac hypertrophy induced by aortic constriction of sixty days duration. The dogs showed no evidence of cardiac pump failure in that there were no signs of edema, and ventricular filling pressures were normal, as were plasma norepinephrine levels and renin activity. Left ventricular mass was increased approximately fifty percent. Length-tension curves obtained from the left ventricle with a strain gauge arch were depressed, indicating that this model of pressure overload was associated with reduced basal myocardial contractile state. However, the reduced contractile state was not yet manifest in signs of cardiac pump failure. The dogs were accordingly judged to be in the compensated state (28). When either isoproterenol or norepinephrine (29) was given by intravenous injection, the associated increase in myocardial contractile state was less in the hypertrophied heart than in the normal heart (Figure 5). As seen in the dogs with heart failure (Figure 3), this blunted contractile response was not associated

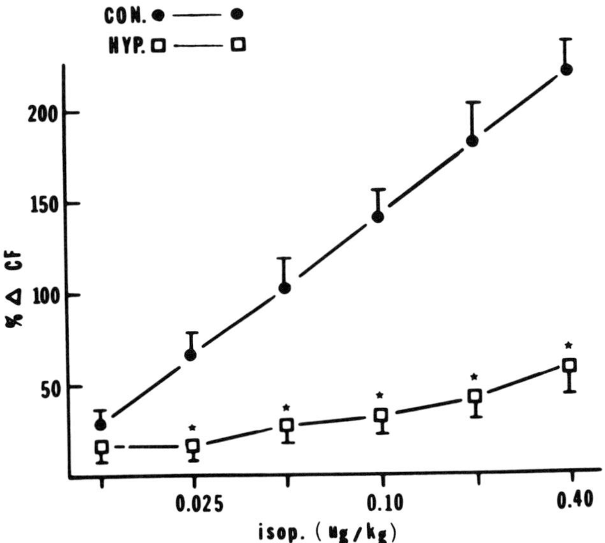

FIGURE 5. Response of left ventricular contractile force to isoproterenol in dogs in the normal state (Norm) and following the induction of pressure overload hypertrophy in these same dogs (Hyp). (From Newman, W.H. and Webb, J.G. Am. J. Physiol. 238:H134, 1980, with permission of the American PhysiologicalSociety.)

with a reduction in the response of either heart rate or blood pressure.

A similar pattern of response has been recorded from rats with cardiac hypertrophy due to two-kidney-one-clip renal hypertension (30). As shown in Figure 6, the increment in left ventricular $dP/dt/P_{40}$ obtained from the _in situ_ heart in response to graded infusion of isoproterenol was less in the hypertrophied heart than in the sham-operated controls. The increment in heart rate produced by isoproterenol was not different between the rats with renal hypertension and the shams. A reduced inotropic response

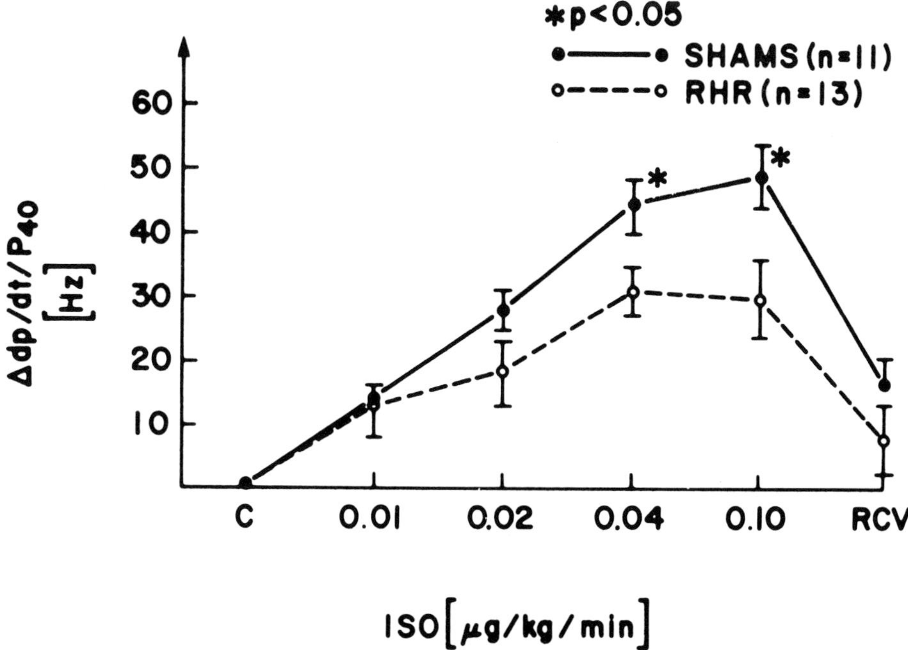

FIGURE 6. Inotropic response measured as the change in left ventricular dP/dt of the hypertrophied hearts of rats with renal hypertension and the appropriate sham controls to isoproterenol. (From Saragoca, M.A. and Tarazi, R.C. Hyperten. 3II:171; 1981 with permission of the American Heart Association Inc.)

but normal chronotropic response to isoproterenol was also seen in isolated hypertrophied hearts from rats with renal hypertension (31). On the other hand, dogs with cardiac hypertrophy from one-kidney-one-clip hypertension showed no reduced response of left ventricular dP/dt to norepinephrine infusions (32). Although these hypertensive dogs had cardiac hypertrophy, basal myocardial contractile state was normal (32). In studies of the contractile response of the hypertrophied heart of rats with spontaneous hypertension, the positive inotropic effect of isoproterenol was found to be blunted when dose-response curves were obtained from the _in situ_ heart (33). In contrast, normal dose-response curves were obtained when these hypertrophied hearts were isolated and perfused (34). Therefore, as observed for hearts in failure, it appears that the hypertrophied comp-ensated heart may also show a blunted inotropic responsive-ness to β-agonists. However, loss of this response may depend on the model studied, the timing of the study with respect to the onset of hemodynamic overload, and the basal contractile state of the heart as well as many other factors. If heart failure induced by hemodynamic overload is viewed as the end of a continuum from normal through a compensated state to failure, then studies at a single point in this time frame may not reveal this deficit in myocardial respon-siveness.

5.   Responsiveness of the Failing Heart to Glucagon.

Both the positive inotropic and positive chronotropic actions of β-agonists are thought to be the consequence of a β-adrenergic receptor mediated activation of the sarco-lemmal adenylate cyclase system. This enzyme system may be activated by mechanisms other than the β-adrenergic receptor. Glucagon, for instance, produces a positive inotropic and chronotropic event in association with an activation of the membrane adenylate cyclase system; however, the increase in contractility and heart rate as well as the activation of cyclase cannot be blocked with a β-adrenergic receptor antagonist such as propranolol. That is, glucagon probably activates adenylate cyclase through a receptor which is distinct from the β-adrenergic receptor. Studies of the contractile response of the failing heart to agents such as glucagon and β-agonists can be used to gain insight into the responsiveness of this important enzymatic pathway that is involved in adjusting the inotropic responsiveness of the myocardium.

The initial studies with glucagon in the failing heart were performed on isolated papillary muscles obtained from cats with right ventricular failure due to chronic pulmonary banding (19). Dose-response curves of tension development showed that increasing concentrations of glucagon in the muscle bath produced dose-dependent increases in contractility in normal muscle but that glucagon was without effect in the failing muscles (Figure 7). An absence of glucagon responsiveness has also been seen in studies of the contractile state of papillary muscles obtained from failing human hearts (35,36). In dogs with heart failure, increases in left ventricular contractile force produced by glucagon injections were reduced when compared to normal, although the chronotropic response was not blunted (20).

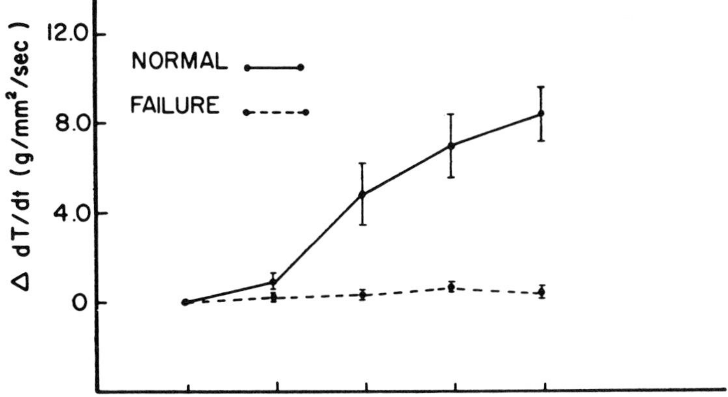

FIGURE 7.   Changes in the rate of tension development produced by glucagon in papillary muscles obtained normal cats and cats with heart failure. (From Gold, H.K., _et al_. J. Clin. Invest. 49:999, 1970 with permission of the American Society of Clinical Investigation.)

It therefore appears that positive inotropism associated with activation of the adenylate cyclase system by agents other than β-receptor agonists may also be blunted in the failing myocardium.

6.   <u>Responsiveness of the Failing Heart to Digitalis</u>.
Digitalis produces an inotropic response that is independent of activation of the adenylate cyclase system which makes it different from any of the positive inotropic agents so far discussed. In further contrast to those agents previously discussed its positive inotropic action appears to be independent of an increase in transarcolemmal calcium influx through the calcium channel that conducts the slow inward current (37-39). Digitalis may produce its inotropic effect by combining with its receptor, the sarcolemmal Na^+-K^+ATPase (40), and consequently increasing intracellular calcium through a Na^+-Ca^{2+} exchange mechanism (41). Studies with digitalis permit examination of the integrity of another pathway to increased inotropic state in the failed heart. Vatner <u>et al</u>. (42), studied conscious dogs with right heart failure from chronic tricuspid insufficiency and pulmonic stenosis and found that in the failure state the inotropic effect of ouabain was potentiated. Right ventricular dP/dt/P and myocardial segment length shortening velocity were increased to a greater extent by a 20 µg/kg dose of ouabain in the failed state than in the normal state. In our studies of either pressure overload hypertrophy or volume overload heart failure we found that the inotropic response to digitalis was unchanged from the control state (21,26). For instance in normal dogs 30 µg/kg of ouabain produced a 35 ± 5% increase in left ventricular contractile force, and when these same dogs where in failure this dose produced a 34 ± 3% increase in contractile force (21) (Figure 8). On the other hand, in these same dogs, 0.1 µg/kg of isoproterenol produced a 171 ± 6% increase in contractile force in the control state which fell to 38 ± 5% when heart failure

developed. The same type of results comparing contractile responsiveness to isoproterenol with ouabain was seen in dogs with compensated pressure overload hypertrophy (26) and has been reported in rats with cardiac hypertrophy from renal hypertension (31). Thus, in contrast to those agents which act through the adenylate cyclase system, the inotropic effect of digitalis does not appear to be reduced in the failing heart.

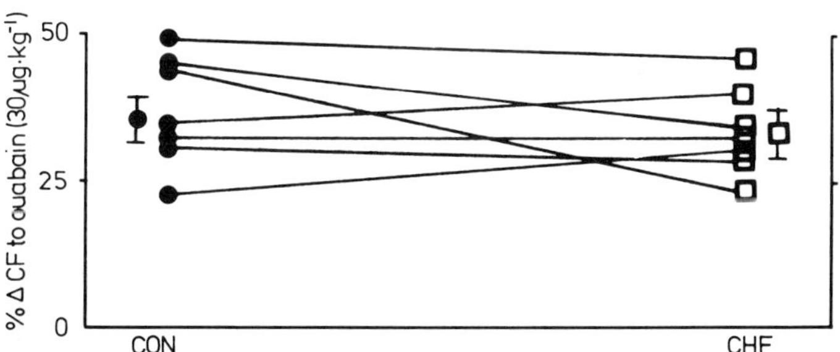

FIGURE 8. Individual response of left ventricular contractile force to ouabain in seven dogs in the control state and during heart failure (CHF). (From Newman, W.H., and Webb, J.G. Cardiovasc. Res. 14:530, 1980 with permission of the British Medical Journal.)

<u>Summary</u>:

The failing heart exhibits depressed inotropic responsiveness both to activation of the sympathetic nervous system and to direct administration of β-adenergic agonists. This blunted inotropic response does not necessarily extend to other consequences of adrenergic receptor activation such as increased heart rate or changed blood pressure. Further the loss of inotropic responsiveness to β-adrenergic agonists may not be indicative of a defect in all cellular pathways which lead to increased contractility since the inotropic response of the failing heart to digitalis is not reduced.

REFERENCES

1. Newman W, Bush ML: Evaluation of drug-induced alterations in myocardial contractility. In: Wilkerson, RD
   (ed) Cardiac pharmacology. Academic Press, New York,
   1981, pp 53-73.
2. Alousi AA, Dobreck HP: Amrinone. In: Scriabine A.
   (ed) New Drugs Annual: Cardiovascular drugs. Raven
   Press, New York, 1983, pp 259-276.
3. Braunwald E, Ross J, Sonnenblick EH: Mechanisms of
   contraction in the normal and failing heart. 2nd ed.
   Little, Brown and Co., Boston, 1976, pp 309-356.
4. Chidsey CA, Braunwald E, Morrow AG, Mason DT: Myocardial norepinephrine content in man: Effects of
   reserpine and of congestive heart failure. New Engl J
   Med (269): 653-658, 1963.
5. Chidsey CA, Braunwald E, Marrow AG: Catecholamine
   excretion and cardiac stores of norepinephrine in
   congestive heart failure. Am J Med (39): 442-451,
   1965.
6. Chidsey CA, Kaiser GA, Sonnenblick EH, Spann JF,
   Braunwald E: Cardiac norepinephrine stores in experimental heart failure in the dog. J Clin Invest (43)
   2386-2393, 1964.
7. Spann JF, Chidsey CA, Braunwald E: Reduction of
   cardiac stores of norepinephrine in experimental heart
   failure. Science (145): 1439-1441, 1964.
8. Spann JF, Buccino RA, Sonnenblick EH, Braunwald E:
   Contractile state of cardiac muscle obtained from cats
   with experimentally produced ventricular hypertrophy
   and heart failure. Circulat Res (21): 341-354, 1967.
9. Vogel JHK, Jacobowitz D, Chidsey CA: Distribution of
   norepinephrine in the failing bovine heart: Correlation of chemical analysis and fluorescence microscopy.
   Circulat Res (24): 7184, 1969.
10. Angelakos ET, Carballo LC, Daniels JB, King MP, Bajuz
    E: Adrenergic neurohumors in the hearts of hamsters
    with hereditary myopathy during cardiac hypertrophy
    and failure. IN: Bajuze and Rona A (eds) Myocardio-
    logy: Recent Advances in Studies of Cardiac Structure
    and Metabolism, Vol I, University Park Press, Baltimore,
    1972, pp 262-278.
11. Covell JW, Chidsey CA, Braunwald E: Reduction of
    cardiac response to postganglionic nerve stimulation
    in experimental heart failure. Cirulat Res (19):
    51-56, 1966.
12. Chidsey CA, Sonnenblick EH, Morrow AG, Braunwald E:
    Norepinephrine stores and contractile force of papil-
    lary muscles from the failing human heart. Circulat
    Res (33) 43-51, 1966.
13. Goldstein RE, Bieser GD, Stampfer M, Epstein SE:
    Impairment of autonomically mediated heart rate control
    in patients with cardiac dysfunction. Circulat Res
    (36): 571-578, 1975.

29. Newman WH, Ellison DM: A differential effect of ouabain and β-agonists on contractility and lactic acid production in the hypertrophied heart. Eur J Pharmacol (68): 437- 442, 1980.
30. Saragoca MA, Tarazi RC: Left ventricular hypertrophy in rats with renovascular hypertension: Alterations in cardiac function and adrenergic responses. Hypertension (3-II): 171-176, 1981.
31. Ayobe MH, Tarazi RC: Beta-receptors and contractile reserve in left ventricular hypertrophy. Hypertension (5-I): 192-197, 1983.
32. Broughton A, Konner PI: Basal and maximal inotropic state in renal hypertensive dogs with cardiac hypertrophy. Am J Physiol (245): H33-H41, 1983.
33. Saragoca M, Tarazi RC: Impaired contractile response to isoproterenol in the spontaneously hypertensive rat. Hypertension (3): 380-385, 1981.
34. Noresson E, Thoren P, Halback - Nordlander M: Performance on the hypertrophied left ventricle in spontaneously hypertensive rats. Effects of adrenergic stimulation. Acta Physiol Scand (114): 497-504, 1982.
35. Parmley WW, Chuck L, Matloff J: Diminished responsiveness of the failing human myocardium to glucagon. Cardiol (55): 211-217, 1970.
36. Goldstein RE, Skelton CL, Levey GS, Glancy DL, Beiser GD, Epstein SE: Effects of chronic heart failure on the capacity of glucagon to enhance contractility and adenyl cyclase activity of human papillary muscles. Circulat (44): 638-648, 1971.
37. McDonald TF, Nawrath H, Trautwein W: Membrane currents and tension in cat ventricular muscle with cardiac glycosides. Circulat Res (37): 674-682, 1975.
38. Josephson I, Sperelakis N: Ouabain blockade of inward slow current in cardiac muscle. J Molec Cell Cardiol (9): 409-418, 1977.
39. McCans JL, Lindenmayer GE, Munson RG, Evans RW, Schwartz A: A dissociation of positive staircase (Bowditch) from ouabain induced positive inotropism. Circulat Res (35): 439-447, 1974.
40. Schwartz A, Lindenmayer GE, Allen JC: The sodium-potassium adenosine triphosphatase: Pharmacological, physiological and biochemical aspects. Pharmacol Rev (27): 3-134, 1975.
41. Langer GA: Relationship between myocardial contractility and the effects of digitalis on ionic exchange. Fed Proc (36): 2231-2234, 1977.
42. Vatner SF, Braunwald E: Effects of chronic heart failure on the inotropic response of the right ventricle of the conscious dog to a cardiac glycoside and to tachycardia. Circulation (50): 728-734, 1974.

14. Thomas JA, Marks BH: Plasma norepinephrine in congestive heart failure. Am J Cardiol (41): 223-243, 1978.
15. Epstein SE, Braunwald E: The effects of beta adrenergic blockade on patterns of urinary sodium excretion. Studies in normal subjects and in patients with heart disease. Ann Intern Med (65): 2027, 1966.
16. Gaffney TE and Braunwald E: Importance of the adrenergic nervous system in the support of circulatory function in patients with congestive heart failure. Am J Med (34): 320-324, 1963.
17. Waagstein F, Hjalmarson A, Varnaus-Kas E, Wallentin I: Effect of chronic beta-adrenergic receptor blockade in congestive cardiomyopathy. Br Heart J (37): 1022-1036, 1975.
18. Swedberg K, Hjalmarson A, Waagstein F, Wallentin J: Beneficial effects of long-term beta blockade in congestive cardiomyopathy. Br Heart J (44): 117-133, 1980.
19. Gold HK, Prindle KH, Levey GS, Epstein SE: Effects of experimental heart failure on the capacity of glucagon to augment myocardial contractility and activate adenyl cyclase. J Clin Invest (49): 999-1006, 1970.
20. Newman WH: Volume overload heart failure: Length-tension curves, and response to β-agonists, Ca^{2+} and glucagon. Am J Physiol (235): H690-H700, 1978.
21. Newman WH, Webb JG, Privitera PJ: Persistence of myocardial failure following removal of chronic volume overload. Am J Physiol (243): H876-H883, 1982.
22. Newman WH: A depressed response of left ventricular contractile force to isoproterenol and norepinephrine in dogs with congestive heart failure. Am Heart J (93): 216-221, 1977.
23. Newman WH, Webb JG: A differential inotropic responsiveness to isoprenaline and ouabain in dogs with heart failure. Cardiovasc Res (14): 530-536, 1980.
24. Newman WH, Frankis MB, Halushka PV: Increased myocardial release of prostacyclin in dogs with heart failure. Cardiovasc Pharmacol (5): 194-201, 1983.
25. Zucker IH, Gilmore JP: Depressed cardiac response to catecholamines in dogs with chronic volume oveload. Circulat (56 III): 54, 1977.
26. Pinsky WW, Lewis RM, Hartley CJ, Entman ML: Permanent changes of ventricular contractility and compliance in chronic volume overload. Am J Physiol (237): 575-583, 1979.
27. Bristow MR, Ginsburg R, Minobe W, Cubiccotti RS, Sageman WS, Lurie W, Billingham ME, Harrison DC, Stinson EB: Decreased catecholamine sensitivity and β-adrenergic receptor density in failing human hearts. New Engl J Med (307): 205-211, 1982.
28. Newman WH, Webb JG: Adaptation of the left ventricle to chronic pressure overload: Response to inotropic drugs. Am J Physiol (238): H134-H143, 1980.

29. Newman WH, Ellison DM: A differential effect of ouabain and β-agonists on contractility and lactic acid production in the hypertrophied heart. Eur J Pharmacol (68): 437- 442, 1980.
30. Saragoca MA, Tarazi RC: Left ventricular hypertrophy in rats with renovascular hypertension: Alterations in cardiac function and adrenergic responses. Hypertension (3-II): 171-176, 1981.
31. Ayobe MH, Tarazi RC: Beta-receptors and contractile reserve in left ventricular hypertrophy. Hypertension (5-I): 192-197, 1983.
32. Broughton A, Konner PI: Basal and maximal inotropic state in renal hypertensive dogs with cardiac hypertrophy. Am J Physiol (245): H33-H41, 1983.
33. Saragoca M, Tarazi RC: Impaired contractile response to isoproterenol in the spontaneously hypertensive rat. Hypertension (3): 380-385, 1981.
34. Noresson E, Thoren P, Halback - Nordlander M: Performance on the hypertrophied left ventricle in spontaneously hypertensive rats. Effects of adrenergic stimulation. Acta Physiol Scand (114): 497-504, 1982.
35. Parmley WW, Chuck L, Matloff J: Diminished responsiveness of the failing human myocardium to glucagon. Cardiol (55): 211-217, 1970.
36. Goldstein RE, Skelton CL, Levey GS, Glancy DL, Beiser GD, Epstein SE: Effects of chronic heart failure on the capacity of glucagon to enhance contractility and adenyl cyclase activity of human papillary muscles. Circulat (44): 638-648, 1971.
37. McDonald TF, Nawrath H, Trautwein W: Membrane currents and tension in cat ventricular muscle with cardiac glycosides. Circulat Res (37): 674-682, 1975.
38. Josephson I, Sperelakis N: Ouabain blockade of inward slow current in cardiac muscle. J Molec Cell Cardiol (9): 409-418, 1977.
39. McCans JL, Lindenmayer GE, Munson RG, Evans RW, Schwartz A: A dissociation of positive staircase (Bowditch) from ouabain induced positive inotropism. Circulat Res (35): 439-447, 1974.
40. Schwartz A, Lindenmayer GE, Allen JC: The sodium-potassium adenosine triphosphatase: Pharmacological, physiological and biochemical aspects. Pharmacol Rev (27): 3-134, 1975.
41. Langer GA: Relationship between myocardial contractility and the effects of digitalis on ionic exchange. Fed Proc (36): 2231-2234, 1977.
42. Vatner SF, Braunwald E: Effects of chronic heart failure on the inotropic response of the right ventricle of the conscious dog to a cardiac glycoside and to tachycardia. Circulation (50): 728-734, 1974.

13

NEW INOTROPIC DRUGS FOR THE TREATMENT OF HEART FAILURE

RICHARD A. GOLDSTEIN

Treatment of congestive heart failure consists of to salt restriction, diuretics, digitalis glycosides and recently, vasodilators. However, reports indicate that the prognosis of heart failure is similar to that of most solid cancers (1). Oral inotropic therapy has been limited to digitalis glycosides for nearly 200 years. Nevertheless, there is still considerable controversy over the efficacy of the drug for acute and chronic failure. Several studies suggest that withdrawal of digitalis does not change the clinical status of most patients (2,3). Fleg _et al_ reported in a double blinded placebo controlled trial that oral digoxin did not increase exercise tolerance or improve left ventricular function (4). In addition, the high frequency of digitalis toxicity has prompted a search for safer, more potent agents to increase contractility. In this paper, the inotropic agents under investigation will be reviewed (Table 1).

Table 1: New Inotropic Agents

β_1 agonists:
 Prenalterol
 ICI 118, 587
 TA-064
β_2 agonists:
 Pirbuterol
 Salbutamol
Bipyridines:
 Amrinone
 Milrinone
Benzimidazoles:
 Sulmazol (ARL 115 BS)

HEMODYNAMIC EFFECTS OF INOTROPIC AGENTS

In general, contractility is decreased in end stage heart failure.
The etiology of this abnormality is still unknown but appears to be
related to a disturbance in the availability of calcium to myofibrillar
proteins. Another potential factor is depletion of endogenous
myocardial catecholamines that make the heart less responsive to
adrenergic stimulation. An ideal inotropic agent would restore
contractility to normal both at rest and during exercise without
adverse effects on the peripheral circulation.

Figure 1 is a schematic representation of the effects that a
selective inotropic agent could have on perfusion, edema and pulmonary
congestion.

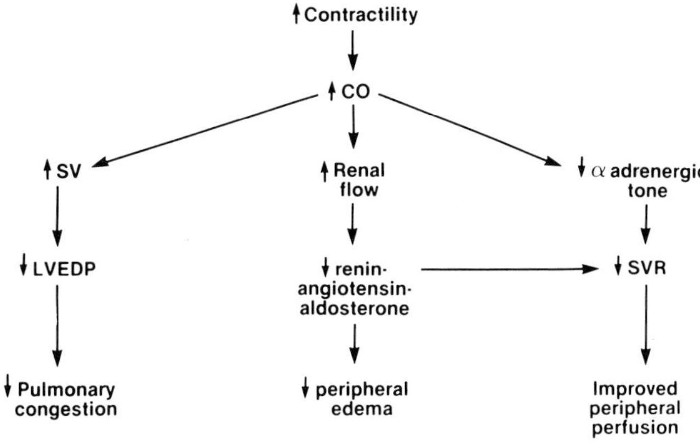

Figure 1: Clinical Effects of a Selective Inotropic Agent
SV = Stroke volume, LVEDP = left ventricular end-
diastolic pressure, CO = cardiac output and SVR =
systemic vascular resistance. The small arrows
indicate an increase (↑) or decrease (↓) in the
parameter.

The effect of inotropic drugs on oxygen supply and demand need to be considered since many patients with heart failure have co-existant coronary artery disease. If cardiac output is restored to normal, systemic vascular resistance (afterload) and left ventricular filling pressure (preload) are reduced. These changes would decrease oxygen demand. A decrease in left ventricular filling pressure would also increase coronary perfusion pressure which is approximated by the difference between diastolic arterial pressure and left ventricular end diastolic pressure. In contrast, an increased contractile state would be expected to increase oxygen demand but this change is usually accompanied by a proportional increase in coronary flow.

SPECIAL CONSIDERATIONS IN THE EVALUATION OF NEW INOTROPIC AGENTS

The development of new drugs for heart failure generally starts with limited animal toxicity and efficacy studies followed by dose ranging in normal volunteers based on non-invasive measurements. The next phase of studies are done in patients with refractory heart failure. Patients with symptoms refractory to conventional treatment have a mortality of close to 90% during the first two months from reaching that status and virtually all patients are dead within a year (5). This disease state in addition to its poor prognosis is associated with serious ventricular ectopy, anorexia, nausea, hepatic congestion, hypotension, and dizziness. Therefore interpretations of side effects related to these drugs may be inaccurate unless an adequate pre-drug observation period was obtained since very few of these studies have control groups.

Investigators and clinicians often have unreasonable expectations for therapy in this seriously ill population. Whereas resting hemodynamics may be improved, exercise intolerance and symptoms may persist. Since chronic heart failure is an end stage of heart disease, therapy is directed to prolonging life, improving the quality of life and minimizing the risk of associated events rather than at reversal of the underlying pathophysiology. However, as of this writing, no agent has been found that achieves these goals.

Most of the studies to be discussed in this paper were done with small groups of patients who were studied for short periods of time.

Objective data is restricted primarily to hemodynamic observations at rest and/or exercise tolerance based on time to fatigue or oxygen uptake. Changes in these parameters have not been shown to improve longevity or productivity in these patients. Other problems with these studies are listed in Table 2. Recently, several double blinded long term studies have been initiated which should help define the role of these drugs for heart failure.

Table 2:   Problems with assessment of new inotropic agents

1. Small number of patients in studies
2. Short study durations
3. Severity of illness
4. Adequate absorption?
5. Poor objective end points to assess the quality of life
6. Disease progression
7. Cause of death (Electrical or pump failure)
8. Uncertain FDA requirements for demonstrating efficacy and safety

MECHANISM OF ACTION OF INOTROPIC AGENTS

A feature common to all inotropic agents is an increase in calcium availability to cardiac myofibrils. Digoxin exerts its inotropic effect by inhibition of the Na-K ATPase pump. The increased intracellular sodium resulting from this inhibition exchanges for extracellular calcium by a Na-Ca transport system. Digoxin is rather limited in this capacity since its narrow toxic-therapeutic ratio prohibits significant adjustments in dose.

The catecholamines bind to β_1 receptors which increase intracellular cAMP via adenyl cyclase (6). The mechanism by which cAMP influences contractility is unclear although it appears to increase calcium binding, increase calcium entry through the slow calcium channel and facilitate the release and uptake of calcium by the sarcoplasmic reticulum. The latter effect may improve left ventricular compliance and thus decrease pulmonary congestion. There have also been agents developed which act primarily on β_2 receptors and produce a decreased afterload by peripheral arterial vasodilation(7). These drugs have been classified as inotropes since they also appear to stimulate β_1 receptors. Tuttle, while at Lilly laboratories, set out to synthesize a catecholamine with selective inotropic effects such that tachycardia, arrhythmias, and alterations in vascular resistance would not occur(8). The resultant compound, dobutamine, approved for use in 1978 by the FDA, offered several advantages over other catecholamines used for heart failure since its arrhythmogenicity is low compared to other catecholamines. It affects both peripheral α and β_2 receptors with a slightly dominant β_2 effect that favors vasodilatation. In clinical studies, the drug was capable of increasing cardiac output from 25-50% and produced decreases in left ventricular filling pressure and systemic vascular resistance (9,10). Most studies have reported a 5-10% increase in heart rate and minimal effects on arterial pressure. Its short half-life (2 minutes) makes it a useful agent for patients with low cardiac output and elevated left ventricular filling pressure. Studies comparing it to digoxin showed a 33% increase in cardiac index with dobutamine versus 9% with digoxin (11). In patients with acute myocardial infarction and failure, no changes in infarct size or the incidence of arrythmias occurred (12). Similarly, pulmonary venous congestion and systemic resistance were decreased by dobutamine but not digoxin (11). However, it is only available as an intravenous drug and there may be tolerance to its effects within 48 hours due to down regulation of beta receptors.

Figure 2 illustrates the chemical structures of the new inotropic agents. Prenalterol is the most studied of the new β_1 agonists. However, the pharmaceutical company sponsoring its development has withdrawn the drug from further studies. Similarly, pirbuterol, a β_2 agonist, has been withdrawn from investigation by its sponsor because of a higher incidence of death in comparison with a reference population of patients with heart failure. Although neither of these drugs were optimal agents, many investigators feel that their demise as a potential therapy for heart failure may have been premature.

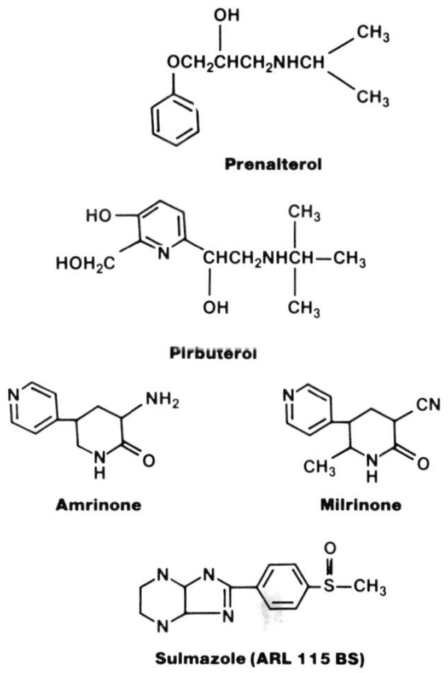

Figure 2:   Chemical structure of new inotropic drugs

Amrinone and milrinone are bipyridine derivatives that appear to
work primarily by inhibiting phosphodiesterase activity and thus
elevate cyclic AMP indirectly (13). There is still some question in
the literature about whether this is the primary inotropic effect of
the drug since there is a report of disparity in the sequence of cAMP
elevation and increased calcium flux (14). It is clear that these
drugs do not affect beta receptors or the Na-K ATPase pump and thus
represent a unique class of drugs.

Sulmazol (ARL115BS) is under clinical investigation in Europe.
Its principal mechanism of action is also believed to be inhibition of
phosphodiesterase and thus its actions may be related to elevation of

cAMP (15). A recent study indicated that in membrane free preparations, it increases the affinity of myofibrils for calcium which may contribute to its effect (16).

CLINICAL EFFECTS OF NEW INOTROPIC AGENTS

In the remainder of this paper, clinical studies using these drugs will be reviewed. The preliminary studies involved in dose ranging of most of these agents was done in normal volunteers whose absorption of oral derivatives would be expected to be higher than in patients with severe heart failure. There is a paucity of information about blood levels of drugs after intravenous or oral administration and thus the effect of a given dose may vary considerably. Additional information about the animal and clinical pharmacokinetics are often sequestered in files within the pharmaceutical industry and thus unavailable to the author.

Table 3 is an overview of the newer inotropic drugs that have been studied most extensively. The plus and minus signs each represent a report of a 10% increase or decrease respectively in the literature. Since the optimal doses of these drugs are not established, some effects may be underestimated.

Table 3: Relative effects of inotropic agents

	Prenalterol*	Pirbuterol*	ARL115BS	Amrinone	Milrinone
CI	+ +	+ + +	+ +/+ + +	+ + +	+ + + +
SVR	−	− − −	− −	− − −	− − −
PCW	−	−	− −	− −	− −
HR	+ +	+	+	0	0
AP	0	0/−	−	0	0
Tolerance	?	yes	?	No	No
Side effects	palpitations, arm pulsations	palpitation, nausea, tremor arrythmias	?	Thrombocytopenia (∿11%) Nausea, anorexia, ?hepatocellular toxicity (1-2%)	

* − withdrawn from investigation by sponsor

Prenalterol

Prenalterol, a β_1 agonist, is effective intravenously and orally. It significantly increases cardiac output and decreases left ventricular filling pressure while slightly increasing heart rate (17, 18). Arterial pressure is not effected. Intravenously it has been administered as a single bolus of 75-225 µg/kg or as a series boluses. The effects are seen within 10 minutes and the drug has a 2 hour half-life after intravenous administration. Eighty-five percent is excerted as a sulphate conjungate with the remainder excreted unchanged. In Sweden, the drug has been used to reverse the deleterious effects of beta blocking agents in patients with acute myocardial infarction. Preliminary studies have not shown significant effects on myocardial oxygen consumption with hemodynamically effective doses (17). Oral therapy is given as 10-100 mg every 8 hours with a bioavailability of approximately 45%. Most studies have reported increases in cardiac output of about 25% (17).

Pirbuterol

Oral pirbuterol, a β_2 agonist, has been administered as a 20-30 mg dose every 8 hours (19, 20). Its peak effect is seen in 2-5 hours and it has a half-life of 2.7 hours. The agent increases cardiac output by approximately 35% and is associated with a 10-20% decrease in pulmonary capillary wedge pressure. However, Colucci reported tolerance to the hemodynamic effects of the drug within one month and an increased frequency of ventricular arrythmias (21). Investigation of this drug has been abandoned as of this writing.

Amrinone

Amrinone has been studied extensively over the last five years. It is effective in both intravenous and oral forms. Most studies demonstrate improved hemodynamics including increased cardiac output and decreased systemic vascular resistance and left ventricular filling pressure (22-24). The pharmacokinetics are shown below in Table 4.

Table 4: Amrinone pharmacokinetics

	Dose	IV
Dose	75-300	10-30
	mg every 8 hrs	µg/kg/min
Onset of Action	30-60 min	5 min
Peak Effect	1-3 hr	10 min
Half Life	5 hr	30-40 min
Duration of Action	4-8 hr	2 hr

Several investigators have reported significant increases in exercise tolerance after oral amrinone. For example, in patients with severe heart failure, exercise capacity increased from 5.9 minutes to 11.5 minutes. Cardiac output increased by 50% and LVFP decreased by 20% (25). The effects on hemodynamics and exercise performance were maintained after 6-8 weeks and withdrawal of drug resulted in symptomatic and hemodynamic deterioration at rest. Similarly, Weber reported significant improvement in aerobic exercise performance that was maintained at restudy four weeks into therapy (26).

The side effects of the drug have been previously outlined in this paper but deserve additional comment. Leier recently suggested that there was a significant number of serious side effects in patients receiving 100 mg every 8 hours (27). The major side effects including a transient "viral-like" illness and increased ectopy at rest and during exercise. We have just completed a study of the electrophysiologic and hemodynamic effects of amrinone in 15 patients with heart failure. Holter monitoring was done for 24-48 hours prior to and after initiation of amrinone (off other cardio-active drugs) (28). Electrophysiologic and right heart catheterizations were performed. Patients were then maintained on oral therapy in doses of 75-200 mg three times daily and monitored electrocardiographically for up to 48 hours. We found that atrial effective refractory period was shortened and 1:1 maximal AV node conduction was enhanced after intravenous administration of amrinone sufficient to increase cardiac output by 30%, decrease left ventricular filling pressure by $\geq$5mm Hg or a maximal dose of 20µg/kg/min was given. There was a high prevalance of ventricular ectopy in our patients before drug, but ventricular

effective refractory period and inducibility of ventricular tachycardia
were not affected. On oral therapy there was no significant changes in
the frequency of extrasystoles or ventricular tachycardia.

Several important questions remain about the utility of oral
amrinone especially in light of the high incidence of thrombocytopemia.
A multicenter long term double blinded placebo controlled trial is
ongoing that should resolve questions about the effect on longevity,
quality of life and significance of side effects. The intravenous form
has been given preliminary approval by the FDA.

Milrinone

Milrinone is a derivative of amrinone. It is about 20 times as
potent as amrinone and treatment to date has not demonstrated the
thrombocytopenia associated with amrinone. The oral form of the drug
peaks at one hour and its effects last 4 hours. The half-life has been
estimated at 1½ hours.

Baim recently reported a group of 20 patients treated with
intravenous and oral milrinone (29). Intravenous drug was given as a
bolus of 25μg/kg followed by one or two additional boluses of 50μg/kg.
Cardiac index increased by 50% and left ventricular filling pressure
decreased by 33%. The hemodynamic effect was maintained for 24 hours
by a continuous infusion of 1 μg/kg/min. Subsequently, patients were
started on oral milrinone in doses of 5-7.5 mg every 4 hours while
awake. Ten patients were followed for more than six months and had
maintained hemodynamic efficacy as measured by radionuclide ejection
fraction and NYHA clinical class improved from 3.4 to 2.6.
Mechanistically, its inotropic effects were confirmed by demonstrating
a significant increase in dP/dt.

Maskin et al reported improved maximal oxygen uptake after four
weeks of oral milrinone therapy from 9.0 to 11.6 ml/kg/min. Withdrawal
of drug in this study and that of Sinoway et al was associated with
deterioration of symptoms that was reversed when therapy was
re-started (30, 31).

This drug appears to be the most promising of the agents
investigated so far. Few side effects have been reported and include
headaches in one patient and transient hypotension. Additional data is

necessary to further demonstrate its safety and efficacy prior to approval for routine use.

Sulmazol (ARL115BS)

Sulmazol has been studied primarily in Europe for the last few years. Thormann et al have studied the effects of a 2-3 mg/kg intravenous bolus. The drug's peak effect occur 10-15 minutes after intravenous therapy and lasted for at least 25 minutes (32). Cardiac output rose by 30% and pulmonary capillary wedge pressure fell by 30%. In patients with coronary artery disease, myocardial oxygen consumption was increased by 33% but was accompanied by an increase in coronary sinus flow of 39%. There was no clinical or metabolic evidence of induction of ischemia in these patients during drug administration.

Sulmazol has also been studied in oral doses of 200mg given every eight hours (33). The onset of action was determined by changes in ejection fraction measured by echocardiography. An effect was seen at 40-60 minutes that was maximal by 120 minutes. Patients were followed for four days and continued efficacy was apparent. Studies are still ongoing with this drug in both intravenous and oral forms.

SUMMARY

The long term treatment of heart failure with inotropic agents has been limited to digitalis glycosides. Several new agents have been shown to improve cardiac output by 25-50% in contrast to 7-15% with digoxin. The drugs all appear to decrease pulmonary congestion - a clinical parameter that digitalis does not consistently affect. Further studies conducted with appropriate controls are required to define the role and efficacy of these drugs.

ACKNOWLEDGEMENTS

Richard A. Goldstein, M.D. is an Assistant Professor of Medicine at the University of Texas Medical School and Graduate School of Biomedical Sciences, Houston, TX. This work is funded in part through an NIH New Investigator Research Award and a grant from the American Heart Association - Texas Affiliate. The author wishes to thank Jeanette Upshaw for preparing the manuscript.

221

REFERENCES

1. Franciosa JA, Wilen M, Ziesche S, Cohn JN: Survival in men with severe chronic left ventricular failure due to either coronary heart disease or diopathic dilated cardiomyopathy. Am J Cardiol (51): 831-836, 1983.
2. Hull SM, Mackintosh A: Discontinuation of maintenance digoxin therapy in general practice. Lancet (II): 1054-1055, 1977.
3. Dobbs SM, Kenyon WI, Dobbs RJ: Maintenance digoxin after an episode of heart failure: placebo-controlled trial in outpatients. Br Med J (1): 749-752, 1977.
4. Fleg JL, Gottlieb SH, Lakatta EG: Is digoxin really important in treatment of compensated heart failure? A placebo-controlled crossover study in patients with sinus rhythm. Amer J Med (73): 244-250, 1982.
5. Jamieson SW, Oyer PE, Bieber CP, Stinson EB, Shumway NE: Transplantation for cardiomyopathy: A review of the results. Heart Transplantation (2): 28-31, 1982.
6. Osnes JB, Skomedol T, Oye I: On the role of cyclic nucleotides in the heart muscle contraction and relaxation. Prog Pharmacol (4): 47-62, 1980.
7. Dawson JR, Bayliss J, Norell MS, Canepa-Anson R, Kuan P, Reuben S, Poole-Wilson PA, Sutton GC: Clinical studies with beta$_2$ adrenoceptor agonists in heart failure. Eur Heart J (3, Suppl D): 135-141, 1982.
8. Tuttle RR, Mills J: Dobutamine: Development of a new catecholamine to selectively increase cardiac contractility. Circ Res (36): 185-196, 1975.
9. Leier CV, Heban PT, Huss P, Bush CA, Lewis RP: Comparative systemic and regional hemodynamic effects of dopamine and dobutamine in patients with cardiomyopathic heart failure. Circ (58): 466-475, 1978.
10. Mikulic E, Cohn, JN, Franciosa JA: Comparative hemodynamic effects of inotropic and vasodilator drugs in severe heart failure. Circ (56): 528-533, 1977.
11. Goldstein RA, Passamani ER, Roberts R: A comparison of digoxin and dobutamine in patients with acute infarction and cardiac failure. N Engl J Med (803): 846-850, 1980.
12. Gillespie TA, Ambos HD, Sobel BE, Roberts R: Effects of dobutamine in patients with acute myocardial infarction. Am J Cardiol (39): 588-594, 1975.
13. Honerjäger P, Schäfer-Korting M, Reiter M: Involvement of cyclic AMP in the direct inotropic action of amrinone. Biochemical and functional evidence. Naunyn-Schmiedebergs Arch Pharmacol (318): 112-120, 1981.
14. Alousi AA, Farah AE, Lesher GY, Opalka CJ: Cardiotonic activity of amrinone Win 40680 (5-amino-3,4'-bipyridin-6(1H)-one). Circ Res (45): 666-677, 1979.
15. Dahmen M, Greeff K: Analysis of the positive-inotropic activity of the benzimidazole derivate AR-L 115 BS in isolated guinea pig atria. Arzeini-Forsch (Drug Res) (31): 161-165, 1981.
16. Solaro RJ, Rüegg: Stimulation of Ca^{++} binding and ATPase activity of dog cardiac myofibrils by AR-L 115BS, a novel cardiotonic agent. Circ Res (51): 290-294, 1982.

17. Hjalmarson A, Abelardo N, Waagstein E: Effects of prenalterol in congestive heart failure. Eur Heart J (3) (Suppl D): 115-121, 1982.
18. Kirlin PC, Pitt B: Hemodynamic effects of intravenous prenalterol in severe heart failure. Am J Cardiol (47): 670-675, 1981.
19. Canepa-Anson R, Dawson JR, Frankl WS, Kuan P, Sutton GC, Reuben S, Poole-Wilson PA: Beta$_2$ adrenoceptor agonists. Pharmacology, metabolic effects and arrhythmias. Eur Heart J (3) (Suppl D): 129-134, 1982.
20. Awan NA, Evenson MK, Needham KE, Evans TO, Hermanovich J, Taylor CR, Amsterdam E, Mason DT: Hemodynamic effects of oral pirbuterol in chronic severe congestive heart failure. Circ (63): 96-101, 1981.
21. Colucci WS, Alexander W, Mudge GH, Rude R, Holman BL, Wynne J, Grossman W, Braunwald E: Acute and chronic effects of pirbuterol on left ventricular ejection fraction and clinical status in severe congestive heart failure. Am Heart J (102): 564-568, 1981.
22. Benotti JR, Grossman W, Braunwald E, Davolos DD, Alousi AA: Hemodynamic assessment of amrinone. A new inotropic agent. N Eng J Med (299): 1373-1377, 1978.
23. LeJemtel TH, Keung E, Sonnenblick EH, Ribner HS, Matsumoto M, David R, Schwartz W, Alousi AA, Davolos D: Amrinone: A new non-glycosidic, Non-adrenergic cardiotonic agent effective in the treatment of intractable myocardial failure in man. Circ (59): 1098-1104, 1979.
24. Siskind SJ, Sonnenblick EH, Forman R, Scheuer J, LeJemtel TH: Acute substantial benefit of inotropic therapy with amrinone on exercise hemodynamics and metabolism in severe congestive heart failure. Circ (64): 966-973, 1981.
25. Maskin CS, Forman R, Klein NA, Sonnenblick EH, LeJemtel TH: Long-term amrinone therapy in patients with severe heart failure. Drug-dependent hemodynamic benefits despite progression of the disease. Am J Med (72): 113-118, 1982.
26. Weber KT, Andrews V, Janicki JS, Wilson JR, Fishman AP: Amrinone and exercise performance in patients with chronic heart failure. Am J Cardiol (48): 164-168, 1981.
27. Leier CV, Dalpiaz K, Huss P, Hermiller JB, Magorien RD, Bashore TM, Unverferth DV: Amrinone therapy for congestive heart failure in outpatients with idiopathic dilated cardiomyopahy. Am J Cardiol (52): 304-308, 1983.
28. Naccarelli GV, Gray EL, Dougherty AH, Hanna JF, Goldstein RA: Amrinone: Electrophysiologic effects. Circ (68) (Suppl III): III-128, 1983.
29. Baim DS, McDowell AV, Cherniles J, Monrad ES, Parker JA, Edelson J, Braunwald E, Grossman W: Evaluation of a new bipyridine inotropic agent-milrinone-in patients with severe congestive heart failure/ N Engl J Med (309): 748-756, 1983.
30. Maskin CS, Sinoway L, Chadwick B, Sonnenblick EH, LeJemtel TH: Sustained hemodynamic and cllinical effects of a new cardiotonic agent, WIN 47203, in patients with severe congestive heart failure. Circ (67): 1065-1070.
31. Sinoway LS, Maskin CS, Chadwick B, Forman R, Sonnenblick EH, LeJemtel TH: Long-term therapy with a new cardiotonic agent, WIN 47203: Drug-dependent improvement in cardiac performance and

progression of underlying disease. JACC (2): 327-331, 1983.
32. Thormann J, Kramer W, Schlepper M: Hemodynamic and myocardial energetic changes induced by the new cardiotonic agent, AR-L 115, in patients with coronary artery disease. Am Heart J (104): 1294-1302, 1982.
33. Thormann J, Kramer W, Schlepper M, Gottwick M: AR-L115BS in the treatment of heart failure. Eur Heart J (3) (Suppl D): 87-95, 1982.

14

TRANSITION TO CARDIAC FAILURE IN SPONTANEOUSLY HYPERTENSIVE
RATS.

J.M. PFEFFER and M.A. PFEFFER

1.   INTRODUCTION

In response to the chronic imposition of a pressure overload, the heart increases the number of its contractile units
and the amount of its connective tissue. This parallel
increase of myocardial fibers permits the ventricle to develop
the augmented tension required to eject blood against an
increased resistance while maintaining the stress of the
individual fibers within normal limits. Despite this initial
compensatory phase in which ventricular performance is sustained, overt cardiac decompensation may supervene in the
face of an unrelenting pressure overload in spite of further
increases in cardiac mass. In our previous studies of the
female spontaneously hypertensive rat (SHR), we observed a
compensated phase in which forward output was sustained from
a moderately hypertrophied left ventricle and a decompensated
phase in which forward output was markedly reduced despite
left ventricular dilatation and further hypertrophic growth
(1,2,3,4). The present study was undertaken to identify
those aspects of cardiac performance which might define more
clearly the transition phase to cardiac failure in the SHR.

2.   METHODS

Hemodynamic studies were performed on female SHR and
normotensive Wistar rats (NWR) at 6,12,18, and 24 months of
age. The basic surgical preparation has been described in
detail previously and is presented here in brief (2,4,5).
Following induction of anesthesia with ether, a tracheostomy
was performed and ventilation and anesthesia then were maintained by a positive pressure respirator connected in series

to an ether drip apparatus. Catheters were placed in the
right carotid artery and jugular vein for continuous monitoring
of systemic arterial and right atrial pressures, respectively,
and into the left femoral vein for infusions. A mid-sternal
thoracotomy exposed the ascending aorta around which an
electromagnetic flow probe (2.0 or 2.5 mm i.d.) was placed
for continuous measurement of mean ascending aortic blood
flow (cardiac output less coronary blood flow). Calculations
of total peripheral resistance were obtained by dividing the
difference between mean arterial and right atrial pressures
by cardiac output. Baseline hemodynamic measurements were
obtained every two minutes over a stable ten minute period,
then averaged.

To assess the maximal pumping capacity of the left
ventricle, Tyrode's solution was infused at a rate of 40 ml/
min/kg for 45 seconds, during which time cardiac output
increased to, then was sustained at a maximal level despite
further elevations of right atrial pressure. Calculations
of maximal stroke work were obtained by multiplying stroke
volume (cardiac output divided by heart rate) times mean
arterial pressure times a conversion factor of 0.0136 and of
maximal minute work by multiplying stroke work by heart rate.
Following return of all hemodynamic variables to baseline
levels, the flow probe was removed and the arterial catheter
advanced into the left ventricle for continuous monitoring of
phasic pressures. To determine the maximal pressure generating
capacity of the left ventricle, the ascending aorta was briefly
(1 second) occluded by a previously placed suture and developed
pressure was calculated (peak systolic minus end-diastolic
pressure).

The heart was excised following arrest with KCl, separated
into right ventricle and left ventricle plus septum, and these
components were weighed separately.

3.   RESULTS

Table 1. The body weight of the SHR was significantly
less than that of NWR from 6 to 18 months of age, but this
difference in weight no longer existed at 24 months of age.

Ventricular weights and blood flow variables were indexed for body weight because of the difference between strains. The right ventricular weight to body weight ratio of the SHR increased with age such that this ratio was increased in 24 month old SHR (P < 0.01) compared to 6 month old SHR as well as compared to 24 month old NWR. The right ventricular weight to body weight ratio of the NWR remained constant with age. The ratio of left ventricular weight to body weight of SHR was always significantly greater than that of NWR and increased with age to the extent that it was 75 percent greater than that of NWR at 24 months of age. This ratio in the NWR was unchanged from 6 to 18 months of age, but increased thereafter to a significant (P < 0.025) value at 24 months compared to 6 months of age.

Table 1. Body and Ventricular Weights of Female Normotensive and Spontaneously Hypertensive Rats.

	6 months	12 months	18 months	24 months
n				
NWR	5	6	9	13
SHR	9	12	13	9
BW(g)				
NWR	300 ± 6	295 ± 17	269 ± 8	258 ± 5
SHR	$220 \pm 3^{\ddagger}$	$248 \pm 4^{\dagger}$	$249 \pm 4^{*}$	256 ± 8
RV(mg)				
NWR	147 ± 7	176 ± 11	184 ± 7	188 ± 7
SHR	147 ± 8	196 ± 16	195 ± 7	$232 \pm 8^{\ddagger}$
LV(mg)				
NWR	649 ± 17	655 ± 41	621 ± 17	643 ± 16
SHR	709 ± 27	$846 \pm 16^{\ddagger}$	$1019 \pm 26^{\ddagger}$	$1116 \pm 48^{\ddagger}$
RV/W(mg/g)				
NWR	0.49 ± 0.03	0.61 ± 0.04	0.68 ± 0.03	0.70 ± 0.03
SHR	$0.68 \pm 0.04^{*}$	0.79 ± 0.06	$0.78 \pm 0.03^{*}$	$0.90 \pm 0.03^{\ddagger}$
LV/W(mg/g)				
NWR	2.18 ± 0.11	2.22 ± 0.07	2.32 ± 0.07	2.50 ± 0.06
SHR	$3.21 \pm 0.11^{\ddagger}$	$3.42 \pm 0.07^{\ddagger}$	$4.10 \pm 0.13^{\ddagger}$	$4.37 \pm 0.20^{\ddagger}$

Results are expressed as mean $\pm$ S.E.M. $^{*}P < 0.05$, $^{\dagger}P < 0.01$ $^{\ddagger}P < 0.001$, SHR compared to age-matched NWR.
n, sample size; BW, body weight; RV, right ventricular weight; LV, left ventricular weight.

Table 2. The mean arterial pressure of the SHR was considerably elevated compared to that of NWR until 24 months of age, by which time the blood pressure of the SHR had dropped to a level comparable to that of age-matched NWR. The heart rate of the SHR and NWR was unchanged with age (except for a slower heart rate in the 6 month old NWR) and was not different between strains at each age (except for a faster heart rate in 6 month old SHR compared to age-matched NWR). The cardiac and stroke volume indices of the SHR remained constant from 6 to 18 months of age and were not different from those of NWR during this time period. However, by 24 months of age, the forward output of the SHR was markedly reduced ($P < 0.01$) not only compared to 6 month old SHR, but also compared to 24 month old NWR. Total peripheral resistance index did not change with age in either SHR or NWR, but significant elevations in vascular resistance occurred in SHR at 12 and 18 months of age compared to age-matched NWR.

Figures 1 and 2. The absolute maximal stroke volume (Figure 1) and cardiac output (Figure 2) ejected by the SHR during a volume loading were unchanged from 6 to 18 months of age and also were not different from those of age-matched NWR. However, by 24 months of age these indices of cardiac flow reserve capacity were depressed in 24 month old SHR compared to 6 month old SHR ($P < 0.05$ for cardiac output, but not for stroke volume) and to age-matched NWR ($P < 0.001$). On the other hand, when maximal stroke volume and cardiac output were expressed in relation to left ventricular weight, a reduction ($P < 0.01$) in these flow indices occurred at an earlier age in SHR: at 18 months instead of at 24 months as observed for absolute values of maximal flow. Both the absolute and relative (to left ventricular weight) values of maximal stroke volume and cardiac output did not change from 6 to 24 months of age in NWR.

Table 2. Post-thoracotomy Baseline Hemodynamics of Female Normotensive and Spontaneously Hypertensive Rats.

	6 months	12 months	18 months	24 months
MAP(mmHg)				
NWR	108 ± 3	97 ± 7	96 ± 3	98 ± 6
SHR	$127 \pm 6^{*}$	$142 \pm 5^{\ddagger}$	$119 \pm 6^{\dagger}$	94 ± 11
HR(beats/min)				
NWR	362 ± 9	398 ± 17	408 ± 9	400 ± 8
SHR	$417 \pm 9^{\dagger}$	402 ± 13	396 ± 13	388 ± 13
CI(ml/min/kg)				
NWR	212 ± 14	244 ± 26	257 ± 18	252 ± 20
SHR	307 ± 37	267 ± 14	263 ± 19	$175 \pm 9^{\dagger}$
SI(ml/kg)				
NWR	0.59 ± 0.05	0.64 ± 0.05	0.63 ± 0.06	0.62 ± 0.04
SHR	0.73 ± 0.08	0.66 ± 0.03	0.66 ± 0.04	$0.46 \pm 0.03^{\dagger}$
TPRI[**]				
NWR	0.51 ± 0.03	0.42 ± 0.05	0.38 ± 0.03	0.40 ± 0.04
SHR	0.47 ± 0.06	$0.54 \pm 0.03^{*}$	$0.46 \pm 0.02^{*}$	0.54 ± 0.08

Results are expressed as mean $\pm$ S.E.M. *$P < 0.05$, [†]$P < 0.01$, [‡]$P < 0.001$, SHR compared to age-matched NWR.
MAP, mean arterial pressure; HR, heart rate; CI, cardiac index; SI, stroke volume index; TPRI**, total peripheral resistance index ($mmHg \cdot ml^{-1}/min \cdot kg^{-1}$).

<u>Figures 3 and 4.</u> The absolute stroke and minute work performed by the SHR from 6 to 18 months of age was equal to or greater ($P < 0.01$) than that of age-matched NWR, but by 24 months of age the work output of the SHR was less than that of 6 month old SHR ($P < 0.001$) and of age-matched NWR ($P < 0.001$). When maximal stroke and minute work were expressed in relation to left ventricular weight, these variables for the 6 and 12 month old SHR were similar in value to those for age-matched NWR. However, work output per gram of left ventricle was markedly reduced at 18 and 24 months of age in SHR compared to both 6 month old SHR ($P < 0.01$ and $P < 0.001$, respectively) and to age-matched NWR ($P < 0.01$ and $P < 0.001$, respectively).

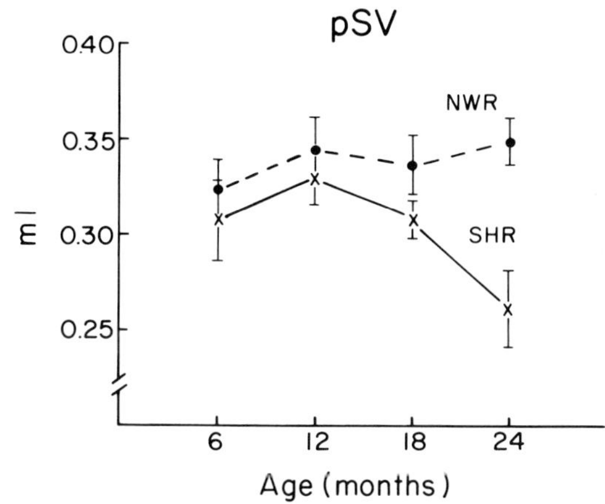

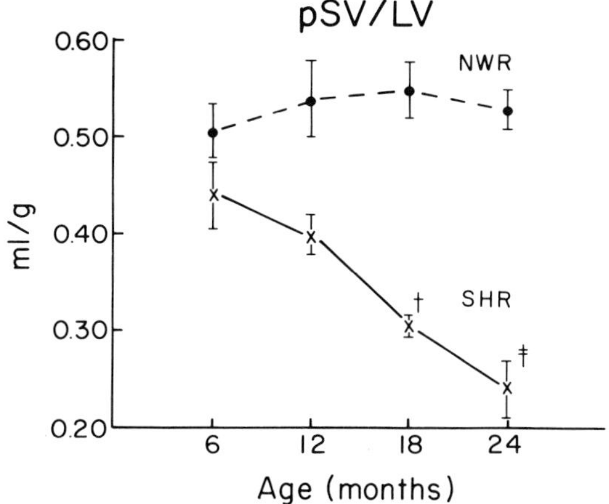

FIGURE 1. The absolute (upper panel) and relative to left ventricular weight (lower panel) maximal stroke volume attained during a volume loading with Tyrode's solution in female SHR and NWR at 6,12,18, and 24 months of age.

Figure 5. The SHR developed greater (P < 0.001) pressures than did the NWR during aortic occlusion at 6(290±7 vs 223±7 mmHg, respectively), 12(283±6 vs 226±8 mmHg, respectively), and 18(296±7 vs 233±5 mmHg, respectively) months of age, but by 24 months of age the SHR was no longer capable of generating greater pressures than the NWR (260+11 vs 246+5 mmHg, respectively). When the relationship between developed pressure and the ratio of left ventricular weight to body weight was determined, a significant association between these two variables occurred if the 24 month old SHR were excluded: Dev P= 152 mmHg + 37 LV/W, r= 0.81, P < 0.001. As can be seen in Figure 5, three of the nine 24 month old SHR fell within the normal relation of pressure and left ventricular weight, whereas the remainder fell downward and to the right of the relation.

4.   DISCUSSION

The process by which the heart adjusts to a continuous stress and which eventuates in an increased mass was described by Meerson as a continuous progression of three stages (6). The first stage is characterized by an augmented force of contraction developed per unit of myocardial mass (stage of increased hyperfunction). At this point, the total force developed is more than adequate to meet the increased demand. With progression to the second stage the number of myocardial contractile units increases so that the total force developed by the heart is increased, but the force developed per contractile unit apparently remains normal (stage of stable hyperfunction). Meerson termed the third stage one of "gradual exhaustion" in which the ability of each contractile unit is decreased, even though total force development might be normal or decreased. By the end of this stage, the myocardium eventually is no longer able to meet the demands placed upon it and cardiac failure supervenes.

One of the important etiologic factors in the development of congestive heart failure is systemic hypertension. During sixteen years of observation in the Framingham Study, 75 percent of the new cases of congestive heart failure had antecedent hypertension, many of which did not have prior myocardial infarction or clinical evidence of coronary artery disease (7). The documentation of the transition from the compensated to the decompensated phases of cardiac hypertrophy in patients with systemic arterial hypertension is most difficult since investigative evaluation usually is not undertaken until clinical symptoms of cardiovascular abnormalities are readily apparent. Nonetheless, in echocardiographic (8-11) and cardiac catheterization (12,13) studies of patients with systemic hypertension and ventricular hypertrophy, phases of both compensated and depressed cardiac performance have been observed.

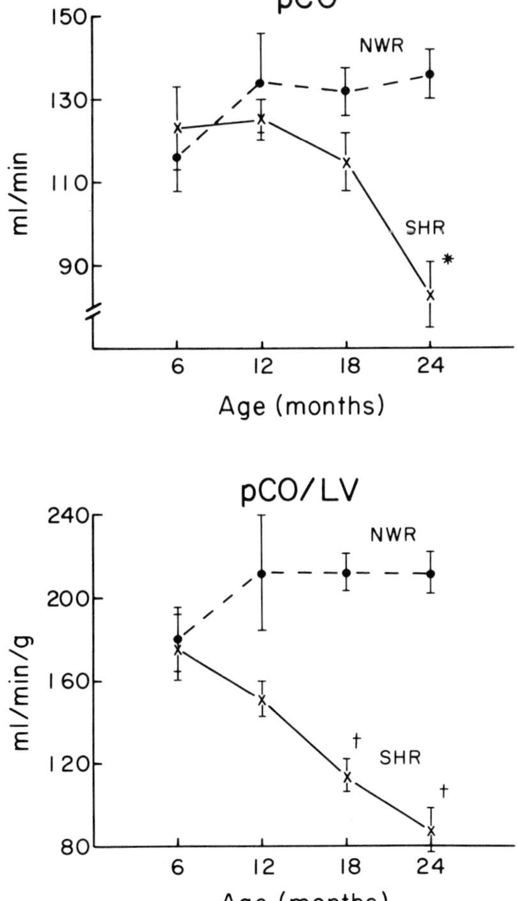

FIGURE 2. The absolute (upper panel) and relative to left ventricular weight (lower panel) maximal cardiac output attained during a volume loading with Tyrode's solution in female SHR and NWR at 6,12,18, and 24 months of age.

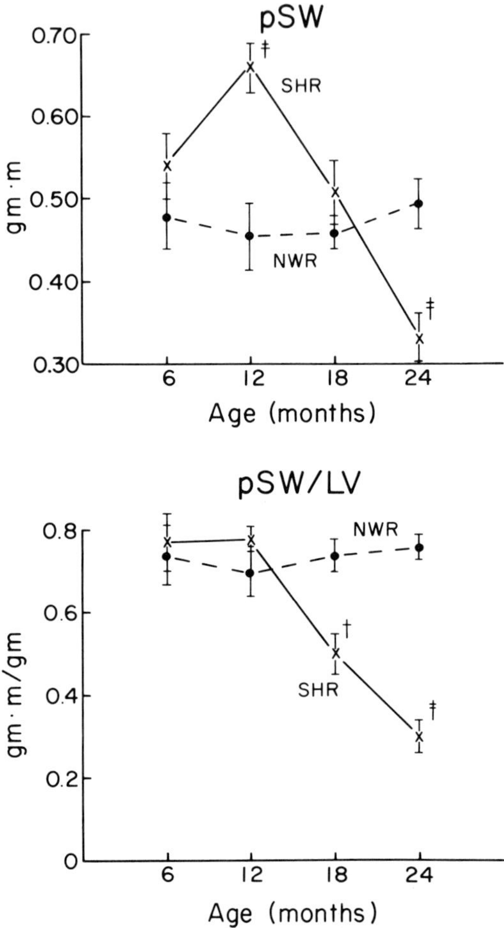

FIGURE 3. The absolute (upper panel) and relative to left ventricular weight (lower panel) maximal external stroke work attained during a volume loading with Tyrode's solution in female SHR and NWR at 6,12,18, and 24 months of age.

In an animal model of genetic hypertension, the SHR, we have identified both a stable phase of moderate ventricular hypertrophy, in which cardiac performance is maintained, and a phase of severe left ventricular hypertrophy, in which ventricular dysfunction is marked (1-5,14,15). In these studies, cardiac performance was assessed under baseline and stressed (volume loading to obtain maximal stroke volume and cardiac output) conditions. A reduction in the baseline and maximal forward output of female SHR was consistently observed at 24 months of age, but not earlier - at 18 months of age. On the other hand, a depression in myocardial contractile state, as assessed by the ejection fraction index - afterload relation, was observed by Mirsky et al. in 18 month old female SHR, a depression that was even more pronounced in 24 month old female SHR (16).

To more fully define the transition to cardiac failure in the SHR, we related the maximal forward output and external work generated during a volume loading procedure to left ventricular mass. In current unpublished studies of male Wistar rats with streptozotocin-induced diabetes or experimentally-produced arterio-venous fistulae, we have observed a phase of compensation in which forward output is normal or increased and myocardial contractiltiy is relatively preserved (as assessed by the ejection fraction-afterload relation). Although the diabetic rats were quite different in body and ventricular weights compared to their age-matched controls, their maximal stroke volumes in relation to left ventricular weight were similar in value: controls, 0.47±0.02 ml/g and diabetics, 0.47±0.04 ml/g. Comparable values of maximal stroke volume per gram of left ventricle (0.45±0.03 ml/g) also were observed in shunted rats despite a 46 percent (0.877 and 1.28 g, controls and shunted rats, respectively) increase in left ventricular weight. In the present study, the relation of maximal stroke volume and ventricular weight in female rats was similar to that of the above mentioned male rats over a wide range of ages (0.50 to 0.55 ml/g from 6 to 24 months of age).

Because the addition of cardiac mass in a concentric form of left ventricular hypertrophy should permit the development of more total force even though force per contractile unit remains normal (Meerson's second stage), we examined the relationship between the maximal pressure developed during an aortic occlusion and the ratio of left ventricular weight to body weight (Figure 5). Only in the 24 month old SHR, in which baseline systemic arterial pressures and forward output were reduced, was there a lack of association between maximal force development and cardiac mass. Our previous observations of a modest depression in myocardial contractility in 18 month old female SHR (16) suggests that maximal pressure generating capacity thus may not be a sensitive enough indicator for the initial phase of cardiac failure.

In compensated pressure overload states, forward output is maintained in the face of the hemodynamic burden imposed. Thus, we examined the relation of external stroke and minute work, which incorporate both flow and pressure generating abilities, to left ventricular weight. At 6 and 12 months of age, the forward output of female SHR was similar to that of age-matched NWR and systemic arterial pressure was higher such that maximal external work was similar to or greater than that of NWR. This increased work output was in relation to the increase in cardiac mass - the maximal stroke and minute work per gram of left ventricle of 6 and 12 month old SHR were similar to those of age-matched NWR. By 18 months of age, however, a further increase in cardiac mass did not further augment external work capacity despite a maintenance of forward output and pressure generating capacity. Absolute stroke and minute work were similar to those of age-matched NWR but, when related to left ventricular weight, were considerably reduced compared to 18 month old NWR. In 24 month old SHR, in which both pumping and pressure generating capacities were impaired, work output was markedly reduced.

In summary, in the SHR with long standing hypertension, a phase is reached in which the further addition of myocardial contractile units no longer maintains an augmented work capacity. This depression in the relation between work output and left ventricular mass occurs at a time when a modest depression in myocardial contractility is observed and thus may be an important hemodynamic variable which heralds the early onset of cardiac failure.

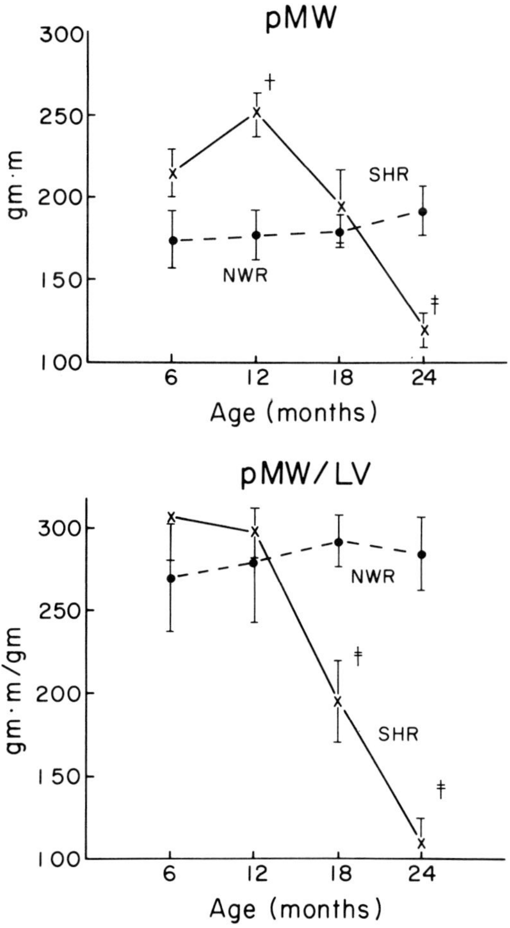

FIGURE 4. The absolute (upper panel) and relative to left ventricular weight (lower panel) maximal external minute work attained during a volume loading with Tyrode's solution in female SHR and NWR at 6,12,18, and 24 months of age.

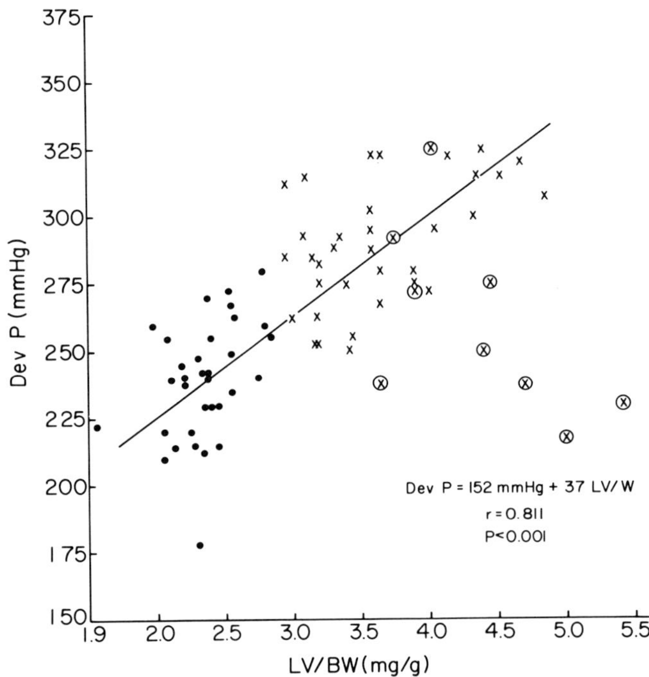

FIGURE 5. The relationship between maximal pressure developed during aortic occlusion and the ratio of left ventricular weight to body weight of female SHR (X) and NWR (●) at 6,12, 18, and 24 (excluding SHR) months of age. The 24 month old SHR are depicted as ⊗.

REFERENCES

1. Pfeffer JM, Pfeffer MA, Fletcher P, Braunwald E: Alterations of cardiac performance in rats with established spontaneous hypertension. Am J Cardiol (44): 994-998, 1979.
2. Pfeffer JM, Pfeffer MA, Fletcher P, Fishbein MC, Braunwald E: Favorable effects of therapy on cardiac performance in

spontaneously hypertensive rats. Am J Physiol (242): 776-784, 1982.
3. Pfeffer JM, Pfeffer MA, Mirsky I, Braunwald E: Regression of left ventricular hypertrophy and prevention of left ventricular dysfunction by captopril in the spontaneously hypertensive rat. Proc Natl Acad Sci (79): 3310-3314, 1982.
4. Pfeffer JM, Pfeffer MA, Braunwald E: Development of left ventricular dysfunction in the female spontaneously hypertensive rat. In: Alpert NA (ed) Perspectives in cardiovascular research. Myocardial hypertrophy and failure. Raven Press, New York, 1983, pp 73-84.
5. Pfeffer MA, Pfeffer JM, Frohlich ED: Pumping ability of the hypertrophying left ventricle of the spontaneously hypertensive rat. Circ Res (38): 423-429, 1976.
6. Meerson FZ: A mechanism of hypertrophy and wear of the myocardium. Am J Cardiol (15): 755-760, 1965.
7. Kannel WB: Role of blood pressure in cardiovascular morbidity and mortality. Prog Cardiovasc Dis (27): 5-24, 1974.
8. Dunn FG, Chandraratna P, de Carvalho JGR, Basta LL, Frohlich ED: Pathophysiologic assessment of hypertensive heart disease with echocardiography. Am J Cardiol (39): 789-795, 1977.
9. Karliner JS, Williams D, Gorwit J, Crawford MH, O'Rourke RA: Left ventricular performance in patients with left ventricular hypertrophy caused by systemic arterial hypertension. Br Heart J (39): 1239-1245, 1977.
10. Savage DD, Drayer JIM, Henry WL, Mathews EC, Ware JH, Gardin JM, Cohen ER, Epstein SE, Laragh JH: Echocardiographic assessment of cardiac anatomy and function in hypertensive subjects. Circulation (59): 623-632, 1979.
11. Takahashi M, Sasayama S, Kawai C, Koturi H: Contractile performance of the hypertrophied ventricle in patients with systemic hypertension. Circulation (62): 116-126, 1980.
12. Strauer BE: Ventricular function and coronary hemodynamics in hypertensive heart disease. Am J Cardiol (44): 999-1006, 1979.
13. Nichols AB, Sciacca RR, Weiss MB, Blood DK, Brennan DL, Cannon PJ: Effect of left ventricular hypertrophy on myocardial blood flow and ventricular performance in systemic hypertension. Circulation (62): 329-340, 1980.
14 Pfeffer JM, Pfeffer MA, Fishbein MC, Frohlich ED: Cardiac function and morphology with aging in the spontaneously hypertensive rat. Am J Physiol (237): H461-468, 1979.
15. Pfeffer JM, Pfeffer MA, Fletcher P, Braunwald E: Impaired cardiac performance in rats with long-term spontaneous hypertension. In: Strauer BE (ed) The heart in hypertension. Springer-Verlag, Berlin, 1981, pp 389-398.
16. Mirsky I, Pfeffer JM, Pfeffer MA, Braunwald E: The contractile state as the major determinant in the evolution of left ventricular dysfunction in the spontaneously hypertensive rat. Circ Res (53): 767-778, 1983.

ACKNOWLEDGMENTS

Supported in part by a grant #HL 28238 from the NHLBI of the National Institutes of Health. Dr. J. Pfeffer is the recipient of a Research Career Development Award #HL 01186 from the NHLBI of the National Institutes of Health. Dr. M. Pfeffer is the recipient of an Established Investigatorship of the American Heart Association.

15

EXERCISE AND PRESSURE-OVERLOAD INDUCED HYPERTROPHY IN DOG

H. LOWELL STONE AND LOUIS A. SORDAHL

INTRODUCTION

It has long been recognized that various forms of exercise can lead
to cardiac enlargement (1,2). What is not known, is whether all cardiac
enlargement is deleterious or if a state of "physiologic" enlargement can
exist that is fundamentally different from that associated with pathologic
enlargement (3). Cardiac enlargement occurs in response to a variety of
stimuli (Fig. 1). Myocardial hypertrophy associated with pathological
enlargement has been shown to be altered by imposition of exercise training (4) which suggests that differences exist in the responses to physiologic
and pathologic load (Fig. 1). Cardiac enlargement due to exercise training

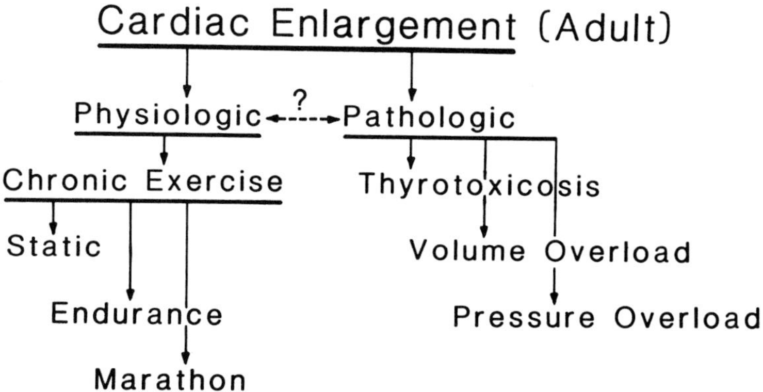

FIGURE 1. Various stimuli resulting in cardiac enlargement.

A. CARDIAC ENLARGEMENT-PHYSIOLOGIC

    1. Increase in Ventricular Mass (7-20%)
    2. Increase in End-Diastolic Volume (End. and Mar.)
    3. Altered Neural Reflexes
    4. Biochemical Changes Small (Except Swimming Rat)
        a. Altered Ca^{++} Movement
        b. Mitochondrial Membrane Changed
        c. Slight Change in S.R.
        d. No Change in Mitochondrial Enzymes
        e. No Change in Contractile Proteins

B. CARDIAC ENLARGEMENT-PATHOLOGIC
    (Pressure Overload)

    1. Increase in Ventricular Mass (up to 100%)
    2. Small or No increase in End-Diastolic Volume
    3. Altered Neural Reflexes
    4. Biochemical Changes can be Large
        a. Altered Ca^{++} Movement
        b. Mitochondrial Alterations
        c. Change in Contractile Proteins
    5. Can Lead to Failure

FIGURE 2. (A) Characteristics of cardiac enlargement in response to exercise training. (B) Characteristics of cardiac enlargement to pressure-overload.

(Fig. 2A) can be characterized by increases in ventricular mass of up to 20% over control with significantly increased end-diastolic volume (endurance and marathon). In contrast, enlargement associated with pressure-overload (Fig. 2B) is characterized by increases in ventricular mass of up to 100% with little or no increases in end-diastolic volume. Altered neural reflexes are associated with both physiologic and pathologic enlargement (Fig. 2), but these changes are not well understood and significant qualitative and quantitative differences may exist between the two types of hypertrophy. Changes in myocardial biochemistry following exercise training by treadmill running have not been dramatic while large changes have been observed in pressure-overload hypertrophy (Fig. 2). Perhaps one of the most significant features that contrasts these two types of myocardial enlargement is the development of contractile failure in pressure-overload hypertrophy (Fig. 2B). Myocardial failure, of course, represents an end point in the response to pressure-overload hypertrophy. To determine if significant differences exist between physiologic (exercise training) and pathologic (pressure-overload) myocardial enlargement, the appropriate approach is to make comparisons at a point where similar degrees of cardiac enlargement exist. A comparative study was therefore undertaken to determine if significant differences could be found between hearts similarly enlarged by either physiologic (exercise training) or pathologic (pressure-overload) stimuli.

METHODS

Mongrel dogs were surgically instrumented under sterile, aseptic conditions (5). Briefly, a Doppler flowprobe was placed around the left circumflex coronary artery, a Konigsberg pressure transducer inserted into the left ventricle via a stab incision at the apex and indwelling catheters placed in the left atria and coronary sinus in order to determine myocardial oxygen consumption. A hydraulic occluder was placed on the ascending aorta in order to produce pressure-overload to the heart during the experimental studies. All leads were exteriorized on the neck and the animals allowed three weeks recovery from surgery prior to any experimental interventions.

The experimental protocol was as follows: 1) each animal was subjected to a submaximal exercise test by treadmill running (5) without the aortic occluder inflated. Heart rate, left ventricular pressure (mmHg), dP/dt (mmHg per sec), coronary blood flow (cm per sec) and myocardial oxygen consumption (ml O_2 per min) were determined during the treadmill test. This constituted the Control (C, ●-●) experiments; 2) the following day the hydraulic occluder on the ascending aorta was inflated to produce an elevation in left ventricular systolic pressure of 40 mmHg and the animal again subjected to the treadmill test. This is the Control-Occluded (C-O; O-O) data; 3) the aortic occlusion was then chronically maintained at

40 mmHg elevation in LV systolic pressure for two weeks. At the end of this time, the treadmill test was again performed with the aortic occlusion still applied, Occluded-Occluded (O-O; Δ-Δ) and a day later with the aortic occlusion released, Occluded-Control (O-C; ▲-▲) data. The animals were then sacrificed and the left ventricular mass determined gravimetrically. Left ventricular tissue samples were taken for studies of mitochondria from these hearts. Mitochondria were isolated and respiratory and calcium transport activities determined by previously published techniques (6). Left ventricular tissue from normal or sham-operated animals served as control for the mitochondrial studies. It should be noted that each animal served as its' own control in these studies.

RESULTS AND DISCUSSION

Table 1 shows the increases in left ventricular weight in the pressure-overloaded dog (LVH) compared to control data (Normal). The increases in left ventricular weight following exercise (Excercise T) are taken from the data of Wyatt and Mitchell (7). Significant increases are seen in both experimental groups compared to the appropriate control. The percentage increase in LV weight was comparable between the two groups, but the percentage of LV mass divided by body weight was larger in the LVH group.

Table 1. Body weights and left ventricular weights in normal, exercise trained, and LVH dogs.

	Normal Dogs (n=9)	Exercise T. (n=7)	LVH (n=6)
Body Weight (kg)	18.7±0.4	13-25	17.4±0.8
Left Ventricle + Septum Weight (gms)	82±2	91±8[+] (9%)	94±7[+] (15%)
LV+S/BW (gms/kg)	4.42±0.12	4.8±0.3[+] (7%)	5.38±0.33[+] (22%)

[+]P<0.05 compared to appropriate control data
Exercise T data from Wyatt and Mitchell (Ref. 7).

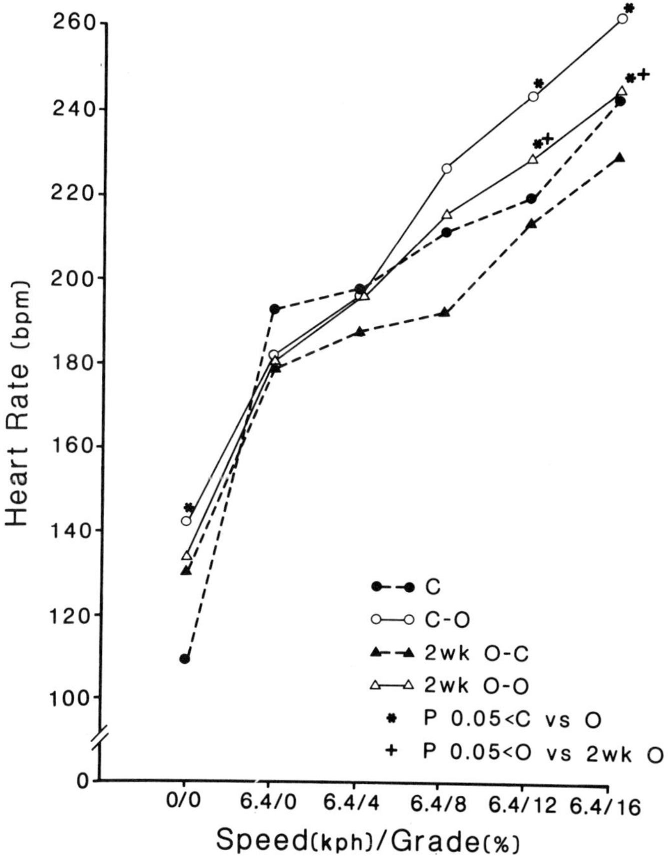

FIGURE 3. Heart rate responses of control and hypertrophic dog hearts
to treadmill running with and without partial aortic occlusion applied.
C, closed circles, control; C-O, open circles, control with aortic
occlusion; O-C, closed triangles, chronically overloaded heart after two
weeks of occlusion with occlusion removed; O-O, open triangles, chronically
overloaded heart after two weeks with occlusion still applied. See Methods
for further details.

However, it should be pointed out that this degree of increase in heart

weight to body weight ratio was relatively small compared to the maximum

values that have been reported.

Fig. 3 shows the heart rate responses to treadmill running before

(C and C-O, circles) and after two weeks of chronically imposed pressure-overload (O-C and O-O, triangles). At the higher work loads (Fig. 3; 6.4/12 to 6.4/16) the control with aortic occlusion imposed (open circles) exhibits a significant elevation in heart rate compared to the control without an acute pressure overload (closed circles). After two weeks of pressure-overload, a significantly higher heart rate is seen in the animals with the aortic occlusion still in place (open triangles) compared to the animals in which the aortic occlusion has been removed (closed triangles). What was more striking was that after two weeks of chronic overload, and with the aortic occlusion still imposed (open triangles), a significant decrease in heart rate was found compared to the initially occluded control (open circles). This suggests that the small enlargement (Table 1; LVH) in left ventricular mass resulted in a reflex alteration in the control of heart rate. The reduction in heart rate from acute to chronic pressure-overload seen are similar in magnitude to those observed in exercise trained dogs following 8 to 10 weeks of training (5). However, the heart rate response to exercise in this study (Fig. 3) was evoked in only two weeks of pressure-overload. This raises the interesting question of the relationship between myocardial mass and the control of heart rate during exercise.

Fig. 4 indicates that expected differences in left ventricular systolic pressure are seen between hearts with aortic occlusion (open symbols) compared during treadmill running to the same hearts without the load imposed (closed symbols). More importantly, are the unconnected open and closed circles at the bottom of Fig. 4 showing no changes in left ventricular end diastolic pressure in either circumstance. The fact that no changes in LVEDP are occurring indicates that myocardial function was not compromise

Fig. 5 shows that no changes occurred in dP/dt regardless of the state of the heart or the additional load placed on it during exercise. This indicates that after two weeks of pressure-overload and a 20% increase in

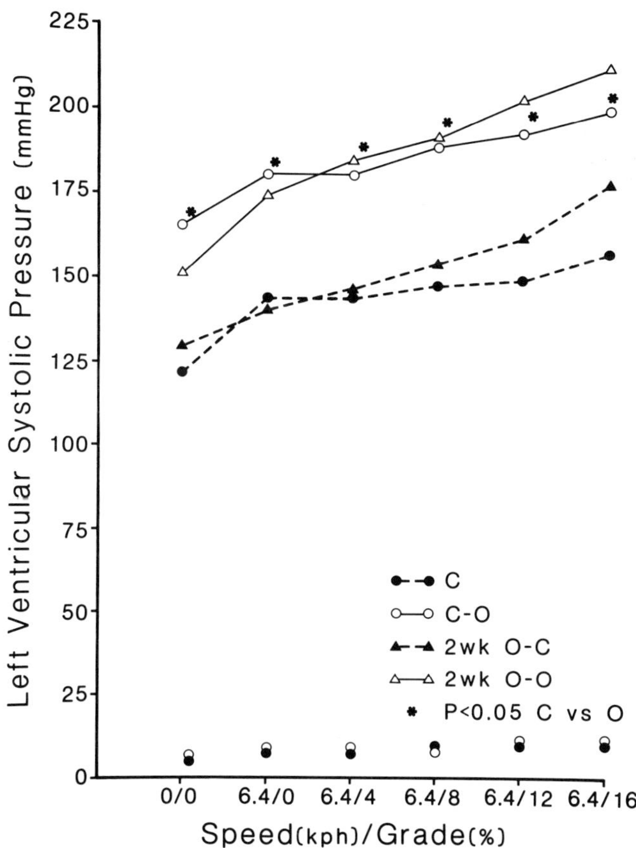

FIGURE 4. LV systolic pressures of control and hypertrophic dog hearts during treadmill running. Connected symbols same as Fig. 3. Unconnected circles at bottom indicate no changes in LV end-diastolic pressure before (open circles) or after two weeks of chronic pressure overload (closed circles).

left ventricular mass (Table 1, LVH), no apparent alteration in myocardial contractility was detectable during exercise (Fig. 5). Previous studies (5) measuring dP/dt max in exercise trained hearts revealed a significant increase in contractility after the exercise trained state was achieved (8-10 weeks). The lack of changes in dP/dt max seen in Fig. 5 should be contrasted with Fig. 3 which suggests that increased ventricular mass can

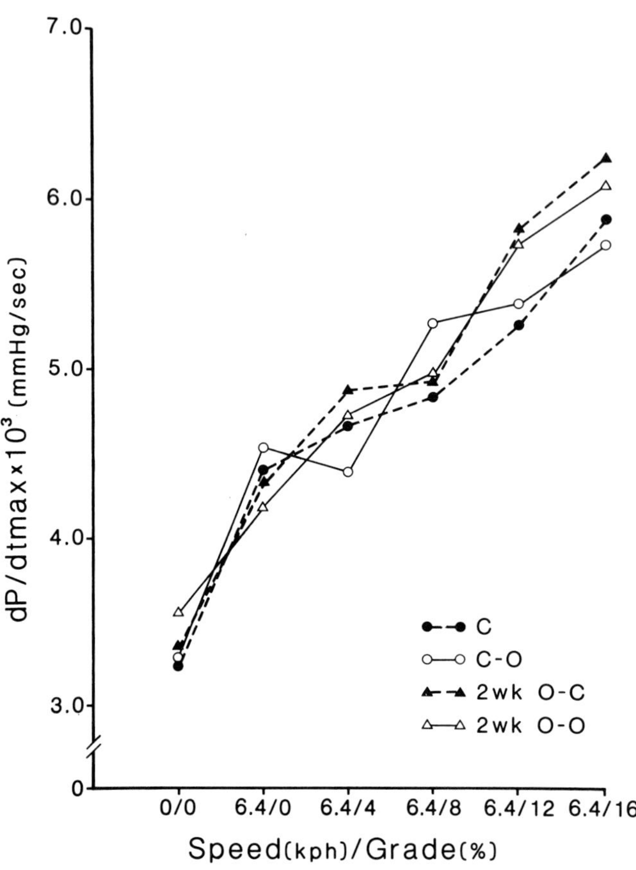

FIGURE 5. Measurements of dP/dt max during treadmill running. Symbols same as Fig. 3.

affect reflex control of heart rate. However, the data in Fig. 5 and previous observations in the exercise trained heart (5) indicate that increase in mass per se is not responsible for an increase in the contractile properties of the exercise trained heart. These differences might be explained by differential synthesis of myosin isoenzymes as reported by Scheuer, et al. (4) or could be due to alterations in intracellular calcium metabolism following exercise training (6). At present, these possibilities are only

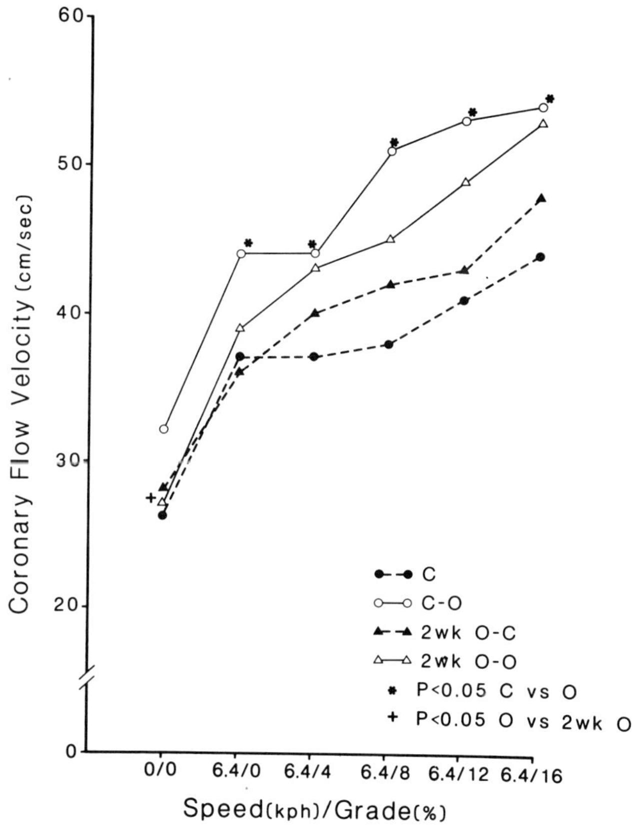

FIGURE 6.   Coronary flows during treadmill running.   Symbols same as Fig. 3.

speculative, but offer avenues for further research effort.

Significant increases in coronary blood flow were observed in initial controls with aortic occlusion (Fig. 6; open circles) compared to the controls without aortic occlusion (Fig. 6; closed circles).   The initial acute systolic pressure elevation produces the marked rise in coronary blood flow seen in the occluded controls (Fig. 6; open circles).   However, after two weeks of pressure-overload no differences in coronary blood flow was seen with (Fig. 6; open triangles) or without the aortic occlusion

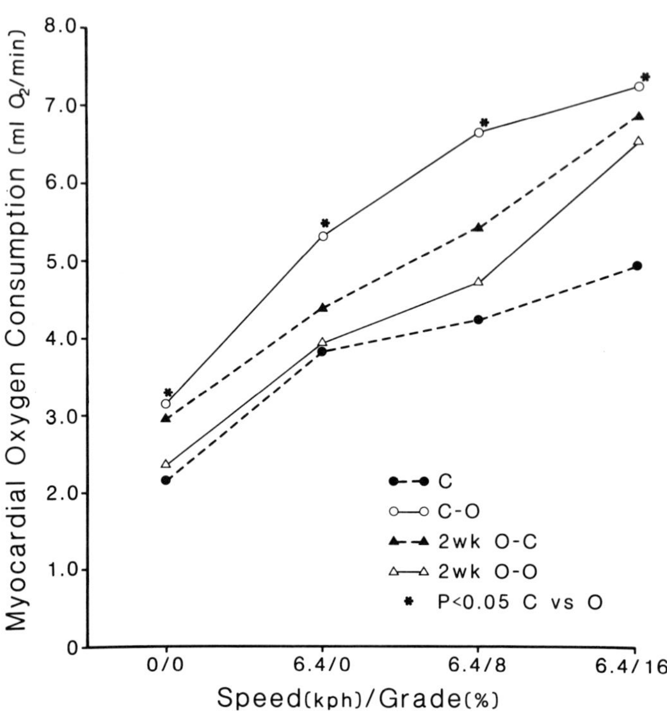

FIGURE 7. Myocardial oxygen consumption during treadmill running. Symbols same as Fig. 3.

imposed (Fig. 6; closed triangles). Fig. 6 also shows that at rest a significant difference (+) in coronary blood flow existed between the two week pressure-overloaded heart (open triangles) and the control (open circles with the aortic occlusion imposed. No differences were seen in the control (closed circles) and two week pressure-overloaded heart (closed triangles) when the aortic occlusion was not in place. Similar results were obtained in exercise trained dogs (5).

Expected increases in myocardial oxygen consumption were seen, at rest and during exercise, in control with aortic occlusion (Fig. 7; open circles) compared to the initial controls without occlusion imposed (Fig. 7; closed circles). However, these differences disappear following two weeks of systolic pressure-overload (Fig. 7; open and closed triangles). The data in Fig. 7 are consistent with the measurements of coronary blood flow (Fig. 6) where no significant increases in flow were observed following two weeks of pressure-overload with or without the aortic occlusion imposed (Fig. 6; open and closed triangles). The lack of a difference after two weeks of pressure-overload probably reflects the normalization of wall tension to the increased pressure load and the decrease in exercise heart rate (Fig. 3).

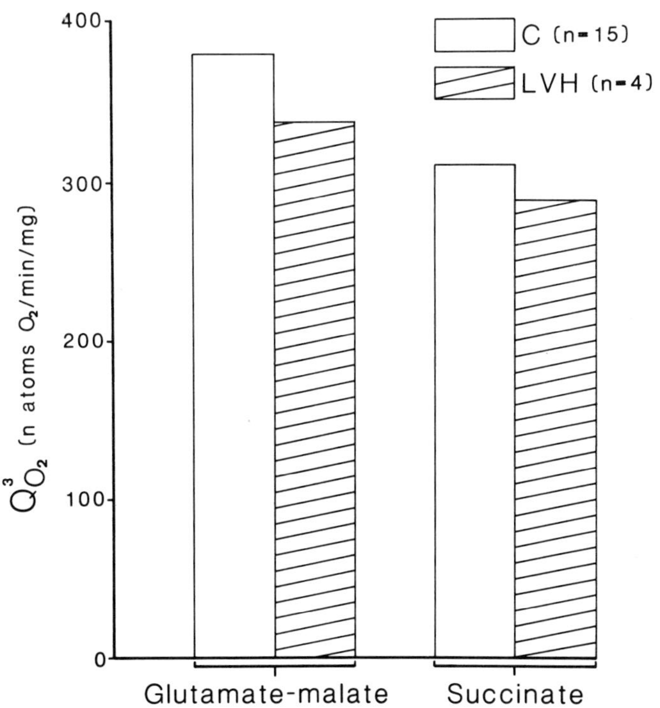

FIGURE 8. Mitochondrial respiratory activity (State 3) in Control (C) and hypertrophied dog hearts (LVH). See Methods for additional details.

Mitochondria isolated from the left ventricles of the hypertrophied hearts exhibit no significant changes in phosphorylating respiration (State 3) compared to controls (Fig. 8). This was true for both NADH-linked (Fig. 8; glutamate-malate) and succinate-linked respiration. It is curiously interesting that mitochondrial respiration in hypertrophied myocardium is consistently lower, although not significantly, compared to control (Fig. 8). At rest, both coronary blood flow (Fig. 6) and myocardial oxygen consumption (Fig. 7) in the two week pressure-overloaded hearts with aortic occlusion still in place (Figs. 6 and 7; open triangles) are essentially the same as the initial, unloaded controls (Figs. 6 and 7; closed circles). Whether or not any correlation exists between these observations remains

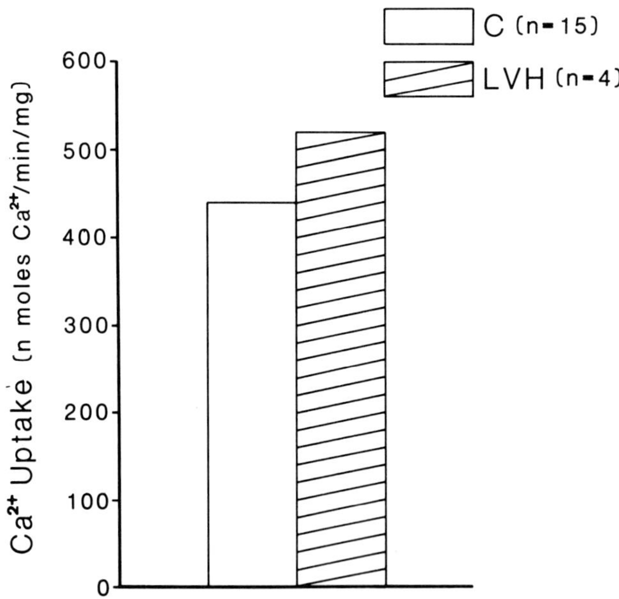

FIGURE 9. Rates of mitochondrial calcium uptake in Control (C) and hypertrophied dog hearts (LVH). Succinate was used as substrate for respiration-driven uptake. Additional details in Methods.

to be determined. Mitochondrial, respiratory-substrate (succinate

supported calcium uptake was also not significantly changed in two week

pressure-overloaded hearts compared to controls (Fig. 9). The mitochon-

drial data obtained from these two week pressure-overloaded dog hearts

is similar in many respects to data obtained from cat hearts in the early

stages of hypertrophy (8). In the previous studies (8), mitochondrial

respiratory activity remained unchanged during the first six weeks after

imposition of a severe pressure-overload. However, rates of mitochondrial

calcium uptake exhibited increases compared to control after three weeks

of pressure-overload which persisted throughout the six week period (8).

Subtle changes in mitochondrial calcium transport have also been found in

exercise trained hearts, the significance of which remains to be determined

(6). Recently, Nuutinen et al. (9) proposed that mitochondrial oxidative

phosphorylation constitutes a regulatory link between myocardial oxygen

consumption and coronary blood flow. A principal feature of this suggested

regulatory mechanism involves the relative energy state of the cell as

reflected in the [ATP]/[ADP] [P_i] ratio (9). Many factors, intrinsic and

extrinsic, can alter this ratio depending on the metabolic requirements

of the heart. Further studies will be necessary to elucidate these

relationships.

In summary, there are differences in the physiological response to

exercise between animals with hypertrophy caused by exercise training and

pressure-overload. These differences are probably a direct result of the

imposed stimulus for the hypertrophy and likely represent different origins

at the cellular level. It would seem reasonable to postulate that a major

difference exists in the autonomic nervous system control of the circula-

tion in the two conditions. This is an area that has been little explored in pathological hypertrophy and deserves further study.

ACKNOWLEDGEMENTS

The authors wish to thank Mr. Gerald Todd for assistance during these studies and Ms. Helen Amato in preparing the manuscript. Portions of this work were supported by grant #22154 from NIH.

REFERENCES

1. Stone HL: The heart and exercise training. In Hearts and Heart-Like Organs, Vol. 2, Academic Press, New York, 1980, pp 389-418.
2. Blomqvist CG, Saltin B: Cardiovascular adaptations to physical training. Ann. Rev. Physiol. (45): 169-189, 1983.
3. Alpert NR: Perspectives in Cardiovascular Research, Vol. 7, Raven Press, New York, 1983, pp 1-720.
4. Scheuer J, Malhotra A, Hirsch C, Capasso J, Schaible TF: Physiologic cardiac hypertrophy corrects contractile protein abnormalities associated with pathologic hypertrophy in rats. J. Clin. Invest. (70): 1300-1305, 1982.
5. Stone HL: Cardiac function and exercise training in conscious dogs. J. Appl. Physiol.: Respirat. Environ. Exercise Physiol. (42): 824-832, 1977.
6. Sordahl LA, Asimakis GK, Dowell RT, Stone HL: Functions of selected biochemical systems from the exercised-trained dog heart. J. Appl. Physiol.: Respirat. Environ. Exercise Physiol. (42): 426-431, 1977.
7. Wyatt HL, Mitchell JH: Influences of physical training on the heart of dogs. Circ. Res. (35): 883-889, 1974.
8. Sordahl LA, Williams JF, Potter RD: Mitochondrial energetics during early hypertrophy of cat ventricular myocardium exhibiting depressed contractile function. Circulation (56): 232, 1977.
9. Nuutinen EM, Nishiki K, Erecinska M, Wilson DF: Role of mitochondrial oxidative phosphorylation in regulation of coronary blood flow. Amer. J. Physiol. (243): 159-169, 1982.

16

DO THE LIMITS OF MOLECULAR ADAPTATIONS INDUCE FAILURE OF THE HYPERTROPHIED HEART?

K. SCHWARTZ, J.J. MERCADIER, L. RAPPAPORT, J.L. SAMUEL, D. CHARLEMAGNE, L. LELIEVRE and B. SWYNGHEDAUW.

1. INTRODUCTION

Increased pressure or volume loading of the heart induces two different types of adaptational mechanisms, cardiac hypertrophy and increased efficiency of contraction, due, respectively, to quantitative and qualitative changes in the genetic expression of the cardiac cell. Both mechanisms are useful adaptations which enable the ventricular chambers to sustain chronic hyperfunction and which allow the heart to develop a normal tension to the detriment of its velocity. In this view, heart failure appears less as a disease than as a process in which the limits of myocardial adaptation have been overcome (see 1 for review). Improving our understanding of the mechanisms responsible for myocardial adaptation will thus help to elucidate the basis for the altered performance and for the transition from compensated hypertrophy to failure. This is one reason why a great number of investigations are now concentrating on the compensatory phase.

To date, the molecular transitions which have been most frequently studied are those of myosin isozymes, which account for the reduction in myofibrillar, actomyosin and myosin ATPase, and for the reduction in maximum velocity of shortening (see 2 and 3 for review). The aims of the present study are (i) to more precisely characterize the temporal regulation of this isozymic change and to determine whether there are species differences (human versus rat studies), and (ii) to describe two new molecular changes, one at the level of the microtubular network and the other on the sarcolemma, involving Na^+-K^+ ATPase. The animal model used was a pressure overload induced in rats by placing a constricting band around the aorta (4,5).

2. ISOMYOSINS

The heterogeneity of ventricular myosin was first demonstrated by Hoh et al. (6) on a special non-dissociating pyrophosphate gel which allows the myosin, a water insoluble protein, to migrate in its native state. Three

isomyosins were separated under these experimental conditions, V1, V2 and V3. V1 and V3 are homodimers of α and β myosin heavy-chains ($\alpha\alpha$ and $\beta\beta$ respectively), while V2 is believed to be an heterodimer (7, 8). V1 has the highest Ca^{2+}-ATPase activity and V3 the lowest. In all animal species, myosin is predominantly V3 during fetal life, and V1 appears around the time of birth (2, 8, 9). Adult rats are mostly V1, while adult rabbits contain approximately 70 % V3 and 30 % V1 (3, 8, 9, 10, 11). An extensive body of evidence now supports the concept that, in rats and rabbits, an isomyosin redistribution from V1 to V3 occurs in response to increased hemodynamic loading (see 2 and 3 for reviews, and Figure 1). These changes have important functional implications, since maximal speed of shortening is linearly correlated to myosin ATPase (see 13 for review) or to isomyosin composition (14, and Figure 2), and since the rate of heat production during one contraction is greater with V1 than with V3 (15). Reappearance of the fetal isomyosin in rats (2) and rabbits (3), is thus now commonly assumed to be a useful adaptation in response to a chronic increase in cardiac work.
When and where in the myocardium is this adaptational mechanism triggered ? To answer this question, it was necessary to localize each isomyosin at the level of individual muscle fiber, and, for this purpose, antibodies that specifically distinguish V1 and V3 were prepared (2, 16, 17). In pressure overloaded rat myocardium, isomyosin V3 appears earlier in subendocardial than in subepicardial layers (17) and is synthesized in the same myocytes which already contain V1 (16). This latter finding was recently confirmed by Weisberg et al. (18), who described a histochemical method which also distinguishes V1 and V3. Within each cell, both isomyosins are identically distributed (16, 19). Figure 3 shows an example of the structural linkage between V1 and V3.

We have now used the same highly sensitive immunological approach to precisely determine at what time after aortic stenosis V3 can be detected. Cardiac overload was induced in 25-day old rats (4). At this developmental stage, the animals possess only the V1 isoform (6,9), and it is thus easy to follow first appearance of the V3 isomyosin. At various intervals after aortic constriction, ventricular myocytes were isolated and labeled by double indirect immunofluorescence with antibodies specific of the V1 or the V3 isoforms (16). The labeling of the myocyte population varied as a function of time after surgery (Table 1).

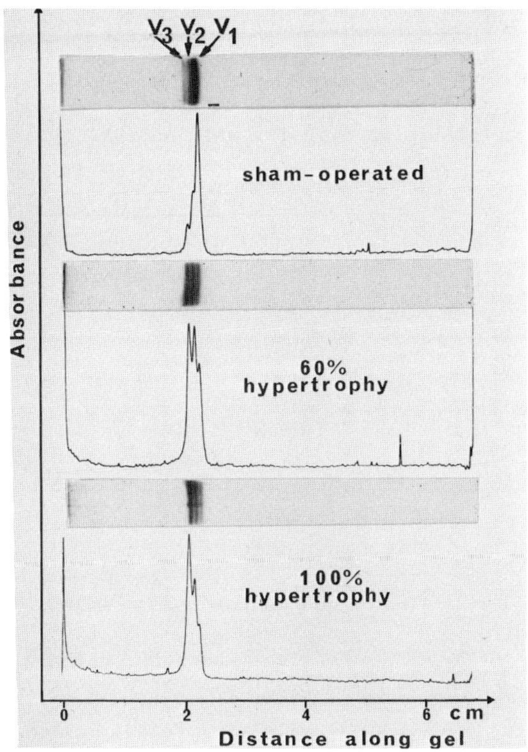

Figure 1. Electrophoretic patterns and densitometric profiles for native myosins from ventricles of one normal and two hypertrophied hearts. Reprinted from Lompré et al. (12), by permission from Nature, vol. 282, n° 5734 pp 105-107. Copyright (c) 1979 Macmillan Journals Limited.

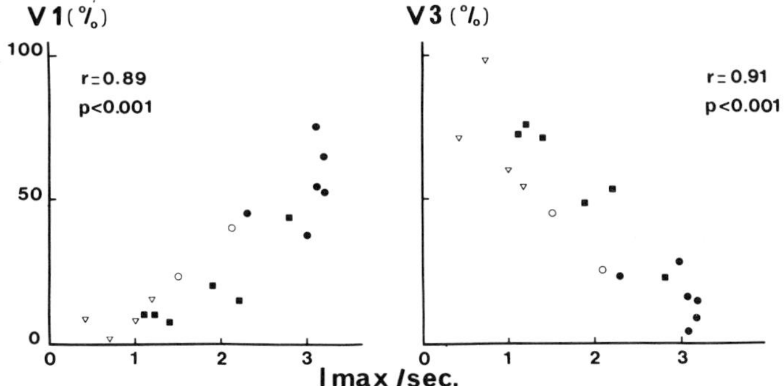

Figure 2. Relationship between the maximum velocity of shortening and the relative amount of myosin isoenzymes V1 and V3 in isolated papillary muscles from control and operated rats. Reprinted from Schwartz et al. (14), by permission of the Journal of Molecular and Cellular Cardiology, vol. 13, pp 1071-1075. Copyright : Academic Press. Inc. (London) Ltd.

Table 1 : Labeling of isolated myocytes with anti-V3 myosin immunoglobulins.

| Rats | Percent of labeled myocytes at days after surgery | | | |
	3	5	9	13
Sham-operated	0	0	0	4 ± 1
Aortic-operated	2 ± 1	15 ± 2	29 ± 5	52 ± 4

- values are means of 3-4 experiments.
- An average of 200 cells were counted for each sample.

At day 0, 100 % of myocytes from sham-operated animals were labeled only with the anti-V1 immunoglobulins. After 13 days, 4 % of the myocytes were labeled with anti-V3. These data, in full agreement with previous studies (16) indicated that the age-dependent synthesis of V1 (10) can be detected with this method even at 4-5 weeks of age. After stenosis, the percentage of the myocyte population containing V3 isomyosin increased much more rapidly than in the sham-operated animals (Table 1). The difference between the populations of myocytes from overloaded and control hearts became truly significant 5 days after stenosis. A homogeneous and similar repartition of both isomyosins was consistently observed, indicating that even at the onset of increased V3 synthesis, there was no preferential localization of the new isoform. Thus, in rats, a change in the genetic expression of myosin is observed as soon as 2 days after the increase in myocardial work. It remains to be determined whether this adaptative mechanism is triggered concomitantly with the increase in protein synthesis which leads to cardiac growth.

Can the isomyosin concept be expanded to the human heart ? Under gel electrophoresis in non denaturing conditions, human myosin migrates like rat V3 (8, 9, 20, 21). No differences were detected in the electrophoretic properties (20, 21), peptide maps and ATPase activities (20) of normal and hypertrophied hearts. Recent immunological studies performed in our laboratory with monoclonal and polyclonal antibodies confirmed that human myosins are

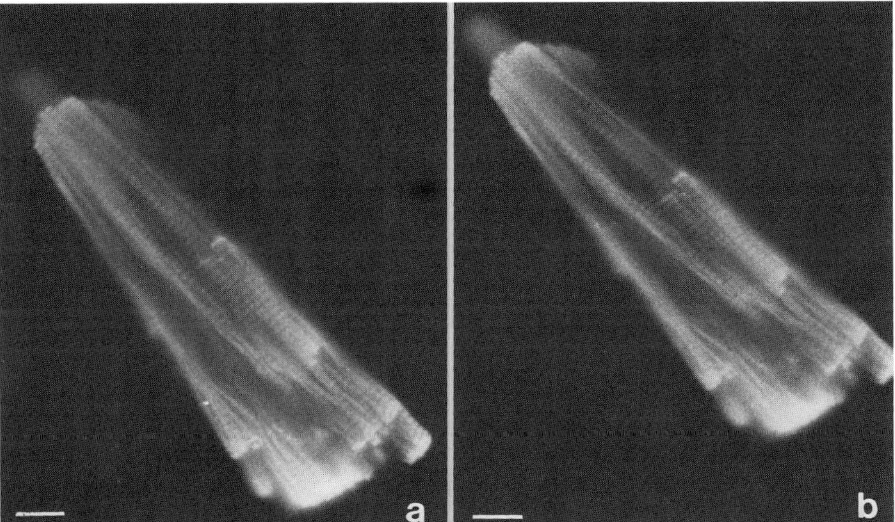

Figure 3. Double indirect immunofluorescence micrograph of a myocyte isolated from a rat heart myocyte. Labeling with anti-V1 isomyosin immunoglobulins revealed by rhodamin (part a) and with anti-V3 isomyosin immunoglobulins revealed by fluorescein (part b). Reprinted from Samuel et al. (16), Circulation Research, vol. 52, pp 200-209 by permission from the American Heart Association, Inc. bar = 10 um.

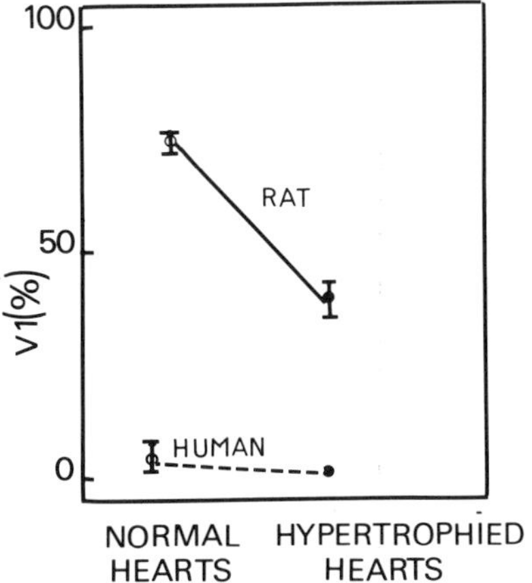

Figure 4. Comparative amounts of isomyosin V1 in rat and human ventricles.

composed mainly of a V3 type (HV3), but also contain some V1 isoform (HV1) (21). Quantification of this HV1 form was then performed by a simple enzyme-linked immunosorbent assay (22). Comparative analysis of the isomyosin distribution of normal and hypertrophied rat and human hearts is shown in Figure 4. In rats, the initial level of V1 is high (75 %) .It decreases to an average of 40 % in most cases, but in large hypertrophies and cardiac insufficiency, values of 5 to 10 % are often observed. In humans, the initial level is low (from 0 to 10 %) with an exception at 15%. In pressure - overloaded human hearts, there is indeed a decrease, as in rats, but this decrease is quantitative small, and is not accompagnied by a significant decrease in myosin ATPase activities (21). Our data thus indicate that in man isomyosin shifts exist but that they contribute little, if at all, to adaptation to chronic mechanical overload.

3. MICROTUBULES

In skeletal muscle, microtubules appear to play a role in cell growth (23) and in the assembly of sarcomeres during myogenesis (24). Cell growth is an early response to an increase in cardiac work, since, after 5 to 6 days, hear weight is already increased by 40 to 50 % (see 1 for review). Are microtubule involved in this induced cell growth ? Studies of their structures have been markedly hampered by the fact that, in muscle cells, microtubules are a minor component within predominantly sarcomeric structures: the percentage of the microtubules' major component, tubulin, is 1000 fold less than in brain (25). Moreover, cardiac myocytes account for approximately 75 % of the heart mass, and the other non muscular cells, fibroblasts for example, contain rather hig levels of tubulin. Immunolabeling of isolated cardiac myocytes with specific anti-tubulin immunoglobulins enabled us to overcome these difficulties and to identify the microtubule pattern of cardiocytes (25). As shown in Figure 5a, microtubules in rats are normally organized around the nuclei with important concentrations at the poles, showing extensions in the cone and in the cytoplasm as loosely organized loops. This pattern was markedly modified afte aortic constriction (Figure 5b). As early as 2 days after aortic stenosis in adult rats, 20 % of the myocytes showed microtubules organized in thick array roughly parallel to the long axis of the cell. Such a reorganization of the microtubule pattern was never observed when myocytes were purified from rat heart at different stages of development, at a time when the percentage of

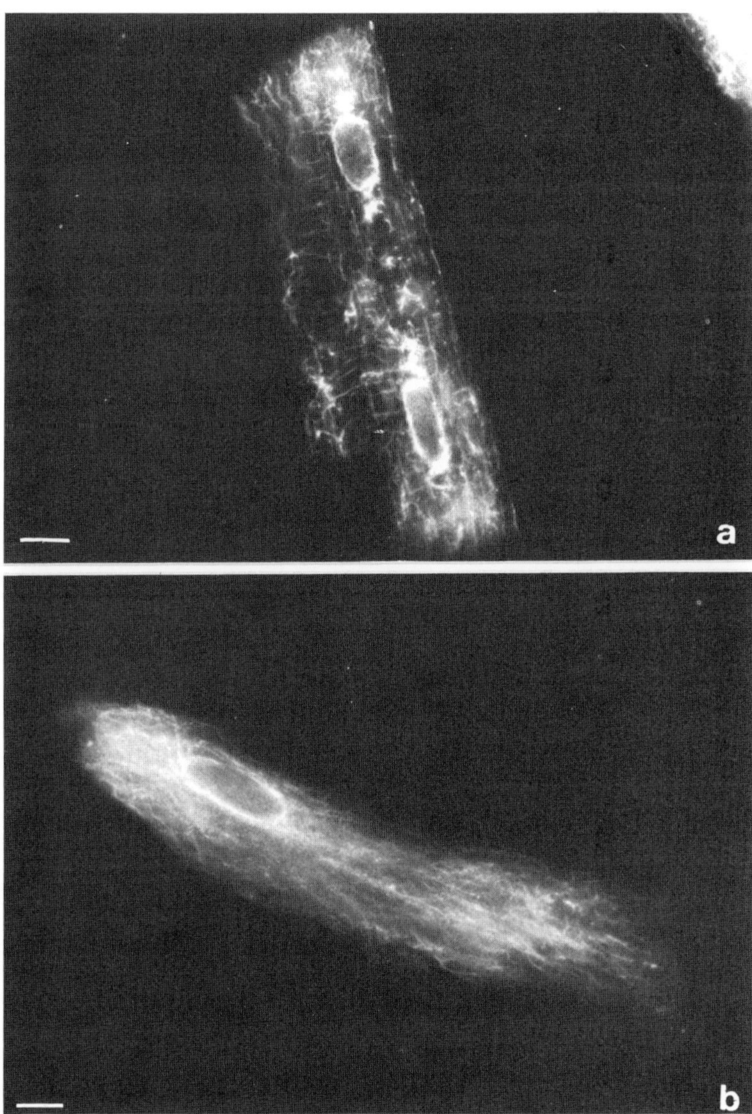

Figure 5. Fluorescence micrographs of the microtubular network in cardiac myocytes isolated fom a sham-operated rat (part A) and a pressure overloaded rat (part B). Note, in B, the increase in staining and the reorganization of microtubules as thick arrays in the axis of the cell (bar = 10 um).

myocytes labeled with a-V3 immunoglobulins was shown to slowly increase from 0 (3 weeks) to 45 % (10 weeks) (16). These results suggest that the reorganization of microtubules may interfere with the onset of some adaptational processes of myocytes to overload, but not in the shift in synthesis of a new isoform of myosin. In vitro reorganization of microtubules implies molecular modifications in tubulin or microtubular associated proteins (MAP), or both. This remains to be determined in our in vivo system.

The question then is to estimate the relative importance of such reorganization of the microtubule pattern and this role. In other types of cells, microtubules are implicated in mitosis, intracellular transport, maintenance of cell shape and motility. In skeletal muscle, microtubules seem to be implicated in the growth of muscle (23) and in the assembly of sarcomeres (24). We have shown, in a previous work, that the shape of myocytes from adult rat heart does not depend on the integrity of the microtubule network (25). It is possible that the reorganization of the microtubule network which we describe here favors a change in the transfer of proteins or organelles throughout the cytoplasm during induced growth of myocytes. On the other hand, a similar type of reorganization of the microtubule network has been described in myocytes cultured in the presence of cAMP and has been associated with a decrease in contractility of the cells (26). The decrease in contractility assessed by Vmax observed during rat heart overload is mainly secondary to the neosynthesis of the V3 - isomyosin . It may be hypothesized that a reorganization of the microtubule network activates the appearance of and/or enhances the decreases in contractility of the myocytes. To date, while microtubules are evident in heart, their involvement in the development of cardiac hypertrophy is not clear.

4. Na^+, K^+-ATPase

The mechanisms by which digitalis increases the force of contraction in normal heart have not been fully elucidated (27), but it is generally accepted that the primary target of the cardiac glycosides is the Na^+, K^+-ATPase (for a review see ref. 29). Indeed, the sensitivities of the cardiac Na^+, K^+-ATPases to inhibition by ouabain have been shown to correlate with the pharmacologically active ouabain concentrations in various species (27, 28), including rat (29, 30).

On the other hand, the response to the use of digitalis varies with the

disease and an excellent response is noted in patients with hypertensive heart
disease, valvular aortic stenosis or regurgitation (31). The question arises
as to whether, in rat cardiac muscle adapted to pressure overload, an
alteration of Na^+, K^+-ATPase functions may account for the increased
sensitivity observed in the whole tissue. Regarding Na^+, K^+ ATPase
activities in hypertrophied heart preparations from different species, highly
conflicting results have been pubqlished (32-35). Enzyme activity was found to
be either increased (32), normal (33, 34) or decreased (35). This
contradictory information can be easily explained by the superimposition of
particular enrichment methods in sarcolemmal vesicles (but with very low
yields) upon different pathological or adaptative models. We comparatively
analyzed the specific activity and the ouabain-sensitivity of the Na^+,
K^+-ATPases present in sarcolemmal vesicles from normal and hypertrophied
hearts.

Highly enriched sarcolemma fractions were isolated by the method of Mansier
et al. (36). Briefly, the isolation procedure is based upon (1) a
Ca^{2+}-free perfusion of the cardiac muscle prior to homogenization (2) an
addition of alkali salts to stop the hypotonic lysis, and (3) four
differential centrifugations. The full (patent plus latent) Na^+,
K^+-ATPase activity was 110 - and 75 - fold in purified normal and
hypertrophied heart preparations, respectively. The highest specific activity
which could be detected in sarcolemmal vesicles from hypertrophied hearts was
half that found in normal cardiac sarcolemma preparations, i.e : 120 ± 20
versus 246 ± 18 umol./h x mg. However, this result should take into account
a difference in enzyme or sarcolemma labilities. Indeed, the distributions of
the enzymatic activity along with the purification steps differed between
normal and hypertrophied tissues. A step associated with a 5-fold purification
of the enzyme in normal heart appeared to inactivate about 50 % of the enzyme
in membranes fom hypertrophied heart. Bearing these limitations in mind, we
studied the ouabain - sensitivity of the Na^+, K^+-ATPase assayed at
different degrees of sarcolemma vesicle purification. The results are
illustrated in Table 2. Assayed in native and opened vesicles from
hypertrophied hearts, the Na^+, K^+-ATPase activity was found to be
completely inhibited at 10^{-6}M ouabain. In normal heart preparation which
served as a basis for comparison under the same experimental conditions the
inhibition never exceeded 63 ± 13 % at 10^{-7}M - 10^{-6}M (30, 32). In

hypertrophied preparations, the amount of drug which half maximally inhibited
the activity (IC_{50}) was found to lie in the range 0.8 to 3.2 x 10^{-9}M.
This value represented a 4 to 15-fold enhancement in sensitivity with respect
to the high sensitivity enzyme form (IC_{50} = 1.2 $\pm$ 0.2 x 10^{-8}M) found
in normal heart treated under the same conditions (i.e , a Ca^{2+}-free
perfusion) (29). These results demonstrate that the very high sensitivity of
the hypertrophied heart to cardiac glycosides is associated with the
identification, in highly enriched sarcolemma fractions, of an active Na^{+},
K^{+}-ATPase form ten-fold more sensitive to ouabain than that of normal
heart.

Table 2. Comparative properties of the sarcolemma-bound Na^{+}, K^{+}-ATPase in
hypertrophied and normal rat hearts.

		Na^{+}, K^{+}-ATPase		
Type of heart	Specific activity (umol.Pi/h x mg)	Sensitivity to ouabain		
		Active enzyme form	Per cent activity associated with	IC50
Hypertrophied 72 - 127 %	95 $\pm$ 22	H.S. + L.S.	85 - 100 % + LD - 15 %	0.8 - 3.2 $\pm$ 10^{-9}M ✱
Normal	57 $\pm$ 7	H.S. + L.S.	55 $\pm$ 15 % 45 $\pm$ 7 %	1.2 $\pm$ 0.2 10^{-8}M 3 $\pm$ 1 x 10^{-5}M

Both heart types were perfused with a Ca^{2+}-free buffer.
H.S. : high sensitivity - L.S. : low sensitivity.
✱ : The very low residual activity did not allow IC50 determination IC50 :
ouabain concentration to half - maximally inhibit the Na^{+}, K^{+}-ATPase
Form.
L.D. : limit of detection

Nevertheless, such high sensitivity to ouabain could result from severe
membrane alterations occurring during the membrane isolation procedure (37).
In fact, we previously showed (29) that, in normal rat heart, a Ca^{2+}-free
perfusion increased the enzyme yield and revealed a Na^{+}, K^{+}-ATPase
form highly sensitive to ouabain. This active form was undetectable in heart

maintained at 2mM Ca^{2+} (25,34, 35) but was still able to bind ^{3}H
ouabain with high affinity (38, 39). Such a role of calcium chelators, already
reported in non muscle cells (40-44), is not a disadvantage but reveals a
difference at the Na^{+}, K^{+} pump level between normal and hypertrophied
rat hearts. This has been suggested by a number of electrophysiological
studies (45, 46). The differences observed at the sarcolemmal level between
the Na^{+}, K^{+}-ATPase active forms in normal and hypertrophied hearts may
be interpretated in terms of isoenzymic forms. This hypothesis is consistent
with the metabolic alterations noted in both the myosin-ATPase and the
creatine-Phosphokinase systems. Alternatively, the membrane environment may
play a role (39, 44). A single class of enzyme molecules may express one or
two sensivities to ouabain depending on interactions with inner face membrane
proteins.

5. CONCLUSION

The challenge for the clinician is to prevent transition from compensatory
hypertrophy to heart failure. Can the molecular changes described in the
present paper, together with the shift in creatine kinase isozymes found by
Ingwall and Fossel (47), be useful to meet this challenge ? In rats, there is
good experimental evidence to hypothesize that cardiac failure occurs when the
isomyosin transition to V3 is complete. Appropriate experimental approaches
should, in the near future, allow confirmation of this hypothesis. At the
present time, Na^{+}, K^{+}-ATPase and CPK changes are not sufficiently well
documented to determine whether they are true adaptational mechanisms, or
whether they contribute to depressed mechanical performance. It is clear
however that these two enzymes are involved in the chronic response of the
cardiac myocyte to new functional requirements, and as such, they are both
candidates for characterizing the transition period. For myosin and creatine
kinase, a striking feature is that, in rats, adaptation of the adult heart to
an increase in cardiac work is mediated through synthesis of a fetal or
neonatal isoform. Does this mean that cardiac hypertrophy induced in adult
animals mimics normal ontogenic development ? Or that extra components can be
added to already differentiated cells only if they undergo the normal
differentiation process ? A third point is the microtubular reorganization
described here. This reorganization is an early and transitory phenomenon,
concerning only part of the myocyte population. Unless similar morphological

changes are found later during the development of cardiac hypertrophy, it seems unlikely that they could contribute to our knowledge of the transition period. Nevertheless,they provide new insights into the biology of cardiac overload, since this is the first report of a response at the cytoskeleton level. The final salient feature is that the biochemical markers which can be used to define an adaptational process vary from one animal species to the other. Isomyosin changes seem to have important functional significance in rats and rabbits, but not in humans. In contrast, creatine-kinase changes have recently been found in humans. Thus, it is apparent that both human and animal studies are even more necessary, not only for their unquestionable applicability to human disease, but also for a complete understanding of the hypertrophic process.

6. ACKNOWLEDGMENTS

We are grateful to S. Sartore and S. Schiaffino (University of Padova) for the gift of the antibody specific of the V3 isomyosin. We thank C. Wisnewsky, P. Bouveret and F. Marotte for expert technical assistance, and P. Cagnac for secretarial work.

REFERENCES

1. Swynghedauw B, Delcayre C: Biology of cardiac overload. Pathobiology Annual (12): 137-183, 1982.

2. Schwartz K, Lompré AM, Bouveret P, Wisnewsky C, Whalen RG: Comparison of rat cardiac myosins at fetal stages in young animals and in hypothyroid Adults. J Biol Chem (257): 14412-14418, 1982.

3. Chizzonitte RA, Everett AW, Clark WA, Jakovcic S, Rabinowitz M, Zak R: Isolation and characterization of two molecular variants of myosin heavy chain from rabbit ventricle. J Biol Chem (257): 2056-2065, 1982.

4. Bugaisky LB, Zak R: Cellular growth of cardiac muscle after birth. Texas Rep Biol Med (39): 123-128, 1979.

5. Beznak M: Changes in heart weight and blood pressure following aortic constriction in rats. Can J Biochem Physiol (33): 995-1002, 1955.

6. Hoh JFY, Mc Grath PA, Hale PT. Electrophoretic analysis of multiple forms of rat cardiac myosin : Effects of hypophysectomy and thyroxine replacement. J Mol and Cell Cardiol (10): 1053-1076, 1978.

7. Hoh JFY, Yeoh GPS, Thomas MAW, Higginbotom L: Structural differences in the heavy chains of rat ventricular myosin isoenzymes. FEBS Letters (97) : 330-334, 1979.

8. Clark A, Chizzonite RA, Everett AW, Rabinowitz M: Zak R. Species correlations between cardiac isomyosins. J Biol Chem (257): 5449-5454, 1982.

9. Lompré AM, Mercardier JJ, Wisnewsky C, Pantaloni C, D'Albis A, Schwartz K. Species and age-dependent changes in the relative amounts of cardiac myosin isoenzymes in mammals. Developmental Biology (84) : 286-290, 1981.

10. Mercadier JJ, Lompré AM, Wisnewsky C, Samuel JL, Bercovici J. Swynghedauw B, Schwartz K: Myosin isoenzymic changes in several models of rat cardiac hypertrophy. Circ Res (49): 525-532, 1981.

11. Litten RZ, Martin BJ, Low RB, Alpert NR: Altered myosin isozyme patterns from pressure-overloaded and thyrotoxic hypertrophied rabbit hearts. Circ Res (50): 856-864, 1982.

12. Lompré AM, Schwartz K, D'Albis A, Lacombe G, Van Thiem N, Swynghedauw B: Myosin isoenzyme redistribution in chronic heart overload. Nature (282): 105-107, 1979.

13. Scheuer J, Bahn AK: Cardiac contractile proteins. Adenosine triphosphatase activity and physiological function Circ Res (45): 1-12, 1979.

14. Schwartz K, Lecarpentier Y, Martin JL, Lompré AM, Mercadier JJ, Swynghedauw B: Myosin isoenzymic distribution correlates with speed of myocardial contraction. J Mol Cell Cardiol (13): 1071-1075, 1981.

15. Alpert NR. Mulieri LA: Increased myothermal economy of isometric force generation in compensated cardiac hypertrophy induced by pulmonary artery constriction in rabbit Circ Res (50): 491-500, 1982.

16. Samuel JL, Rappaport L, Mercadier JJ, Lompré AM, Sartore S, Triban C, Schiaffino S, Schwartz K: Distribution of myosin isozymes within single cardiac cells. Circ Res (52): 200-209, 1983.

17. Gorza L, Pauletto P, Pessina AC, Sartore S, Schiaffino S: Isomyosin distribution in normal and pressure-overloaded rat ventricular myocardium. Circ Res (49): 1003-1009, 1981.

18. Weisberg A, Winegrad S, Tucker M, Mc Clellan G: Histochemical detection of specific isozymes of myosin in rat ventricular cells. Circ Res (51): 802-809, 1982.

19. Mercadier JJ, Lompré AM, Bouveret P, Samuel JL, Rappaport L, Swynghedauw B Schwartz K: Myosin isoenzymic distribution in hypertrophied rat and human hearts. In : Jacob R, Gülch RW, Kissling G: Cardiac adaptation to hemodynamic overload, training and stress, Steinkopff Verlag, Darmstadt, 1983, pp 104-112.

20. Schier JJ, Adelstein RS: Structural and enzymatic comparison of human cardiac muscle myosin isolated from infants, adults, and patients with hypertrophic cardiomyopathy. J Clin Inv (59): 816-825, 1982.

21. Mercadier JJ, Bouveret P, Gorza L, Schiaffino S, Clark WA, Zak R, Swynghedau, Schwartz K: Myosin isoenzymes in normal and hypertrophied huma ventricular myocardium. Cir Res. (52): 53, 1983.

22. Mercadier JJ, Bouveret P, Wisnewsky C, de la Bastie D, Schwartz K: Simplified methodology using non-competitive Elisa assay for the quantitation of myosin isoforms. In : Avrameas S, Druet P, Masseyeff R. Fedmann G (eds), Immunoenzymatic Techniques, Elsevier, 1983 pp 329-332.

23. Cartwright JJr, Goldstein MA: Microtubules in soleus muscles of the post natal and adult rat. J Ultrastr Res (79) 74-84, 1982.

24. Toyama Y, Forry-schaudies S, Hoffman B, Holtzer H: Effects of taxol and colcemid on myofibrillogenesis. Proc Natl Acad Sci USA (79) 6556-6560, 1982.

25. Samuel JL, Schwartz K, Lompré AM, Delcayre C, Marotte F, Swynghedauw B, Rappaport L: Immunological quantitation and localization of tubulin in adult rat heart isolated myocytes. Eur J Cell Biol (31) : 99-106, 1983.

26. Nath K, Shay JW, Bolley AP: Relationship between dibutyryl cyclic -AMP anc microtubules organization in contracting heart muscle cells. Proc Natl Aca Sci USA (75) 319-323, 1978.

27. Noble D: Mechanism of action of therapeutic levels of cardiac glycosides. Cardiovasc. Res. (14), 495-514, 1980.

28. Akera T, Brody TM: Myocardial membranes : Regulation and function of the sodium pump. Ann Rev Physiol (44), 375-388, 1982.

29. Mansier P, Lelievre LG: Ca^{2+}-free perfusion of rat heart reveals a Na+, K+ -ATPase form highly sensitive to ouabain. Nature (300), 535-537, 1982.

30. Mansier P, Cassidy PS, Charlemagne D, Preteseille M, Lelievre LG: Three Na+, K+ -ATPase forms in rat heart as revealed by K+/ouabain antagonism. FEBS Lett. (153), 357-360, 1983.

31. Spann JF, Hurst JW: Treatment of heart failure, In : Hurst JW, Logue RB, Schlant RC, Wenger NK (eds), The Heart, Mc Graw-Hill Book Company, New-York, 1978, pp. 580-606.

32. Khatter JC, Prasad K: Myocardial sarcolemmal ATPase in dogs with induced mitral insufficiency. Cardiovasc Res (10) 637-641, 1976.

33. Gibson K, Harris P: The distribution of microsomal (Na+ + K+)-ATPase in ra heart and the effect of induced right ventricular hypertrophy and feeding with digitalis sodium and potassium. Cardiovasc Res (4) 6-13, 1970.

34. Swynghedauw B, Bouveret P, Hatt PY: New fractionation scheme for preparation of heart particles. ATPase activity of purified myofibrils in chronic aortic insufficiency in the rabbit. J Mol Cell Cardiol (5), 441-459, 1973.

35. Tomlinson CW, Lee SL, Dhalla NS: Abnormalities in heart membranes and myofibrils during bacterial infective cardiomyopathy in the rabbit. Circ Res (39) 82-92, 1975.

36. Mansier P, Charlemagne D, Rossi B, Preteseille M, Swynghedauw B, Lelievre LG: Isolation of impermeable inside-out vesicles from an enriched sarcolemma fraction of rat heart. J Biol Chem (258) 6628-6635, 1983.

37. Schwalb H, Dickstein Y, Heller M: Interactions of cardiac glycosides with cardiac cells. III. Alterations in the sensitivity of (Na+ + K+)-ATPase to inhibition by ouabain in rat hearts. Biochim Bophys Acta (689) 241-248, 1982.

38. Adams R, et al.: High-affinity ouabain binding site and low-dose positive inotropic effect in rat myocardium. Nature (296) 167-169, 1982.

39. Erdmann E, Philipp G, Schol Z: Cardiac glycoside receptor, (Na+ + K+)-ATPase activity and force of contraction in rat heart. Biochem Pharmacol (29) 3219-3229, 1980.

40. Lelievre LG, Charlemagne D, Paraf A: The modification of (Na+/K+) ATPase sensitivity to ouabain after extraction of membrane constituents distinct from the enzyme. Biochem Biophys Res Commun (72) 1526-1533, 1976.

41. Zachowski A, Lelievre LG, Aubry J, Charlemagne D, Paraf A: Roles of proteins from inner face of plasma membranes in susceptibility of (Na+,K+)-ATPase to ouabain. Proc Natl Acad Sci USA (74) 633-637, 1977.

42. Lelievre LG, Zachowski A, Charlemagne D, Laget P, Paraf A: Inhibition of Na+,K+ ATPase by ouabain : involvement of calcium and membrane proteins. Biochim Biophys Acta (557) 399-408, 1979.

43. Lelievre LG, Piascik MT, Potter JD, Wallick ET, Schwartz A: Specific involvement of calmoduline in the sensitivity of the Na+,K+ - ATPase to ouabain in murine plasmocytoma cells. In the Proceeding on the IIIrd Intl. Na, K-ATPase conf. FB, Forbush and J, Hoffman (Eds) in press. Academic Press.

44. Geny B, Paraf A, Fedon Y, Charlemagne D: characterization of a - actinin - like protein in purified non-muscle cell membranes. Biochim Biophys Acta (692) 345-354, 1982.

45. Houser SR, Freeman AR, Jaeger MJ, Breisch EA, Coulson RL, Carey R, Spann JF: Resting potential changes associated with Na+ - K+ pump in failing heart muscle. Am J Physiol (240) H168-H176, 1981.

46. Keung ECH, Aronson RS: Non-uniform electrophysiological properties and electronic stimulation in hypertrophied rat myocardium. Circ Res (49) 150-158, 1981.

47. Ingwall JS, Fossel ET : Changes in the creatine kinase system in the hypertrophied myocardium of the dog and rat, In : Alpert NR (ed), Myocardial hypertrophy and failure, Raven Press, New York, 1983, pp 601-618.

17

SARCOLEMMAL ALTERATIONS IN CARDIAC HYPERTROPHY DUE TO PRESSURE OVERLOAD IN PIGS*

V. PANAGIA, D.F. MICHIEL, J.C. KHATTER, K.S. DHALLA, P.K. SINGAL and N.S. DHALLA.

1. INTRODUCTION

Sarcolemma is considered to play an important role in raising and lowering the intracellular concentration of calcium for cardiac contraction and relaxation, respectively (1-4). Binding of Ca^{2+} with sarcolemmal membrane in the absence of ATP is considered to represent a superficial store of Ca^{2+}, which is made available for entry during excitation of the myocardial cell, whereas ATP hydrolysis due to activation of Ca^{2+}-ATPase in sarcolemma is believed to provide energy for opening calcium channels to allow the influx of Ca^{2+} (1-4). On the other hand, ATP-dependent Ca^{2+} binding and Ca^{2+}-stimulated Mg^{2+}-dependent ATPase activities of sarcolemma are considered to serve as Ca^{2+}-pump mechanisms for Ca^{2+}-efflux from the myocardial cell (1-4). The adenylate cyclase in sarcolemma has been thought to be involved in increasing Ca^{2+}- influx as well as Ca^{2+}- efflux by phosphorylating calcium channels and Ca^{2+}- pump mechanisms through cyclic AMP-dependent protein kinase system (1,3). Furthermore, sarcolemmal Na^+-K^+ ATPase, which is known to regulate the concentration of Na^+ and K^+, is believed to influence the efflux of Ca^{2+} indirectly through the Na^+-Ca^{2+} exchange mechanism (1,3). Thus any alteration in one or more of these sarcolemmal systems can be conceived to affect Ca^{2+} movements across the myocardial cell membrane and subsequently result in an abnormal heart function.

A great deal of data concerning changes in the adenylate cyclase, Na^+-K^+ ATPase, Ca^{2+}-ATPase and Ca^{2+} binding activities in different experimental models of heart failure (2,3) indicate a defect in the sarcolemmal membrane under pathological conditions. However, only scattered information is available with respect to sarcolemmal changes in cardiac hypertrophy. In

---

* This work was supported by a grant from the Medical Research Council of Canada.

this regard, Tomlinson et al (5) observed a decrease in sarcolemmal Na^+-K^+ ATPase and ATP-independent Ca^{2+} binding activities without any changes in the basal adenylate cyclase or ATP-dependent Ca^{2+} binding activities in hypertrophied rabbit hearts induced by implanting a catheter in the left ventricle through the right carotid artery for 6 days. Furthermore, Lamers et al (6) have reported an alteration of the sarcolemmal function in hypertrophied non-failing hearts because the activities of some of the enzymes associated with this membrane were found to be depressed in heart homogenates after constricting the descending aorta in rabbits for about 4 weeks. Since heart hypertrophy has been shown to be either physiological or pathological in nature (7), it was considered important to gain information concerning sarcolemmal changes at different stages of its development. In this study therefore we have investigated changes in sarcolemmal enzyme and Ca^{2+}-binding activities at two stages of cardiac hypertrophy induced by pressure overload in pigs by banding the aorta for 4 and 8 weeks. Previously, we have shown that the function of isolated muscle from this experimental model was supernormal at 4 weeks but depressed at 8 weeks of aortic constriction and it has been suggested that the cardiac hypertrophy at these times was physiological and pathological in nature, respectively (8).

2. MATERIALS AND METHODS

The left ventricular hypertrophy due to pressure overload was produced in pigs by banding the supravalvular aorta for 4 and 8 weeks as described earlier (8). Sham operated animals under identical conditions were used as control. The animals were assessed hemodynamically but no signs of heart failure were noted (9). Left ventricular tissue was dissected out after sacrificing these animals by a bullet blow on the forehead. Sarcolemmal fraction was isolated and purified by the hypotonic shock-LiBr treatment method described elsewhere (10). The techniques for checking purity of the preparation and for determining the Na^+-K^+ ATPase, Mg^{2+} ATPase, Ca^{2+} ATPase, adenylate cyclase, ATP-independent Ca^{2+} binding, ATP-dependent Ca^{2+} binding and Ca^{2+}-stimulated ATPase activities were same as those employed earlier in this laboratory (11-14). Ouabain sensitive Na^+-K^+ ATPase was determined in the presence of 1 mM ouabain and adenylate cyclase activity was measured in the absence (basal) and presence of 8 mM NaF or 100 µM epinephrine. The methods for determining SDS-gel electrophoresis

and phospholipid composition of the sarcolemmal preparations were same as
used previously (15). The data were analyzed statistically using the
Student't t-test and a P value < 0.05 was taken to reflect a significant
difference.

3. RESULTS

Electron microscopic examination of the sarcolemmal preparations from
control and experimental hearts revealed varying sizes and shapes of
membrane vesicles with cell surface material and the absence of intact
mitochondria or myofibrils. However, marker enzyme studies including
the cytochrome C oxidase and oxalate supported calcium uptake activities
showed 2-3% cross contamination by mitochondrial and sarcoplasmic reticular
fragments. Repeated extraction of the membrane fractions with 0.6 mM KCl,
which is known to remove myofibrils, did not alter the Mg^{2+} ATPase

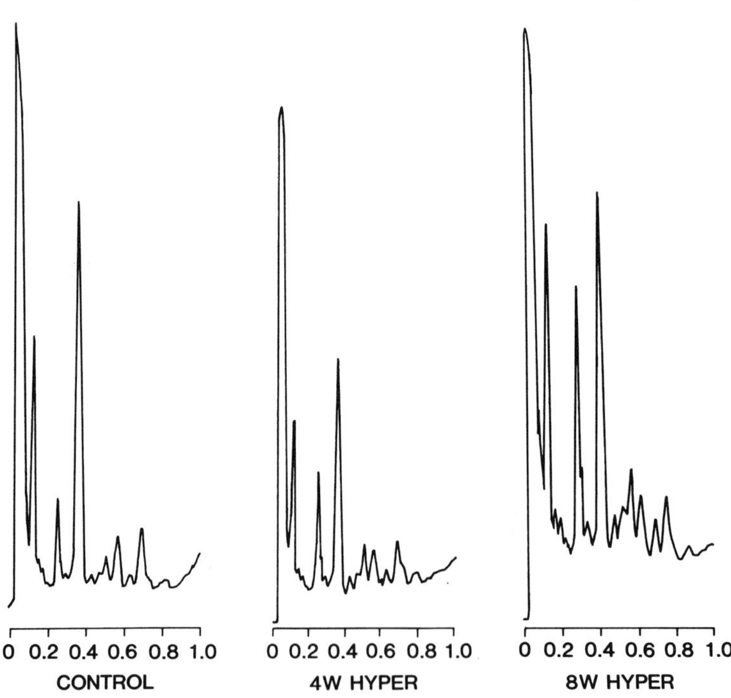

FIGURE 1. SDS-polyacrylamide gel electrophoretic pattern of sarcolemma
from control, 4 weeks (4W HYPER) and 8 weeks (8W HYPER) hypertrophied
pig hearts. Each tracing is a typical for at least 4 to 6 experiments
in each group.

activity. Furthermore, the sarcolemmal preparations from control, 4
weeks and 8 weeks hypertrophied hearts were enriched by 8.1, 8.4 and 8.3
fold with respect to adenylate cyclase activities and 9.8, 9.4 and 9.6
fold with respect to ouabain-sensitive Na^+-K^+ ATPase activities as
compared to these activities in heart homogenate respectively. There were
no qualitative differences in the SDS-gel profiles of the sarcolemmal (Fig. 1)
preparations from control and experimental hearts; however, these preparations showed some quantitative differences in four major peaks in the
gel profile. These results demonstrate that the sarcolemmal preparations
employed in this study contained minimal contamination by other subcellular
organelles and the membrane fractions from control and experimental
hearts were purified to an equal degree. No significant changes in the
phospholipid composition of sarcolemma were observed during the development
of cardiac hypertrophy except that the lysophosphatidylcholine contents
were increased in 8 weeks hypertrophied hearts (Table 1).

TABLE 1. Phospholipid composition of sarcolemmal fractions isolated from
sham control and hypertrophied pig left ventricle. The data for 4 and 8
week sham control were pooled. Each value is a mean ± S.E. of 7 to 8
experiments. * - P < 0.05.

Phospholipid	Sham control	4 week Hypertrophy	8 week Hypertrophy
	nmol lipid Pi/mg protein		
Total Phospholipids	142.5 ± 8.1	151.9 ± 7.4	163.8 ± 11.9
Phosphatidylcholine	47.0 ± 3.4	56.7 ± 4.2	57.6 ± 4.5
Phosphatidylethanolamine	37.5 ± 2.8	44.0 ± 3.0	44.5 ± 3.7
Lysophosphatidylcholine	2.4 ± 0.2	3.0 ± 0.6	4.5 ± 0.6*
Sphingomyelin	9.5 ± 1.4	8.1 ± 1.1	10.2 ± 1.0
Diphosphatidylglycerol	13.6 ± 1.4	13.6 ± 0.6	13.9 ± 2.5
Phosphatidylserine	8.1 ± 0.7	7.2 ± 0.5	9.5 ± 1.7
Phosphatidylinositol	9.9 ± 0.9	7.9 ± 0.8	10.8 ± 1.9
Phosphatidic Acid	3.2 ± 0.5	2.5 ± 0.5	2.8 ± 0.7
Unknowns	11.0 ± 1.9	8.5 ± 1.8	9.4 ± 2.4

The results shown in Table 2 indicate that the basal adenylate cyclase
activity as well as its activation by NaF or epinephrine in sarcolemmal
preparations from 4 weeks hypertrophied heart was not different from control.
On the other hand, sarcolemma from 8 weeks hypertrophied hearts showed a
significant depression in the basal adenylate cyclase activity without any

changes in its stimulation by NaF or epinephrine. The data in Table 3 show a significant depression in the ouabain sensitive Na^+-K^+ ATPase activities at 4 and 8 weeks of aortic constriction. However no changes in the sarcolemmal Mg^{2+} ATPase activities were seen in the hypertrophied

TABLE 2. Cardiac sarcolemmal adenylate cyclase activity in sham control and hypertrophied pig left ventricle. The data for 4 and 8 weeks sham control were pooled. Each value is a mean ± S.E. of 6 to 8 experiments. * - P < 0.05.

Animal Group	Basal adenylate cyclase activity (pmol cyclic AMP/mg/min)	Stimulation (%) by	
		8 mM NaF	100 μM Epinephrine
Sham control	78 ± 5	464	136
4 weeks hypertrophy	73 ± 4	474	133
8 weeks hypertrophy	61 ± 5*	462	138

TABLE 3. Sarcolemmal Mg^{2+} ATPase and Ca^{2+} ATPase activities in sham control and hypertrophied pig left ventricle. The data for 4 and 8 weeks sham control were pooled. Each value is a mean ± S.E. of 6 to 8 experiments. * - P < 0.05.

Animal Group	ATPase activity (μmoles Pi/mg protein/hr)		
	Ouabain sensitive Na^+-K^+ ATPase	Mg^{2+} ATPase	Ca^{2+} ATPase
Sham control	5.6 ± 0.4	6.1 ± 0.3	8.4 ± 0.4
4 weeks hypertrophy	4.3 ± 0.2*	6.3 ± 0.6	9.7 ± 0.3*
8 weeks hypertrophy	3.9 ± 0.5*	7.0 ± 0.7	7.4 ± 0.6

myocardium. The activity of sarcolemmal Ca^{2+} ATPase in the presence of 1.25 mM Ca^{2+} was significantly increased at 4 weeks but was unaltered at 8 weeks of cardiac hypertrophy (Table 3). It should be pointed out that 1 mM ouabain inhibited the sarcolemmal Na^+-K^+ ATPase activity by 60 to 70% and there was no difference in its inhibitory effect on control and experimental preparations. A 100% inhibition of the Na^+-K^+ ATPase activity by ouabain was produced upon treating these membrane preparations with deoxycholate at a detergent/protein ratio of 0.2.

Sarcolemmal Ca^{2+} binding in the absence of ATP was determined at two concentrations of Ca^{2+} and the results are given in Table 4. No change in the high affinity Ca^{2+}-binding site in sarcolemma was evident during cardiac hypertrophy as Ca^{2+} binding activity of the sarcolemma from hypertrophied heart in the presence of 0.1 mM Ca^{2+} was not different from the control value. The low affinity Ca^{2+}-binding sites as determined in the presence of 1.25 mM Ca^{2+} in sarcolemma from 8 weeks hypertrophied heart, unlike that from 4 weeks hypertrophied heart, were significantly increased in comparison to the control value. It was interesting to note that control values for both high and low affinity Ca^{2+}-binding sites in pig heart sarcolemma were low in comparison to those for the rat heart preparations (11,12).

TABLE 4. Sarcolemmal Ca^{2+} binding in the sham control and hypertrophied pig left ventricle. The data for 4 and 8 weeks sham control were pooled. Each value is a mean ± S.E. of 5 to 7 experiments. *- $P < 0.05$.

Animal Group	ATP independent calcium binding (nmoles/mg protein/5 min)	
	0.1 mM Ca^{2+}	1.25 mM Ca^{2+}
Sham control	7.6 ± 1.2	31 ± 4.5
4 week hypertrophy	8.4 ± 1.7	33 ± 6.1
8 week hypertrophy	8.5 ± 1.3	54 ± 4.8*

In another set of experiments, ATP- dependent Ca^{2+}-binding and Ca^{2+}-stimulated ATPase activities were determined. It should be mentioned that the sarcolemmal preparations isolated by the hypotonic shock-LiBr treatment method from rat heart show negligible ATP-dependent Ca^{2+}-binding and Ca^{2+}-stimulated ATPase activity. However, pig heart sarcolemma, like that isolated from rabbit heart (5) was found to exhibit these Ca^{2+}-pump activities. This is most probably due to differences in the proportion of the inside-out membrane vesicles in the sarcolemmal preparations. In this regard it should be pointed out that the inside-out membrane vesicles as estimated by measuring the ouabain sensitive Na^{+}-K^{+} ATPase activity with or without detergent treatment were found to be 30 to 40% in the pig heart in comparison to about 10% in the rat heart sarcolemmal preparations. The data in Table 5 reveal that both ATP-dependent Ca^{2+} binding and Ca^{2+}-stimulated ATPase activities were unaltered in sarcolemma from 4 weeks hypertrophied hearts. However, in 8 weeks of cardiac hypertrophy these Ca^{2+}-pump activities were significantly depressed.

TABLE 5. ATP-dependent sarcolemmal Ca^{2+} binding and Ca^{2+} stimulated ATPase activities in sham control and hypertrophied pig heart left ventricle. The data for 4 and 8 weeks sham control were pooled. Each value is a mean ± S.E. of 4 to 6 experiments. * - $P < 0.05$.

Animal Group	ATP dependent calcium binding (nmoles/mg protein/5 min)	Ca^{2+} stimulated ATPase activity (μmoles Pi/mg protein/hr)
Sham control	51 ± 5	2.8 ± 0.32
4 weeks hypertrophy	47 ± 6	2.9 ± 0.27
8 weeks hypertrophy	23 ± 6*	1.7 ± 0.18*

4. DISCUSSION

In this study we have shown that changes in Na^{+}-K^{+} ATPase, Ca^{2+}-ATPase, Ca^{2+}-stimulated ATPase, adenylate cyclase, ATP-independent Ca^{2+} binding and ATP-dependent Ca^{2+} binding occur at 4 or 8 weeks of cardiac hypertrophy due to pressure overload in pigs. These results suggest some alteration in the sarcolemmal membrane in hypertrophied heart since these changes were not associated with any differences in the sidedness of the membrane vesicles or the degree of cross contamination by other subcellular organelles. It should be pointed out that sarcoplasmic reticular Ca^{2+} pump activity was increased at 4 weeks and decreased at 8 weeks of aortic stenosis in this experimental model, respectively (16). Furthermore mitochondrial Ca^{2+} binding was increased at 8 weeks of cardiac hypertrophy in these animals (17). Thus it appears that heart hypertrophy is not only associated with changes in contractile proteins as commonly reported by several investigators (7,18) but there also occur changes in different membrane systems during the development of cardiac hypertrophy. In addition, alterations in both sarcolemmal and sarcoplasmic reticular membranes seem to occur before those in mitochondria and it is likely that such changes are adaptive in nature since hypertrophy is a compensatory mechanism in response to increased workload on the myocardium.

Although the exact reason for the observed sarcolemmal changes during the development of cardiac hypertrophy is not clear, it is possible that such alterations may be due to changes in the sarcolemmal composition as well as interaction of membrane protein-phospholipid components (19). SDS-gel electrophoretic pattern of hypertrophied heart sarcolemma has revealed some changes in the magnitude of certain protein peaks and this can be taken to suggest alterations in the membrane protein contents. On the other hand, no changes in the major phospholipid contents were observed to occur in hypertrophied heart sarcolemma except that lysophosphatidyl-choline was increased in 8 weeks hypertrophied hearts. Such a change may occur due to the activation of phospholipase A in hypertrophied heart because an increase in lysophosphatidylcholine without any changes in other phospholipids has been shown to occur in heart sarcolemma due to Ca^{2+}-stimulated phospholipase A activity (20). Furthermore, lysophosphatidyl-choline has been reported to inhibit the heart sarcolemma Na^+-K^+ ATPase activity (21).

A depression in the sarcolemmal Na^+-K^+ ATPase and an increase in Ca^{2+}-ATPase activities at 4 weeks of aortic stenosis can be seen to increase in Ca^{2+}-influx through Na^+-Ca^{2+} exchange mechanism and by opening more calcium channels respectively. Such an increase in calcium entry at early stages of cardiac hypertrophy may contribute in explaining the supernormal function of the cardiac muscle observed at 4 weeks of aortic stenosis in pigs (8). On the other hand, an increase in sarcolemmal Ca^{2+} stores, as reflected by an increase in ATP-independent Ca^{2+} binding, and a further depression in Na^+-K^+ ATPase activity may favour increased Ca^{2+}-entry at 8 weeks hypertrophied heart. Increased lysophosphatidylcholine in sarcolemma from 8 weeks hypertrophied heart may also promote Ca^{2+}-influx since this phospholipid has been shown to potentiate Ca^{2+} accumulation in myocardium (22). In addition, Ca^{2+}-efflux at 8 weeks hypertrophied heart may be impaired since ATP-dependent Ca^{2+} binding and Ca^{2+}-stimulated ATPase activities were decreased. Both increased Ca^{2+}-influx and decreased Ca^{2+}-efflux can be seen to result in an intracellular Ca^{2+}-overload which may be considered to determine the transition of physiological hypertrophy at 4 weeks to pathological hypertrophy at 8 weeks of aortic stenosis in pigs (8). A depression in sarcolemmal Ca^{2+}-pump activities at 24 hr of catecho-lamine administration has also been reported to result in pathological heart hypertrophy (23). It should be noted that sarcolemmal changes associated with an increase in calcium entry in 8 weeks of hypertrophied heart are not likely to be due to change in the sarcolemmal adenylate cyclase system since the basal adenylate cyclase activity was decreased and its activation by NaF or catecholamines was unaltered at this stage of cardiac hypertrophy.

5. SUMMARY

Cardiac hypertrophy in pig due to pressure overload induced by aortic stenosis for 4 weeks was associated with a decrease in the sarcolemmal ouabain sensitive Na^+-K^+ ATPase and an increase in Ca^{2+}-ATPase activities. On the other hand, sarcolemma obtained from hypertrophied hearts at 8 weeks of aortic stenosis showed an increase in ATP-independent Ca^{2+} binding and a decrease in basal adenylate cyclase, ATP-dependent Ca^{2+} binding and Ca^{2+}-stimulated ATPase activities in addition to a further depression in the Na^+-K^+ ATPase activity. The magnitude of certain peaks in the SDS-gel electrophoretic pattern was altered but no changes in the sarcolemmal phospholipid composition were seen except that lysophosphatidylcholine contents were increased at 8 weeks hypertrophied hearts. These results have been interpreted to suggest an increase in Ca^{2+}-influx in physiological hypertrophy at 4 weeks of aortic stenosis whereas intracellular Ca^{2+}-overload may occur in pathological hypertrophy due to an increase in Ca^{2+}-influx and a decrease in Ca^{2+}-efflux mechanisms at 8 weeks of aortic stenosis.

REFERENCES

1. Dhalla NS, Ziegelhoffer A, Harrow JAC: Regulatory role of membrane systems in heart function. Can J Physiol Pharmacol (55): 1211-1234, 1977.
2. Dhalla NS, Das PK, Sharma GP: Subcellular basis of cardiac contractile failure. J Mol Cell Cardiol (10): 363-385, 1978.
3. Dhalla NS, Pierce GN, Panagia V, Singal PK, Beamish RE: Calcium movements in relation to heart function. Basic Res Cardiol (77): 117-139, 1982.
4. Bing RJ: The biochemical basis of myocardial failure. Hospital Practice (September): 93-112, 1983.
5. Tomlinson CW, Lee SL, Dhalla NS: Abnormalities in heart membranes and myofibrils during bacterial infective cardiomyopathy in the rabbit. Circ Res (39): 82-92, 1976.
6. Lamers JMJ, Stinis JT, Kort WJ, Hülsman WC: Biochemical studies on the sarcolemmal function in the hypertrophied rabbit heart. J Mol Cell Cardiol (10): 235-248, 1978.

7. Wikman-Coffelt J, Parmley WW, Mason DT: The cardiac hypertrophy
    process. Analyses of factors determining pathological vs physiological
    development. Circ Res (45): 697-707, 1979.
8. Singal PK, Dhillon KS, Panagia V, Dhalla NS: Cardiac muscle function
    during the development of hypertrophy in pigs due to pressure overload.
    In: Jacob R, Gulch RW, Kissling G (eds), Cardiac Adaptation to Hemo-
    dynamic Overload, Training and Stress. Dr. D. Steinkopff, Verlag,
    Darmstadt, 189-196, 1983.
9. Sharma GP, Singal PK, Dhalla NS: Hemodynamic adaptation of the left
    ventricle during aortic stenosis in pigs. J Mol Cell Cardiol (12
    Suppl 1): 151, 1980.
10. Dhalla NS, Anand-Srivastava MB, Tuana BS, Khandelwal RL: Solubilization
    of a calcium dependent adenosine triphosphatase from rat heart
    sarcolemma. J Mol Cell Cardiol (13): 413-423, 1981.
11. Takeo S, Duke P, Taam GML, Singal PK, Dhalla NS: Effects of lanthanum
    on heart sarcolemmal ATPase and calcium binding activities. Can J
    Physiol Pharmacol (57): 497-503, 1979.
12. Dhalla NS, Anand MB, Harrow JAC: Calcium binding and ATPase activities
    of heart sarcolemma. J Biochem (79): 1345-1350, 1976.
13. Harrow JAC, Das PK, Dhalla NS: Influence of some divalent cations
    on heart sarcolemmal bound enzymes and calcium binding. Biochem
    Pharmacol (27): 2605-2609, 1978.
14. Dzurba A, Ganguly PK, Beamish RE, Dhalla NS: Stimulation of calcium
    pump activity in heart sarcolemma by timolol. Can J Physiol
    Pharmacol (61): 240-244, 1983.
15. Alto LE, Dhalla NS: Role of changes in microsomal calcium in the
    effects of reperfusion of Ca^{2+}-deprived rat hearts. Circ Res (48):
    17-24, 1981.
16. Dhalla NS, Alto LE, Heyliger CE, Pierce GN, Panagia V, Singal PK:
    Sarcoplasmic reticular Ca^{2+}-pump adaptation in cardiac hypertrophy
    due to pressure overload in pigs. Europ Heart J: in press, 1983.
17. Pierce GN, Tuana BS, Moffat MP, Singal PK, Panagia V, Dhalla NS:
    Mitochondrial oxidative phosphorylation and calcium transport in
    cardiac hypertrophy due to pressure overload in pigs. This volume.
18. Singal PK, Dhillon KS, Dhalla KS, Sharma GP, Dhalla NS: Contractility
    and myofibrillar adenosine triphosphatase activities in hypertrophied
    pig heart. J Mol Cell Cardiol (12 Suppl 1): 155, 1980.
19. Pierce GN, Kutryk MJB, Dhalla NS: Alterations in Ca^{2+} binding by
    and composition of the cardiac sarcolemmal membrane in chronic
    diabetes. Proc Natl Acad Sci USA (80): 5412-5416, 1983.
20. Owens K, Pang DC, Weglicki WB: Production of lysophospholipids and
    free fatty acids by a sarcolemmal fraction from canine myocardium.
    Biochem Biophys Res Commun (89): 368-373, 1979.
21. Karli JN, Karikas GA, Hatzepavlou PK, Levis Gm, Moulopoulos SN:
    The inhibition of Na^+ and K^+ stimulated ATPase activity of rabbit
    and dog heart sarcolemma by lysophosphatidylcholine. Life Sci
    (24): 1869-1876, 1976.
22. Sedlis SP, Corr PB, Sobel BE, Ahumade GG: Lysophatidylcholine
    potentiates Ca^{2+} accumulation in rat cardiac myocytes. Am J Physiol
    (244): H32-H38, 1983.
23. Dhalla NS, Dzurba A, Pierce GN, Tregaskis MG, Panagia V and Beamish
    RE: Membrane changes in myocardium during catecholamine-induced
    pathological hypertrophy. Perspect Cardiovasc (7): 527-534, 1983.

18

STRUCTURAL ALTERATIONS IN THE HYPERTROPHIED AND FAILING MYOCARDIUM

SANFORD P. BISHOP, D.V.M., PH.D.

1. INTRODUCTION

The increase in size of the heart which occurs in response to a variety of physiological and pathological stimuli is well known and a number of studies have characterized the morphologic features of cardiac hypertrophy. During normal growth of the heart from the early neonatal period when myocyte cell division normally ceases to the adult stage, there is a remarkable increase in heart size and cell volume, ranging from 20 to 40 times, depending on species (1). During this period of rapid cellular hypertrophy, the relative organelle composition of the myocyte remains nearly constant (2,3). Exercise induced cardiac hypertrophy, or physiologic hypertrophy, results in few ultrastructural alterations in the cardiac myocytes or interstitial tissue (4), but is associated with an increase in the capillary concentration in young rats (5-8). Cardiac hypertrophy associated with sustained increase in work load, sublethal ischemia or toxic injury, however, is associated with a variety of structural alterations involving the blood vessels, interstitial tissue, and the myocytes (9-15). Progression of cardiac hypertrophy to myocardial failure is accompanied by further morphologic alterations (9,10,16-19), but these have received much less study than those present in compensated cardiac hypertrophy. This is, in part, due to the paucity of suitable animal models. The purpose of this review is to describe the structural alterations present in the hypertrophied and failing myocardium.

Cardiac hypertrophy is well recognized as a common and nearly constant feature of chronic congestive heart failure. The Framingham Study has underscored the relationship between cardiac hypertrophy and the development of congestive heart failure (20). Electrocardiographic evidence of left ventricular hypertrophy in the Framingham cohort was strongly associated with both ischemic heart disease and hypertension.

Persons with definite electrocardiographic evidence of left ventricular hypertrophy had 10 times the risk of developing congestive heart failure as those with normal electrocardiograms. Although the mechanisms responsible for the conversion of stable hypertrophy to myocardial failure are poorly understood, it is clear that the presence of cardiac hypertrophy is an ominous harbinger of congestive heart failure. In the Framingham study, persons with the largest hearts as indicated by electrocardiographic and radiographic evidence were the most likely to develop congestive heart failure (21). However, heart size is not an absolute predictor of congestive heart failure since we have often noted patients at autopsy with large hearts of over 700 grams without failure, and other hearts with less than two times increase in mass from patients who died in myocardial failure. Since cardiac hypertrophy is a response to a wide variety of stimuli, it is not surprising that not all hypertrophied hearts are equally susceptible to development of congestive heart failure.

Many structural alterations have been identified in nypertrophied myocardium, but the significance of any of these remains conjectural. Identification of specific alterations which could serve as indicators of impending myocardial failure would be of considerable interest from both an experimental point of view and for evaluation of biopsy material from patients. In a recently published study (22), there was a strong correlation between length of survival and the severity of ultrastructural changes in the myocardium of patients who had aortic or mitral valve replacement. Myocardial biopsies were obtained during valve replacement surgery from 44 patients who were then followed for more than 10 years. Early deaths occurred in patients with the most severe ultrastructural changes. These changes included decreased myofibril volume percent from 53 to 31, decreased mitochondrial volume percent from 30 to 23, increased intracellular space from 10 to 30 percent, increased numbers of myelin figures and increased alterations of Z-bands consisting of clumping, fragmentation, and accumulation of irregular extensions of Z-band material. The patients with the most severe changes had the highest incidence of early death due to cardiac failure, and many patients with minimal changes survived longer than 10 years. Therefore, although the extent of cardiac enlargement was not evaluated in this study, there was a good correlation with the severity of ultrastructural alterations and the length of survival. Severe alterations were clearly associated with imminent or irreversible myocardial failure. These authors did not attempt to correlate the ultrastructural changes with the degree of cardiac hypertrophy or the clinical stage of congestive heart failure. Therefore, ultrastructural features of compensated cardiac hypertrophy which might serve as predictors of myocardial failure could not be identified in this study.

2. PATHOLOGIC AND PHYSIOLOGIC HYPERTROPHY

In an attempt to classify various forms of cardiac hypertrophy, the terms physiologic and pathologic hypertrophy have been used to refer to hypertrophy associated with either normal or abnormal function, biochemistry and structure, respectively (23,24). Physiologic hypertrophy generally refers to the increase in cell size associated with functions within the range of normal, including normal growth and exercise. Exercise-induced cardiac hypertrophy may result in up to 30% or more increase in heart mass, but no alterations in myocardial cell structure have been found other than an increase in cell size (4,8), and muscle function and biochemical composition have been reported as either normal or augmented (23,24). Pathologic hypertrophy, on the other hand, is used to refer to enlarged heart muscle cells which do have alterations in structure, function and biochemical composition considered to be detrimental to the cell. It is clear that within the pathologically hypertrophied heart there is a wide range of alterations ranging from barely detectable to very severe. It is also clear that a compensated state of myocardial hypertrophy may exist in which there are alterations in cellular structure, altered biochemical composition and depressed function, but not of sufficient severity as to result in frank congestive myocardial failure. The division between compensated myocardial hypertrophy and decompensated hypertrophy or myocardial failure is not clear, and the point where irreversible changes have occurred is not defined.

An important question is whether hypertrophy proceeds through a series of programmed steps from mild early stages characteristic of physiologic hypertrophy to chronic stable or compensated hypertrophy, and finally to myocardial failure, or alternatively, that physiologic hypertrophy and pathologic hypertrophy are two entirely separate and unrelated processes. Many investigators have used the model of exercise induced cardiac hypertrophy to study various aspects of the process, but there is no evidence that such physiologic hypertrophy ever proceeds on to myocardial failure in the absence of some other induced stress on the heart. Recent studies by Scheuer and coworkers (25) have suggested that exercise induced physiologic hypertrophy may have a protective effect against the debilitating functional and biochemical alterations associated with pathological hypertrophy induced by chronic renal hypertension. In their studies, exercise induced hypertrophy resulted in increased muscle contractility and a shift in myosin ATPase isozymes toward the V1 type associated with faster contractility. When chronic renal hypertension was superimposed on exercise induced hypertrophy in these rats, the contractile function was less depressed, and there was less V3 ATPase isozyme than occurred with renal hypertension alone, although the degree of hypertrophy was greater in animals with both treatments than in either group alone. These studies support the concept that physiologic and pathologic hypertrophy are two separate entities. Whether these results will hold true for other models of pathologic hypertrophy and in other species will require additional testing.

3. BLOOD VESSELS IN CARDIAC HYPERTROPHY
3.1. <u>Large epicardial coronary arteries.</u>

Evaluation of the size of the larger coronary arteries in hypertrophied hearts of both man and experimental animals has produced conflicting results from several investigators. Hutchins et al. (26) confirmed earlier studies by Harrison and Wood (27) and by Lewis and Gotsman (28), that in the absence of significant coronary artery disease, the large coronary arteries of the human heart increase in diameter in proportion to the increase in cardiac mass in hearts up to 1200 grams. Leon and Bloor (29) found that swimming in the rat induced an increase in the coronary vascular bed which paralleled the increase in cardiac mass. These studies were in agreement with previous studies by Tepperman and Perlman (30) and Stevenson et al. (31) who measured the coronary vasculature by corrosion-cast techniques. However, other investigators (32) have demonstrated that some patients have relatively small coronary arteries with increased heart weight and that myocardial infarction is more frequently found at necropsy in this group compared to patients with relatively large coronary vessels. Rodriquez and Robbins (33) found that total coronary capacity as measured by injected barium gelatin mass did not keep pace with the increased heart size in hypertrophied human hearts. Therefore, it appears that in some forms of cardiac hypertrophy, especially that induced by exercise, there is an increase in the size of the major epicardial coronary arteries. However, large vessel size does not keep pace with increase in cardiac mass in all forms of hypertrophy, and may be a contributing factor to reduced delivery of blood to the myocardium under conditions of maximum flow demand.

3.2. <u>Intramyocardial coronary arteries and arterioles.</u>

The intramural arteries and arterioles are subject to intimal and medial changes which may result in narrowing of the lumen. Such changes have been described in a variety of conditions in the human heart including cardiac hypertrophy (for a review, see ref. 34). In experimental animals, O'Keefe (35) has described a thickening of the coronary arterial medial wall in dogs with chronic hypertension induced cardiac hypertrophy. In the spontaneously hypertensive rat, Folkow et al. (36,37) have demonstrated an increase in the wall to lumen ratio in muscular arteries in skeletal muscle. Intimal proliferations are commonly encountered in small coronary arteries of aging SHR (38, personal observations) and also are constant findings in both dogs (39) and humans (40) with congenital subaortic or valvular aortic stenosis. Therefore, several conditions resulting in increased wall stress have been reported to be associated with abnormalities of the resistance vessels in the heart which could be a major factor responsible for the decrease in coronary vascular reserve found in both experimental animals (41,42) and human hearts (43) with hypertrophy due to aortic stenosis. Although good correlative studies of these lesions and presence of myocardial failure have not been done, both man and dogs with aortic valvular or subvalvular stenosis are highly prone to development of irreversible myocardial failure (39,40).

3.3. <u>Capillaries.</u>

Morphologic studies have generally demonstrated a decrease in capillary density in models with pressure overload induced cardiac hypertrophy (44-49). The decreased capillary density is presumably due to an increase in cross-sectional area of the hypertrophied myocyte, which produces a dilution of the number of capillaries per square unit area. Although demonstration of the decrease in capillary density in cardiac hypertrophy is an important finding, only a few studies (50,51) have evaluated capillary vascular space, capillary diameter, or capillary lumen surface area in models of severe cardiac hypertrophy. These measurements, as well as determination of the variability of maximum diffusion distance in hypertrophied myocardium are important measurements to be evaluated. Techniques for their measurement have recently been reviewed by Rakusan (52).

It has been proposed for many years that a factor in the development of myocardial failure is the increased diffusion distance from the capillaries to the energy producing organelles of the hypertrophied myocytes (46,47,53). Many studies have shown that with pressure overload induced cardiac hypertrophy, the number of capillaries does not increase, with resulting increase in intercapillary distance (54). However, this hypothesis assumes that oxygen diffusion through tissue is strictly dependent upon distance and ignores facilitated oxygen transport by myoglobin, or possible preferential location of mitochondria in regions of the myocyte closest to the capillaries. More recent studies by Honig and Goyeski (55) have suggested that diffusion distance is unlikely to be a limiting factor in delivery of oxygen to tissue. A more likely candidate for limitation of oxygen transport is the amount of capillary surface area per unit of tissue. Experimental validation of this hypothesis remains to be obtained.

In volume overload induced myocardial hypertrophy, in contrast to pressure load induced hypertrophy, several investigators have reported an increase in capillary density suggesting a proliferation of endothelial cells and capillaries (5-8,56). Exercise induced cardiac hypertrophy (5-8,56) and dipyridamole induced volume overload in the rat (57) and pig (58) have been shown to cause a proliferation of capillary endothelial cells in the myocardium. With such an increase in capillary density in the myocardium, one might expect a protective effect against the development of myocardial failure. Ljungqvist (59) has demonstrated that rats with cardiac hypertrophy induced by chronic swimming exercise have a smaller infarct size following coronary ligation compared to normal rats or rats with hypertension induced cardiac hypertrophy. On the other hand, other investigators have shown that dogs with pressure overload induced cardiac hypertrophy have larger infarcts and increased mortality following coronary ligation than dogs without cardiac hypertrophy (60,61). Therefore, it appears that exercise induced hypertrophy may have a protective effect against the development of myocardial failure, possibly mediated through the increased number of capillaries, while pressure overload induced hypertrophy increases the risk of acute myocardial infarction.

4. CONNECTIVE TISSUE

The role of connective tissue content in the myocardium in the development of cardiac hypertrophy and particularly, myocardial failure, has been controversial, and there are conflicting reports in the literature. Although commonly believed that connective tissue is increased in the hypertrophied heart, the issue is obscured by the frequent presence of ischemic coronary artery disease in hypertrophied human hearts. Several studies have examined the hydroxyproline content of the hypertrophied heart in the absence of obstructive coronary artery disease, and generally have failed to find increased hydroxyproline content in hypertrophy when compared to age matched controls (62-64). However, some reports have identified a positive correlation of cardiac hypertrophy and interstitial connective tissue (65). In a recent morphometric study of tissue sections, an increase in stainable collagen was found in hypertrophied human hearts. This increased connective tissue was most pronounced in those patients with hypertrophy plus myocardial failure (66).

Evaluation of the connective tissue content is often done by chemical measurement of hydroxyproline content of tissue. However, results must be interpreted with caution since the heart contains other hydroxyproline-containing proteins such as elastin, as well as several molecular species of collagen which vary in hydroxyproline content (67). Nevertheless, useful qualitative information may be obtained from hydroxyproline determinations, and comparison may be made between different regions within the myocardium. Morphologic evaluation of histologically stained collagen provides useful information concerning the distribution of connective tissue in the heart, but the method is less sensitive than hydroxyproline measurement, and is also subject to imprecise specificity. However, morphometric evaluation of stained collagen in tissue sections combined with biochemical determination of hydroxyproline does provide useful information.

In situations considered to represent physiologic hypertrophy, the connective tissue response is absent or mild (68). In most types of congenital heart disease, there is minimal connective tissue proliferation. The exception is aortic valvular or subvalvular stenosis, which is characterized by considerable increase in subendocardial connective tissue in dogs (39) and subendocardial ischemia in man (40). In exercise induced hypertrophy, or that associated with thyroxine, there is no increase in the concentration or content of collagen (4,68-70).

In pressure overload induced experimental cardiac hypertrophy, the amount of connective tissue increase has varied depending on several factors including models used and the length of time hypertrophy was present. Hydroxyproline concentration and content has been shown to be increased in the Spontaneously Hypertensive rat (SHR), particularly in the subendocardial areas of the left ventricle (68,71). Histologic examination of the myocardium of SHR reveals multifocal areas of connective tissue which are seen more frequently in older animals. The increased hydroxyproline levels characteristic of SHR appeared even when hypertension was prevented by neonatal immunosympathectomy with nerve growth factor antiserum, although the development of cardiac hypertrophy was not prevented (72). This study indicates that, in this model at least, collagen deposition is not secondary to hypertension-induced myocardial damage. In another study, Lund et al. (71) found that myocardial hydroxyproline concentration was increased in WKY with hypertension induced by sudden constriction of the abdominal aorta but not in age- and sex-matched SHR despite the fact that blood pressure levels were comparable in both groups. These findings indicate that in the SHR the myocardial connective tissue response to pressure overload lags behind myocyte hypertrophy and that growth of connective tissue is less vigorous than that seen in the aortic constriction model. Earlier studies had also demonstrated an increased hydroxyproline content in the myocardium of animals with acute constriction of the aorta or pulmonary artery (68,69,73,74). However, we (75) have previously shown that with experimentally induced sudden pressure overload in the cat and the rabbit, there is multifocal acute necrosis and replacement fibrosis present as early as one day after banding (Fig. 1). These multifocal areas of fibrosis appear to be an artifact of the experimental model, and not the result of cardiac hypertrophy.

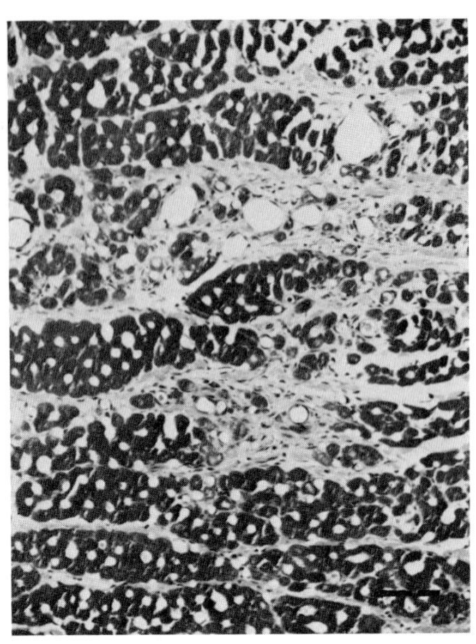

FIGURE 1. Right ventricular free wall of a cat three days after a constricting band was placed on the pulmonary artery. There is focal myocardial necrosis and early replacement fibrosis. Similar lesions were randomly distributed throughout the right ventricular free wall. Gomori aldehyde-fuchsin-trichrome stain. Bar = 100 µm. (Reproduced by permission from the American Heart Association)

In animal models with progressive increase in severity of stenosis such as produced by banding the aorta or pulmonary artery of neonatal or weanling animals, the development of cardiac hypertrophy is often greater than that induced in adult animals, but the amount of connective tissue response has usually been reported as minimal. Fibrosis was not apparent in histologic sections of hypertrophied hearts of dogs with aortic banding from the first week of postnatal life (unpublished observations). Increased hydroxyproline concentration, but not content, has been reported in one study in the cat with progressive pulmonary artery stenosis from weaning (76), but was not found in the rat with aortic banding (77).

In some models of cardiac hypertrophy there is very clearly an increase in the amount of connective tissue in the myocardium. Isoproterenol induced hypertrophy, for example, is associated with increased connective tissue in focal subendocardial areas and increased hydroxyproline associated with a 50 to 60% increase in heart weight (78). In both SHR and the cardiomyopathic hamster there is an increase in connective tissue content compared to non-affected animals of the same species. In SHR, fibrosis increases with age, is multifocal to diffuse and is predominantly subendocardial in distribution (68,79,80). In the myopathic hamster model, fibrosis is multifocal throughout both ventricles, and no further increase in connective tissue occurs after the first few months of age in this model in spite of further increase in heart weight (81). In both SHR and the cardiomyopathic hamster there is decreasing myocardial function with increasing age (82,83), with death due to myocardial congestive failure the eventual outcome in the hamster.

It is reasonable to presume that increased connective tissue content in the heart, particularly if diffusely distributed and surrounding muscle fibers, would result in decreased contractile function and myocardial failure. However, in spite of increased connective tissue content in several animal models and in many human hearts with myocardial failure, there is no direct evidence that increased connective tissue content of the heart is due to cardiac hypertrophy, or that connective tissue plays a role in the development of myocardial failure. Indeed, Schwarz and coworkers (84) failed to find a correlation between increased connective tissue content and diastolic compliance in biopsies from human hearts with hypertrophy due to aortic stenosis. The significance of connective tissue in the development of myocardial failure in the hypertrophied heart, therefore, remains conjectural.

5. MYOFIBERS

During normal growth of the heart and in exercise induced hypertrophy there is a proportional increase in all components of the myocardial cell (2,3). Much attention has been given to identification of structural alterations in the hypertrophied heart in several animal models and in various forms of human myocardial hypertrophy. A number of studies have identified structural alterations in the hypertrophied failing myocardium, but precise identification of those changes associated with compensated hypertrophy versus those found in hypertrophy with failure has been difficult due to a paucity of good animal models and the difficulty of defining the functional limits of compensated and failing myocardium. Structural changes have been identified in the nucleus and other organelles of protein synthesis, the mitochondria, the membrane systems and the contractile apparatus of the myocyte.

5.1. <u>Organelles of protein synthesis.</u>

The nuclear membrane has been noted to have increased folding and tubule formation from the inner membrane in hypertrophied hearts (85). The nucleus is often enlarged in human hearts and polyploidy is increased in both humans (86,87) and in subhuman primates (88). Polyploidy has not been identified in hypertrophy of subprimate species (89-91). The nucleolus has a ribbon-like structure during active development of hypertrophy, and may be multiple, typical of cells actively synthesizing protein. Increased amounts of rough endoplasmic reticulum and prominent Golgi bodies are present in hypertrophying myocardium. However, distinctive abnormalities of these organelles have not been identified with myocardial failure.

5.2. <u>Mitochondria</u>

Mitochondria have been found to be increased in number in cardiac hypertrophy due to thyrotoxicosis (92,93), a condition of increased metabolic activity requiring increased ATP production. In early studies with aortic band induced cardiac hypertrophy in the rat, Meerson (13) reported an initial increase in the volume percent of the myocyte occupied by mitochondria, which returned to normal in compensated cardiac hypertrophy. In later stages of compensated hypertrophy, Meerson identified a decrease in the volume percent mitochondria in hypertrophied myocytes. This decrease in mitochondrial volume percent also occurs in animal models not showing clinical evidence of congestive heart failure such as the SHR (16,79,94), aortic banded (14,15,92) and renal hypertensive rats (10,11,95), and gradually constricted aorta in the rabbit (96). Similarly, there is a decrease in mitochondrial volume percent in hypertrophied human hearts due to aortic stenosis (97) or mitral insufficiency (98). With the development of more advanced stages of cardiac hypertrophy with myocardial failure the number of mitochondria may actually be increased, but the individual mitochondria are smaller than normal with a resulting further decrease in cellular mitochondrial volume percent. The finding of large numbers of small mitochondria by electron microscopy in severely hypertrophied and failing hearts suggests an increased turnover rate of mitochondria with production of immature forms. This is consistent with the finding of reduced mitochondrial protein synthesis in severe hypertrophy (99-101). It might be expected that these immature mitochondria would have decreased ability to produce ATP, a finding reported by some investigators in isolated mitochondria from severely hypertrophied and failing hearts (102,103).

5.3. <u>Contractile apparatus</u>

The organelle ultimately responsible for decrease in contractile function and myocardial failure is the myofibril. The sarcomere, the functional unit of the myofibril, is present in larger numbers in the hypertrophied cell. The cell membranes, including those of the sarcolemma, the intercalated disc, and the sarcoplasmic reticulum, are required to transfer calcium and other ions essential for normal excitation-contraction coupling. Few structural changes have been identified in the sarcoplasmic reticulum or plasma membrane in the hypertrophied or failing myocardium (92), although depressed function has been reported in several models (104).

The intercalated disc has been proposed to have a role in myofibril formation since the 19th century, and more recent electron microscopic evidence supports such a theory (9,79,105). Relatively early in the development of cardiac hypertrophy in several animal models, including progressive pulmonary artery stenosis of dogs (9,105,106), SHR (16), and Goldblatt hypertensive rats (107), an increased folding and tortuosity of the intercalated disc is apparent (Fig. 2). Normally, the longitudinal folding of the intercalated disc is less than 1.0 μm, but in hearts developing hypertrophy, folds greater than 1.0 μm occur. In more advanced stages of hypertrophy the folds may cover the extent of several sarcomere lengths. Loose, unorganized myofilaments are frequently present within the intercalated disc folds, and many are incompletely organized into sarcomeres, suggesting that new sarcomeres are being assembled at the intercalated disc. The expanded folds of the intercalated disc appear to have an increase in myofilament attachment areas (fasciae adherentes), often occuring as multiple short segments. Streaming of the electron-dense material of the filament attachment areas into the adjacent cytoplasm is common. The increased folding often results in redundancies of the disc area with the formation of so-called "multiple intercalated discs" (106). Multiple discs, consisting of repeating units of disc material separated by one to ten sarcomeres, and the increased folds, produce a greater surface area which would be required to augment the assembly of new sarcomeres if

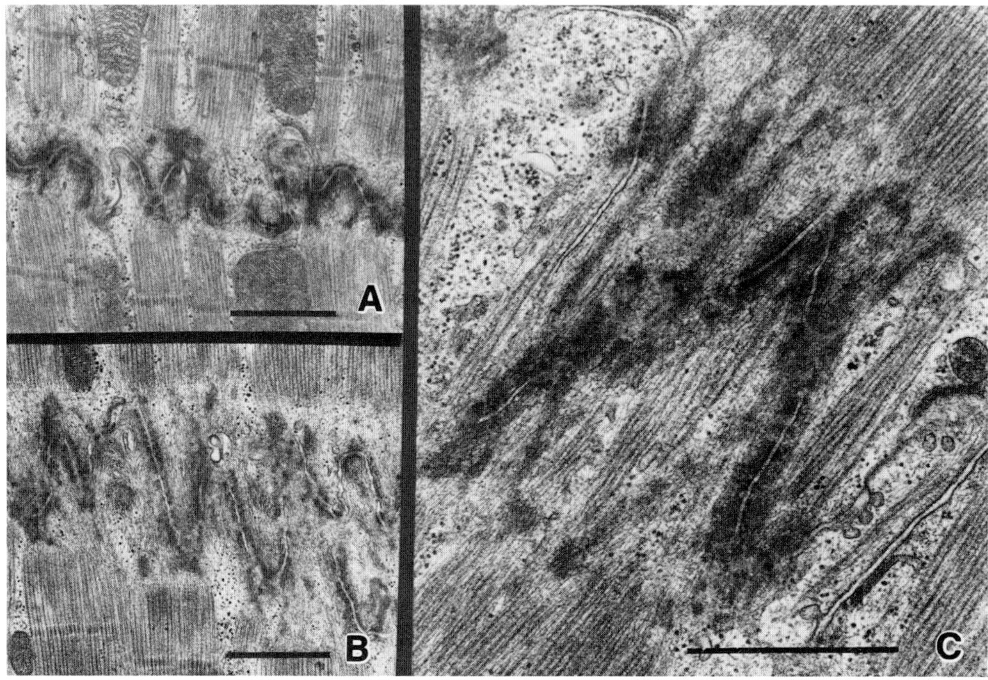

FIGURE 2. A: Intercalated disk from the right ventricle of a normal dog. Bar = 1 µm. B: Intercalated disk from the right ventricle of a dog with developing cardiac hypertrophy due to progressive pulmonary artery stenosis of 4 weeks' duration. Note increased folding. Compare to Fig. 2A. Bar = 1 µm. C: Intercalated disk from the left ventricle an 8-week-old puppy with progressive aortic stenosis due to a band placed on the ascending aorta at 3 days of age. Note streaming of electron-dense material to form Z-lines and numerous thick and thin filaments within the folds, partially organized into sarcomeres. Bar = 1 µm. (Reproduced by permission from Raven Press)

the hypothesis relating intercalated disc myofilament attachment areas to sarcomere assembly is correct. Widened intercalated discs are characteristic of rapidly developing hypertrophy, and appear before functional evidence of myocardial failure is readily detected. In the failing myocardium, such as in older SHR (16) and in dogs with progressive pulmonary artery stenosis (9), the discs become more prominent, and may have folds up to 8-10 microns in width.

Expansion of the Z-line material or Z-line rod body formation occurs in a variety of animals with experimentally induced or naturally occurring hypertrophy and failure (9,16-18,108), and in severely hypertrophied human myocardium (109,110). The expanded Z-lines consist of electron-dense material which may be diffuse in nature, often associated with unorganized sarcomeres (Fig. 3). More often there is a characteristic parallel arrangement of fibrils with an approximate 200-Å spacing. The elctron-dense Z-line material extends in one or both directions from the Z-line and is associated with disruption of the normal uniform lateral register of sarcomeres. Adjacent sarcomeres may be incompletely organized, suggesting an intermediate stage of sarcomere formation. The Z-line expansion may cover areas up to a full sarcomere in length with electron-dense material. The dense material may be incomplete, revealing thin filaments morphologically similar to actin.

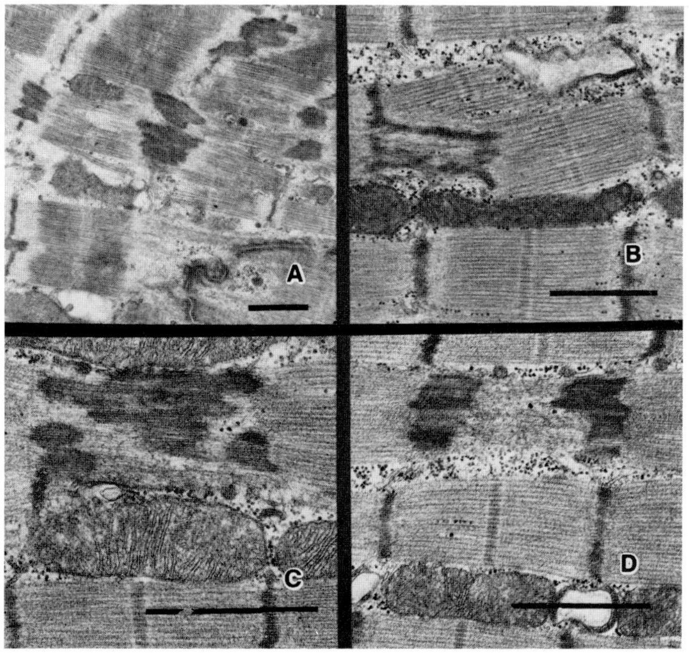

FIGURE 3. Electron micrographs from myocardium of dogs with cardiac hypertrophy and myocardial congestive failure illustrating variations in form of Z-line expansions. A: Multiple symmetrical early expansions of Z-lines. B: Longitudinal displacement of sarcomere by Z-line expansions. C: Z-line expansion to full sarcomere width with partial loss of dense Z-line material. D: Sarcomere with thin filaments but no thick filaments in space between dense Z-line expanions at ends. Bar = 1 μm. (Reproduced by permission from Raven Press)

The expanded Z-line material is found in the myocardium of animals or humans with rapidly developing hypertrophy due to excessive work load. It is a characteristic finding in the hearts of animals with decreased functional capacity such as increased end-diastolic pressure, venous congestion, and fluid accumulation in body space and tissue. It is not present in animal models with mild degrees of hypertrophy such as the aortic-banded rat, or in animals or patients with compensated stages of cardiac hypertrophy. The expanded Z-line appears to be a lesion of pathologic hypertrophy, indicating the presence of myocardial failure.

6. CONCLUSION

The process of enlargement of the heart which occurs during normal growth, during physiological increases in workload such as exercise, and during prolonged overload conditions leading to severe cardiac enlargement and myocardial failure is dynamic and complex. Normally growing cells increase in volume at least 30 times from birth to adulthood, and retain structural intracellular relationship after the neonatal period. With increased functional requirements within the physiologic range, such as exercise, the cells are able to undergo further increase in volume, but cell structural relationships remain proportional. The normal structure of these cells reflects the normal or augmented functional and biochemical properties of these physiologically hypertrophied cells.

In the presence of severe sustained workload as in various disease states, there are structural alterations of the myocardial cells. Whether these structural alterations are merely an extension of the physiologic hypertrophy occurring during normal growth or exercise, or indeed represent a separate process in the cell remains conjectural at the present time. Morphologic changes which occur with prolonged abnormal workloads probably affect all parts of the cell, but are most pronounced in the mitochondria, membranes of the intercalated disc, and the Z-line region of the myofibrils. Mitochondria respond early in the course of pressure overload induced myocardial hypertrophy by an increase in total mass, but in stable stages of hypertrophy return to the normal proportion in the hypertrophied cell. With increasing time, and presumably with the development of early decompensation, the mitochondrial volume density decreases, and in later stages, the mitochondria become small in size although numerous. Increased surface area of the intercalated disc expressed morphologically as increased longitudinal folding, occurs relatively early in the development of sustained workload, and becomes very marked as myocardial failure develops. Expansions of dense Z-line material are found with increasing frequency throughout the severely hypertrophied and failing myocardial cell. These expanded Z-line changes, consisting of electron dense material with a definite periodicity, appear to disrupt the normal lateral alignment of the myocyte and may provide a structural explanation for the decreased functional capacity of the heart. Although the exact role of these Z-line structural alterations remains unclear at the present time, they do appear to be a pathologic marker of failing myocardial tissue. Taken together, these alterations of the mitochondria, intercalated disc and the Z-line, as well as less well characterized changes in other cellular organelles, provide a distinctive morphologic pattern which distinguish the severely hypertrophied and failing heart, or pathologic hypertrophy, from the heart with physiologic hypertrophy associated with normal growth or exercise. Which, if any, of these changes may be associated with irreversible myocardial failure remains to be determined.

ACKNOWLEDGEMENT

This work was supported in part by a grant from the Alabama Heart Association and by National Heart, Lung, and Blood Institute grants RO1HL 23255, RO1HL 27514, Ischemic Heart Disease SCOR P17HL 17667, and Hypertension SCOR P50HL 25451. The author would like to acknowledge the expert assistance of Irene Lynn in the preparation of this manuscript.

References

1.   Zak R: Development and proliferative capacity of cardiac muscle cells. Circ Res (Suppl II) (34-35):II-17-26, 1974.
2.   Page E, Earley J, Power B: Normal growth of ultrastructure in rat left ventricular myocardial cells. Circ Res (Suppl II)(34-35):II-12-16, 1974.
3.   Hirakow R, Gotch T, Watanabe T: Quantitative studies on the ultrastructural differentiation and growth of mammalian cardiac muscle cells. I. The atria and ventricles of the rat. Acta Anat (108):144-152, 1980.
4.   Tomanek RJ, Taunton CA, Liskop KS: Relationship between age, chronic exerise, and connective tissue of the heart. J Gerontol (27):33-38, 1972.
5.   Tomanek RJ: Effects of age and exercise on the extent of the myocardial capillary bed. Anat Rec (167): 55-62, 1970.

6. Ljungqvist A, Unge G: The finer intramyocardial vasculature in various forms of experimental cardiac hypertrophy. Acta Path Microbiol Scand (80):329-340, 1972.

7. Unge G, Carlsson S, Ljungqvist A, Tornling G, Adolfsson J: The proliferative activity of myocardial capillary wall cells in various aged swimming-exercise rats. Acta Pathol Microbiol Scand (87):15-17, 1979.

8. Anversa P, Levicky V, Begi C, McDonald SL, Kikkawa Y: Morphometry of exercised-induced right ventricular hypertrophy in the rat. Circ Res (52):57-63, 1983.

9. Bishop SP, Cole CR: Ultrastructural changes in canine myocardium with right ventricular hypertrophy and congestive heart failure. Lab Invest (20):219-229, 1969.

10. Anversa P, Loud AV Vitali-Mazza L; Morphometry and autoradiography of early hypertrophic changes in the ventricular myocardium of adult rat. An electron microscopic study. Lab Invest (35):475-483, 1976.

11. Anversa P, Loud AV, Giacomelli F, Wiener J: Absolute morphometric study of myocardial hypertrophy in experimental hypertension. II. Ultrastructure of myocytes and interstitium. Lab Invest (38):597-609, 1978.

12. Meerson FZ: The myocardium in hyperfunction, hypertrophy and heart failure. Circ Res (Suppl II) (25):1-163, 1969.

13. Meerson FZ, Zaletayeva TA, Lagutchev SS, Pshennikova MG: Structure and mass of mitochondria in the process of compensatory hyperfunction and hypertrophy of the heart. Exp Cell Res (36):568-578, 1964.

14. Page E, Polimeni PI, Zak R, Earley J, Johnson M: Myofibrillar mass in rat and rabbit heart muscles: Correlation of microchemical and stereological measurements in normal and hypertrophic hearts. Circ Res (30):430-439, 1972.

15. Poche R, DeMello Mattos CM, Rembarz H-W, Stoepel K: Uber das Verhaltnis Mitochondrien zu Myofibrillen in den Herzmuskel Zellen der Ratte bei Druckhypertrophie des Herzens. Virchows Arch Abt A [Pathol Anat] (344):100-110, 1968.

16. Kawamura K, Kashii C, Imamura K: Ultrastructural changes in hypertrophied myocardium of spontaneously hypertensive rats. Jpn Circ J (40):1119-1145, 1976.

17. Schaper J, Thiedemann, KU, Flameng W, Schaper W: The ultrastructure of sarcomeres in hypertrophied canine myocardium in spontaneous subaortic stenosis. Basic Res Cardiol (69):509-515, 1974.

18. Hatt PY, Berjal G, Moravec J, Swynghedauw B: Heart failure: An electron microscopic study of the left ventricular papillary in aortic insufficiency in the rabbit. J Mol Cell Cardiol (1):235-247, 1970.

19. Maron BJ, Ferrans VJ: Ultrastructural features of hypertrophied human ventricular myocardium. Prog Cardiovasc Dis (21):207-238, 1978.

20. Kannel WB, Castelli WP, McNamara PM, McKee PA, Feinleib M: Role of blood pressure in the development of congestive heart failure. The Framingham Study. New Engl J Med (287):781-787, 1972.

21. Kannel WB, Gordon T, Offutt D: Left ventricular hypertrophy by electrocardiogram. Prevalence, incidence and mortality in the Framingham Study. Ann Intern Med (71):89-101, 1969.

22. Slezak J, Geller SA, Litwak RS, Smith Jr H: Long-term study of the ultrastructural changes of myocardium in patients undergoing cardiac surgery, with more than 10 years follow-up. Int J Cardiol (4):153-168, 1983.

23. Scheuer J, Bhan AK: Brief Reviews: Cardiac contractile proteins: Adenosine triphosphatase activity and physiological function. Circ Res (45):1-12, 1979.

24. Wikman-Coffelt J, Parmley WW, Mason DT: The cardiac hypertrophy process: Analyses of factors determining pathological vs physiological development. Circ Res (45):696-707, 1979.

25. Scheuer J, Malhotra A, Hirsch C, Capasso J, Schaible T: Physiologic cardiac hypertrophy corrects contractile protein abnormalities associated with pathologic hypertrophy in rats. J Clin Invest (70):1300-1305, 1982.

26. Hutchins GM, Bulkley BH, Miner MM, Boitnott JK: Correlation of age and heart weight with tortuosity and caliber of normal human coronary arteries. Am Heart J (94):196-202, 1977.

27. Harrison CV, Wood P: Hypertensive and ischemic heart disease: A comparative clinical and pathological study. Br Heart J (11):205-229, 1949.

28. Lewis BS, Gotsman MS: Relation between coronary artery size and left ventricular wall mass. Br Heart J (35):1150-1153, 1973.

29. Leon AS, Bloor CM: Effects of exercise and its cessation on the heart and its blood supply. J Appl Physiol (24):485, 1968.

30. Tepperman J, Perlman D: Effects of exercise and anemia on coronary arteries of small animals as revealed by the corrosion-cast technique. Circ Res (9):576-584, 1961.

31. Stevenson JAF, Feleki V, Rechnitzer P, Beaton JR: Effect of exercise on coronary tree size in the rat. Circ Res (15):265-269, 1964.

32. Wilens SL, Plair CM, Henderson D: Size of the major epicardial coronary arteries at necropsy. JAMA (198):1325-1329, 1966.

33. Rodriquez FL, Robbins SL: Capacity of human coronary arteries. A postmortem study. Circulation (19):570-578, 1959.

34. Geer JC, Bishop SP, James TN: Pathology of small intramural coronary arteries. In: Sommers SC, Rosen PP (ed) Pathology Annual. Part 2. Appleton-Century-Crofts, New York, 1979, pp. 125-154.

35. O'Keefe DD, Hoffman JIE, Cheitlin R, O'Neil MJ, Allard JR, Shapkin E: Coronary blood flow in experimental canine left ventricular hypertrophy. Circ Res (43):43-51, 1978.

36. Folkow B, Hallback M, Lundgren Y, Weiss L: Background of increased flow resistance and vascular reactivity in spontaneously hypertensive rats. Acta Physiol Scand (80):93-106, 1970.

37. Folkow B, Hallback M, Lundgren Y, Weiss L: Structurally based increase of flow resistance in spontaneously hypertensive rats. Acta Physiol Scand (79):373-379, 1970.

38. Ohtaka M: Vectorcardiographical and pathological approach to the relationship between cardiac hypertrophy and coronary arteriosclerosis in spontaneously hypertensive rats (SHR). Jpn Circ J (44):283-293, 1980.

39. Flickinger GL, Patterson DF: Coronary lesions associated with congenital subaortic stenosis in the dog. J Path Bact (93):133, 1967.

40. Lewis AB, Heymann MA, Stanger P, Hoffman JIE, Rudolph AM: Evaluation of subendocardial ischemia in valvar aortic stenosis in children. Circulation (49):987-984, 1974.
41. Rembert JC, Klienman LH, Fedor JM, Greenfield JC, Wechsler AS: Myocardial blood flow distribution in concentric left ventricular hypertrophy. J Clin Invest (21):379-386, 1978.
42. Bache, RJ, Vrobel TR, Ring WS, Emery, RW, Andersen, RW: Regional myocardial blood flow during exercise in dogs with chronic left ventricular hypertrophy. Circ Res (48):76-87, 1981.
43. Marcus M, Doty DB, Hiratzka LF, Wright CB, Eastham CI: Decreased coronary reserve. A mechanism for angina pectoris in patients with aortic stenosis and normal coronary arteries. N Eng J Med (307):1362-1367, 1982.
44. Breisch EA, Houser SR, Carey RA, Spann JF, Bove AA: Myocardial blood flow and capillary density in chronic pressure overload of the feline left ventricle. Cardiovasc Res (14):469-475, 1980.
45. Rakusan K: Quantitative morphology of capillaries of the heart. Number of capillaries in animal and human hearts under normal and pathological conditions. Meth Achievm Exp Path (5):272, 1971.
46. Roberts JT, Wearn JT, Boten I: Quantitative changes in the capillary muscle relationship in human hearts during normal growth and hypertrophy. Am Heart J (21):617-633, 1941.
47. Shipley RA, Shipley LJ, Wearn JT: The capillary supply in normal and hypertrophied hearts of rabbits. J Exp Med (65):29-44, 1936.
48. Turek Z, Grandtner M, Kreuzer F: Cardiac hypertrophy, capillary and muscle fiber density, muscle fiber diameter, capillary radius and diffusion distance in the myocardium of growing rats adapted to a simulated altitude of 3500 m. Pfluegers Arch (335):19-28, 1972.
49. Murray PA, Vatner SF; Reduction of maximal coronary vasodilator capacity in conscious dogs with severe right ventricular hypertrophy. Circ Res (48):25-33, 1981.
50. Rakusan K, Moravec J, Hatt PY: Regional capillary supply in the normal and hypertrophied rat heart. Microvasc Res (20):319-326, 1980.
51. Turek Z, Rakusan K: Log normal distribution of intercapillary distance in normal and hypertrophic rat heart as estimated by the method of concentric circles: its effect on tissue oxygenation. Pflugers Arch (391):17-21, 1981.
52. Rakusan K: Assessment of cardiac growth. In: Zak R (ed) Growth of the Heart in Health and Disease. Raven Press, New York, (in press 1983)
53. Wearn JT: Morphological and functional alterations of the coronary circulation. Harvey Lec 243-270, 1940.
54. Henquell L, Odoroff CL, Honig CR: Intercapillary distance and capillary reserve in hypertrophied rat hearts beating in situ. Circ Res (41):400-408, 1977.
55. Honig CR, Gayeski TEJ: Capillary reserve and tissue O2 transport in normal and hypertrophied hearts. In: Tarazi RC, Dunbar JB (ed) Perspectives in Cardiovascular Research, Vol. 8 Myocardial Hypertrophy and Failure, Raven Press, New York, 1983, pp 249-260.
56. Bloor CM, Leon AS: Interactions of age and exercise on the heart and its blood supply. Lab Invest (22):160-165, 1970.
57. Tornling G, Unge G, Skoog L, Ljungqvist A, Carlsson S, Adolfsson J: Proliferative activity of myocardial capillary wall cells in dipyridamole-treated rats. Cardiovasc Res (12):692-695, 1978.

58. Nakagawa Y, Keisuke T, Katano Y, Matsubara I, Nabata H, Nakazawa M, Hashimoto T, Sakurai H, Ogasawara S, Yokoyama H, Otorii T, Imai S: Development of coronary collateral circulation in miniature swine and effects of several drugs. Jpn J Pharmacol (29):271-284, 1979.

59. Tornling G, Carlsson S, Unge G, Ljungqvist A: The effect of increased cardiac pressure load and volume load on the size of myocardial infarction following coronary artery occlusion. Acta Pathol Microbiol Scand (89):309-312, 1981.

60. Koyanagi S, Eastham C, Marcus ML: Effects of chronic hypertension and left ventricular hypertrophy on the incidence of sudden cardiac death after coronary artery occlusion in conscious dogs. Circulation (65):1192-1197, 1982.

61. Koyanagi S, Eastham C, Harrison DG, Marcus ML: Increased size of myocardial infarction in dogs with chronic hypertension and left ventricular hypertrophy. Circ Res (50):55-62, 1982.

62. Blumgart H, Gilligan DR, Schlesinger MJ: The degree of myocardial fibrosis in normal and pathological hearts as estimated chemically by the collagen content. Trans Assoc Am Physicians (55):313-325, 1940.

63. Montfort I, Perez-Tamayo R: The muscle collagen ratio in normal and hypertrophic human hearts. Lab Invest (11):463-470, 1962.

64. Oken DE, Boucek RJ: Quantitation of collagen in human myocardium. Cir Res (5):357-361, 1957.

65. Fuster V, Danielson MA, Robb RA, Broadbent JC, Brown AL Jr, Elveback LR: Quantitation of left ventricular myocardial fiber hypertrophy and interstitial tissue in human hearts with chronically increased volume and pressure overload. Circulation (55):504-508, 1977.

66. Pearlman ES, Weber KT, Janicki JS, Fishman AP, Pietra GG: Muscle fiber orientation and connective tissue content in the hypertrophied human heart. Lab Invest (46):158-164, 1982.

67. Miller EJ: Biochemical characteristics and biological significance of the genetically distinct collagens. Mol Cell Biochem (130):165-192, 1976.

68. Medugorac I: Myocardial collagen in different forms of heart hypertrophy in the rat. Res Exp Med (Berl) (177):201-211, 1980.

69. Bartosova D, Chvapil M, Korechy B, Poupa O, Rakusan K, Turek Z, Vizek M: Growth of the muscular and collagenous parts of the rat heart in various forms of cardiomegaly. J Physiol (Lond) (200):285-295, 1969.

70. von Knorring EJ, Lindy S, Turto H: Heart volume and myocardial connective tissue during development and regression of thyroxine induced cardiac hypertrophy in rats. Acta Physiol Scand (97):(4)514-518, 1976.

71. Lund DD, Twietmeyer TA, Schmid PG, Tomanek RJ: Independent changes in cardiac muscle fibers and connective tissue in rats with spontaneous hypertension, aortic constriction and hypoxia. Cardiovasc Res (13):39-44, 1979.

72. Cutilletta AF, Erinoff L, Heller A, Low J, Oparil S: Development of left ventricular hypertrophy in young spontaneously hypertensive rats after peripheral sympathectomy. Circ Res (40):428-434, 1977.

73. Buccino RA, Harris E, Spann JF Jr., Sonnenblick EH: Response of myocardial connective tissue to development of experimental hypertrophy. Am J Physiol (216):425-528, 1969.

74. Caspari PG, Newcomb M, Gibson K, Harris P: Myocardial collagen, the effects of right ventricular hypertrophy and its involution induced by changes in atmospheric pressure. Cardiovasc Res (12):173-178, 1978.

75. Bishop SP, Melsen LR: Myocardial necrosis, fibrosis, and DNA synthesis in experimental cardiac hypertrophy induced by sudden overload. Circ Res (39):238-245, 1976.

76. Cooper G,IV, Tomanek RJ, Ehrhardt JC, Marcus ML: Chronic progressive pressure overload of the cat right ventricle. Circ Res (48):488-497, 1981.

77. Julian FJ, Morgan DL, Moss RL, Gonzalez M, Dwivedi P: Myocyte growth without physiological impairment in gradually induced rat cardiac hypertrophy. Cir Res (49):1300-1310, 1981.

78. Stanton HC, Brenner G, Mayfield ED Jr: Studies on isoproterenol-induced cardiomegaly in rats. Am Heart J (77):72-80, 1969.

79. Lund DD, Tomanek RJ: Myocardial morphology in spontaneously hypertensive and aortic-constricted rats. Am J Anat (152):141-152, 1978.

80. Pfeffer MA, Frohlich ED: Hemodynamic and myocardial function in young and old normotensive and spontaneously hypertensive rats. Circ Res (Suppl 1) (32/33):28-35, 1973.

81. Gertz E, Stam AC, Sonnenblick EH: Dissociation of collagen proliferation from hypertrophy in experimental cardiomyopathy. Am J Cardiol (26):634, 1970.

82. Pfeffer J, Pfeffer M, Fletcher P, Braunwald E: Alterations of cardiac performance in rats with established spontaneous hypertension. Am J Cardiol (44):994-998, 1979.

83. Forman R, Parmley WW, Sonnenblick EH: Myocardial contractility in relation to hypertrophy and failure in myopathic Syrian hamsters. J Mol Cell Cardiol (4):203-211, 1972.

84. Schwarz F, Flameng W, Schaper J, Hehrlein F: Correlation between myocardial structure and diastolic properties of the heart in chronic aortic valve disease: Effects of corrective surgery. Am J Cardiol (42):895-903, 1978.

85. Ferrans VJ, Jones M. Maron BJ, Roberts WC: The nuclear membrane in hypertrophied human cardiac muscle cells. Am J Pathol (78):427-460, 1975.

86. Eisenstein R, Wied GL: Myocardial DNA and protein in maturing and hypertrophied human hearts. Proc Soc Exp Biol Med (133):176-179, 1970.

87. Kompmann M, Paddags I, Sandritter W: Feulgen cytophotometric DNA determinations on human hearts. Arch Pathol (82):303-308, 1966.

88. Pfitzer P: Polyploide Zellkerne im Herzmuskel von Affen. Virchows Arch Abt B Zellpath (10):268-274, 1972.

89. Pfitzer P: Polyploide Zellkerne im Herzmuskel von Tieren. Verh Dtsch Ges Pathol (55):801, 1971.

90. Kuhn H, Pfitzer P, Stoepel K: DNA content and DNA synthesis in the myocardium of rats after induced renal hypertension. Cardiovasc Res (8):86-91, 1974.

91. Grove D, Nair KG, Zak R: Biochemical correlates of cardiac hypertrophy. III. Changes in DNA content; the relative contributions of polyploidy and mitotic activity. Circ Res (25):463-471, 1969.

92. Page E, McCallister LP: Quantitative electron microscopic description of heart muscle cells. Application to normal, hypertrophied and thyroxine-stimulated hearts. Am J Cardiol (31):172-181, 1973.
93. McCallister LP, Page E: Effects of thyroxin on ultrastructure of rat myocardial cells: A stereological study. J Ultrastruct Res (42):136-155, 1973.
94. Page E, Oparil S: Effect of peripheral sympathectomy on left ventricular ultrastructure in young spontaneously hypertensive rats. J Mol Cell Cardiol (10):301-305, 1978.
95. Weiner J, Giacomelli F, Loud AV, Anversa P: Morphometry of cardiac hypertrophy induced by experimental renal hypertension. Am J Cardiol (22):909-929, 1979.
96. Goldstein MA, Sordahl LA, Schwartz A: Ultrastructural analysis of left ventricular hypertrophy in rabbits. J Mol Cell Cardiol (6):265-273, 1974.
97. Warmuth H, Fleischer M. Themann H, Achatzy RS, Dittrich H: Feinstrukturell-morphometrische Befunde an der Kammerwand Hypertrophierter Menschlisher linker Ventrikel. Virchows Arch [Pathol Anat] (380):135-147, 1978.
98. Fleischer M, Wippo W, Themann H, Achatzy RS: Ultrastructural morphometric analysis of human myocardial left ventricles with mitral insufficiency. A comparison with normally loaded and hypertrophied left ventricles. Virchows Archiv A [Pathol Anat] (389):205-210, 1980.
99. Sordahl LA: Mitochondrial changes in pressure-overload hypertrophy and failure. In: Alpert NR (ed) Perspectives in Cardiovascular Research, Vol. 7 Myocardial Hypertrophy and Failure. Raven Press, New York, 1983, pp 535-540.
100. Rabinowitz M, Zak R: Biochemical and cellular changes in cardiac hypertrophy. Annu Rev Med (23):245, 1972.
101. Rabinowitz M and Zak R: Mitochondria and cardiac hypertrophy. Circ Res (36):367-376, 1975.
102. Lindenmayer GE, Sordahl LA, Schwartz A: Reevaluation of oxidative phosphorylation in cardiac mitochondria from normal animals and animals in heart failure. Circ Res (23):439-450, 1969.
103. Sordahl LA, McCollum WB, Wood WG, Schwartz A: Mitochondria and sarcoplasmic reticulum function in cardiac hypertrophy and failure. Am J Physiol (224):497-502, 1973.
104. Scheuer J: Alteration in sarcoplasmic reticulum in cardiac hypertrophy. In: Tarazi RC, Dunbar JB (ed) Perspectives in Cardiovascular Research, vol 8: Cardiac Hypertrophy in Hypertension. Raven Press, New York, 1983, pp 111-122.
105. Adomian GE, Laks MM, Morady F, Swan HJC: Significance of the multiple intercalated disc in the hypertrophied canine heart. J Mol Cell Cardiol (6):105-110, 1974.
106. Laks MM, Morady R, Adomian GE, Swan HJC: Presence of widened and multiple intercalated discs in the hypertrophied canine heart. Circ Res (27):391-402, 1970.
107. Wendt-Gallitelli MF, Ebrecht G, Jacob R: Morphological alteration and their functional interpretation in the hypertrophied myocardium of Goldblatt hypertensive rats. J Mol Cell Cardiol (11):275-287, 1979.

108. Bishop SP: Effect of aortic stenosis on myocardial cell growth, hyperplasia, and ultrastructure in neonatal dogs. In: Dhalla NS (ed) Recent Advances in Studies on Cardiac Structure and Metabolism, Vol. 3 Myocardial Metabolism. University Park Press, Baltimore, 1973, pp 637-656.
109. Ferrans VJ, Morrow AG, Roberts WC: Myocardial ultrastructure in idiopathic hypertrophic subaortic stenosis. Circulation (45):769-792, 1972.
110. Legato MJ: Sarcomerogenesis in human myocardium. J Mol Cell Cardiol (1):425-437, 1970.

19

MYOCARDIAL FAILURE - THE MISMATCH OF SUBCELLULAR ADAPTIVE CHANGES[*]

NORMAN R. ALPERT, LOUIS A. MULIERI, RAYE Z. LITTEN, ROBERT GOULETTE, LINDSEY SCHINE. DEPARTMENT OF PHYSIOLOGY AND BIOPHYSICS, UNIVERSITY OF VERMONT COLLEGE OF MEDICINE, BURLINGTON, VERMONT 05405

INTRODUCTION

When myocardial contraction is inadequate or when the circulatory needs of the organism are increased the heart responds by increasing the cardiac output. The short term response to a deficient cardiac output is mediated mainly by the Frank-Starling mechanisms (change in sarcomere length) (1,2) and an increase in both the heart rate (3) and sympathetic tone (4). A prolonged increase in demand (hypertensive heart disease, aortic or pulmonary stenosis, arterio-venous fistula, valvular insufficiency, thyrotoxicosis, exercise) is met by myocardial hypertrophy. If the myocytes did not hypertrophy, con- gestive heart failure would occur (5,6,7). The increase in mass is not the arithmetic addition of identical subunits. Reorganization occurs at the organ, cellular and subcellular level leading to a spectrum of outcomes ranging from compensated hypertrophy to congestive heart failure. Further- more, in the compensated hypertrophied heart there are a range of responses from the slow contraction produced by pressure overload to the speeding up of the response in thyrotoxicosis.

We speculate that, in compensated hypertrophy, the heart uses a reper- toire of matched functional and molecular changes which recapitulate some of those seen in evolution and development (8). Support for this view is found in the following comparisons: 1) frog versus tortoise skeletal muscles (9,10,11); 2) fast (extensor digitorum longus, EDL), slow (soleus, SOL) and developing mammalian skeletal muscles (12,13); and 3) hearts hypertrophied secondary to thyrotoxicosis (T) versus pressure overload (P)(14). The func- tional and molecular changes of interest are mechanical performance, con- tractile protein ATPase and myothermal economy of isometric force development. Comparing frog with tortoise and EDL with SOL, in the first of each pair, the

*Supported in part by USPHS Grant PHS 28001

maximum velocity of shortening and myosin ATPase are greater while the curvature of the force velocity relationship (high a/P_o), the economy of isometric
force maintenance and time to peak tension are lower (Figs. 1A & 1B)(Table 1)
(9-13,15-18). The similarity of the comparisons above and those found between
pressure overload and thyrotoxic hypertrophy are striking. The P
hypertrophied hearts exhibit a decrease in the maximum unloaded velocity of
shortening, an increase in the force velocity curvature, an increase in

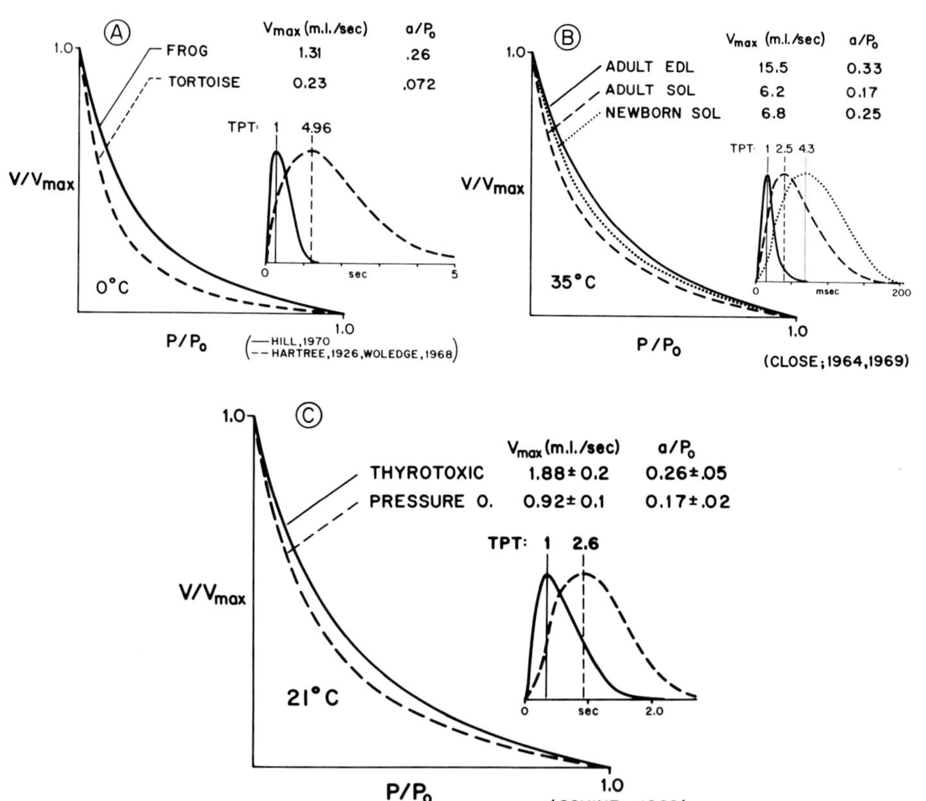

Figure 1. Normalized force velocity curves and isometric twitch records for
for frog and tortoise muscle (A), rat extensor digitorum longus (EDL), adult
and newborn soleus muscle(SOL)(B) and rabbit pressure overload and thyrotoxic
hypertrophied heart papillary muscles (C). Unloaded shortening velocity and
the ratio a/P_o are tabulated in the upper right hand corner. The ratio a/P_o
is inversely related to the force velocity curvature and is derived from the
classic Hill equation $(P + a)(V + b) = b(P_o + a)$ where "a", "b" and "P_o" are
constants for a given muscle (17). (Redrawn from 8)

time to peak tension and an increase in the economy of isometric force
maintenance (Fig. 1C)(Table 1)(14,19). The T hypertrophied hearts show an
increase in maximum velocity of shortening, a decrease in the force velocity
curvature, a decrease in time to peak tension and a decrease in the economy
of isometric force maintenance(Fig. 1C)(Table 1)(14,20).

<u>Table 1</u>

RATIOS OF MECHANICAL, BIOCHEMICAL AND THERMODYNAMIC PARAMETERS

PREPARATIONS	Vmax	a/P_o	TPT	ATPase	Economy
Frog/Tortoise	5.3	3.6	0.20	15.0	0.02
EDL/SOL	2.3	1.9	0.23	2.3	0.17
T/P	2.0	1.5	0.38	2.5	0.50

Where Vmax = maximum velocity of shortening; a/Po = the constants from Hill
equation reflecting the curvature of the force velocity relationship (see
legend Fig. 1); TPT = time to peak isometric tension; ATPase = actin activated
myosin ATPase; Economy = isometric tension/isometric heat rate.

Thus in a number of crucial ways the evolutionary differences seen
between frog and tortoise muscle or the developmental differences seen between
fast and slow muscles are similar to the differences seen between the two
extreme types of compensated myocardial hypertrophy (P vs T). In compensated
hypertrophy the heart uses a multitude of adaptive techniques which parallel
those used by the frog or EDL muscle (thyrotoxic hypertrophy) or those used by
the tortoise or SOL muscles (pressure overload hypertrophy). The specific
adaptation used by the heart seemed to be controlled by the nature of the
stress applied to the myocardium. There are specific coordinated changes in
the excitation contraction coupling (EC) and contractile systems which interact to produce the unique adaptation to the pressure overload or thyrotoxic
stresses. We hypothesized that if the heart is subjected to the pressure
overload and thyrotoxic stresses simultaneously, there would be a mismatch of
these adaptive changes and failure would occur. This hypothesis was tested by
applying various combinations of pressure overload and thyrotoxic stresses.
We found that certain regimens produce heart failure while others resulted in
compensated hypertrophied hearts whose performance characteristics fell on a

line connecting the two extreme types of hypertrophy (pressure overload,
thyrotoxic). In the heart failure preparations there was a mismatch between
the adaptive changes which occurred in the EC coupling system as compared wit
the contractile system.

<u>METHODS</u>

<u>Animal models and experimental plan.</u> The experimental plan was to use a
regimen whereby two distinctly different types of stresses are applied to the
rabbit heart. The stresses chosen, when applied separately, produce differer
models of hypertrophy. They represent the extremes of functional and molecular reorganization of the heart consistant with compensated myocardial hypertrophy. Pressure overload hypertrophy (P) was produced in 1.8 kg rabbits by
threading a spiral monel metal constrictor around the pulmonary artery to
reduce the internal diameter of the right ventricular outflow tract by 67%
(Fig. 2; 19,20). Thyrotoxic hypertrophy (T) was produced by 14 daily injec-

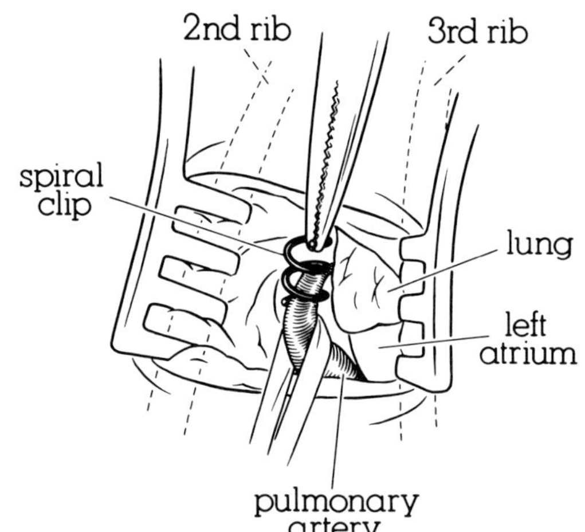

Figure 2. Surgical procedure for producing right ventricular pressure overload by banding the pulmonary artery. Male canadian albino rabbits, weighing
between 1.6 and 2.0 kg, are anaesthetized with methoxyfluorane following
pretreatment with 25mg promethazine HCl and 25 mg/kg sodium pentobarbital.
Succinylcholine is administered intravenously as needed for relaxation. The
thorax is opened through the third intercostal space, the pericardium opened,
the pulmonary artery exposed and a spiral monel metal spring is twisted into
place. The chest is closed and the pneumothorax reduced. Recovery takes
place in a heated recovery chamber ventilated with 95% O_2 and 5% CO_2.

tions of 0.2 mg/kg of L-thyroxine (Sigma)(21). On the days when the body
weight fell below 80% of the value at the start of thyroxine treatment, the
injection was omitted.

The combination of pressure overload and thyrotoxic stress (PT) were
applied by banding the pulmonary artery and then starting the thyroxine
treatment at various times following the surgery (Fig. 3).

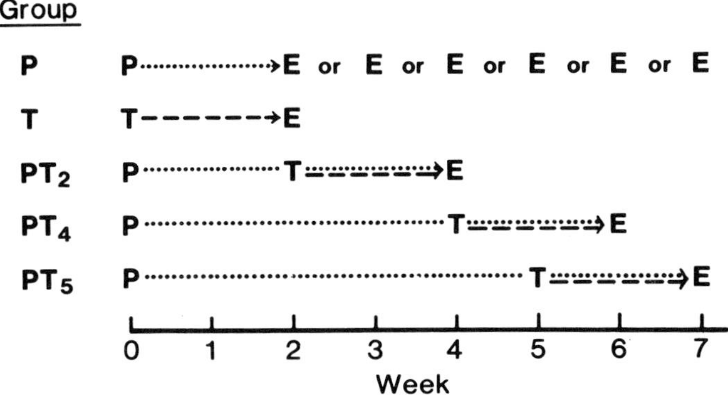

Figure 3. Experimental protocol for the double treated animals. Pulmonary
artery banding and thyroxine treatment are indicated by P and T, respectively
(see text for details). The dotted line represents the period during which
the pulmonary artery outflow tract diameter is reduced. The dashed line
represents the period during which thyroxine is administered. The experiment
is terminated at E and the papillary muscles prepared for myothermal and
mechanical analyses. Thus in the PT$_2$ animals the thyroxine treatment was
started two weeks after the banding of the pulmonary artery and continued for
the standard two week period.

<u>Measurement of right ventricular pressure.</u> The animals were anaesthe-
tized as described for banding the pulmonary artery. An 18 gauge, 2 inch
hypodermic needle is inserted into the right ventricular lumen. The needle is
directed through the epigastric wall and diaphragm into the ventricle. An
Ailtech pressure transducer (MS10-D) and and Beckman Type R dynagraph are used
for recording the pressure.

<u>Preparation of papillary muscles for mechanical and thermal measurements.</u>
Excised hearts, from rabbits stunned by a blow to the base of the skull, were
exsanguinated by washing with oxygenated Krebs solution at 37 C and then
transferred to a dissection chamber at room temperature (23-25 C). A thin
papillary muscle greater than 3.5 mm in length was dissected from the heart
and mounted vertically, base up, on the thermopile surface (22). The tendin-
ous end (bottom) was attached to a stationary glass hook while the cut end
(top) was attached to the isometric capacitance force transducer (23). The
papillary muscle and thermopile frame were then placed in an incubating
chamber which permitted oxygenation, incubation in Krebs solution and on line
calibration. The entire assembly was immersed in a 70 liter water bath and
allowed to equilibrate for one to three hours before the experiment is started. A square wave stimulus (0.2 Hz), 10% above threshold, was applied to the
ends of the muscle during the entire equilibration period and throughout the
experiment. The length of the muscle was adjusted in small increments until
the optimal length is reached (for details see 22).

<u>Measurement of right ventricular weight and actomyosin ATPase activity.</u>
After dissection and removal of the papillary muscle the right ventricular
free wall blotted weights were obtained. Actin activated myosin ATPase
activity of the right ventricular tissue was then measured as previously
described (24).

<u>Myothermal measurements and analyses.</u> The temperature of a muscle is
dependent on the following: 1) the rate of heat production; 2) the combined
thermal capacity of the muscle, the part of the thermopile with which the
muscle is in contact and the Ringer solution adhering to the muscle; and 3)
the rate of heat loss through the various heat loss pathways. Muscle heat
production is a function of resting heat, initial heat and recovery heat.
This study deals only with initial heat. Initial heat was measured from the
oscillating temperature changes seen in the muscle during repetitive stimulation at 0.2 Hz (Fig. 4). The temperature change associated with initial
heat was obtained by turning off the stimulus, allowing the muscle to cool and
extrapolating the falling temperature curve back to the previous temperature
record. This is seen in the dashed line extending the next to the last
temperature record (Fig. 4). The temperature difference between the peak
temperature and the falling base line is the temperature change associated
with initial heat corrected for heat loss. This value was then multiplied by
the thermal capacity of the muscle and adhering Ringers solution obtained by
means of the standard infra-red cool off calibration procedure (22). The

initial heat is the sum of the heat liberation associated with calcium release
and uptake and the heat liberated as a result of myosin cross-bridge head
cycling. Both the calcium (tension independent, TIH) and cross bridge related
(tension dependent, TDH) heats arise from ATP hydrolysis. The initial heat
was partitioned into TIH and TDH by making the initial heat measurements and
then repeating the experiment in 2.5 X hyperosmotic mannitol Krebs solution.
Tension was eliminated under these conditions with no substantial change in
calcium cycling (25). The triggerable heat output obtained in mannitol is, to
a first approximation, the TIH. This value was subtracted from the initial
heat to give the TDH.

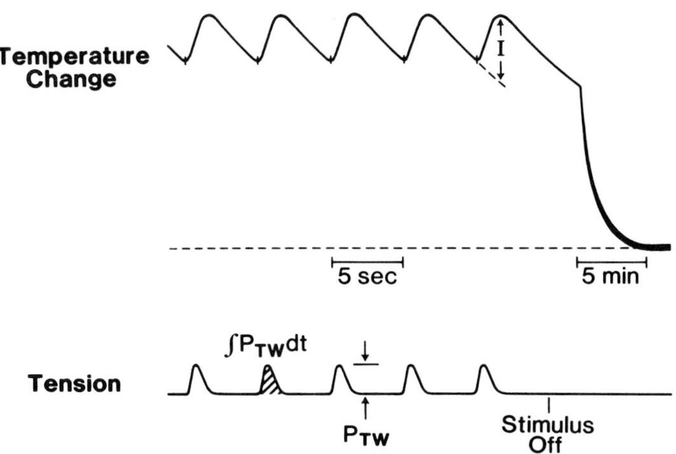

Figure 4. Initial heat measurement from oscillating temperature trace. Above
is a record of the temperature change of papillary muscle contracting
isometrically while below is a record of isometric force production. The
details for analyzing the records are presented in the text.

<u>RESULTS</u>

The appearance of the animals subjected to pressure overload and thyrotoxic stress was normal except for the low body weight and hyperventilation in
the latter group. The animals were alert, moved well and there were no
outward signs of congestive heart failure. The double treated animals were
divisable into two groups. The PT_2 and PT_3 animals exhibited signs of con-

gestive heart failure (the results of the two treatments are combined under
PT_{2-3}). These rabbits were lethargic, appeared cynotic and at sacrifice had
acites fluid in the thorax and abdomen. The appearance of the PT_4 and PT_5
preparations were similar to the T rabbits (PT_4 and PT_5 are combined under
PT_{4-5}).

The right ventricular peak systolic pressure was elevated in all experimental preparations (Table 2). The right ventricular diastolic pressure was
normal in the control (C), PT_{4-5} and T preparations (Table 2). It was slightly but significantly elevated in the P hearts and substantially elevated in
the PT_{2-3} hearts (Table 2). The right ventricular weight (RVW) for the C
hearts was 0.71 g. There was a 194%, 139% and 191% increase in the RVW for
the P, T and double treated preparations, respectively.

TABLE 2

Right Ventricular Pressures (mm Hg)

PREPARATION	C	P	T	PT2-3	PT4-5
Systolic	17	38	31	69	47
Diastolic	1.2	2.2	1.2	4.7	1.3

The peak twitch force and time to peak tension in papillary muscles from
C hearts was 5.90 g/mm^2 and 627 msec, respectively. Peak twitch force was
slightly but not significantly decreased in the P and PT_{4-5} preparations while
it was markedly depressed in the T and PT_{2-3} hearts (Table 3). Time to peak
tension was increased in the P hearts and decreased in the other preparations
(Table 3).

TABLE 3

Peak Twitch Force (P_{TW}) and Time to Peak Tension (TPT) (% C)

PREPARATION	P	T	PT2-3	PT4-5
P_{TW}	93	61	22	88
TPT	143	52	60	77

The tension dependent heat per peak twitch force (TDH/P_{TW}), the tension independent heat per gram of muscle (TIH/g) and the actin activated myosin ATPase for the C hearts were 2.0 u cal/g cm, 0.4 m cal/g and 0.14 u moles Pi/mg min, respectively. The tension dependent heat per unit tension was reduced in the P and elevated in the PT_{4-5} and T preparations (Table 4). In each of these preparations there was a corresponding change in the actin activated myosin ATPase (Table 4). In the PT_{2-3} group the tension dependent heat per unit tension was markedly depressed while the ATPase values were much less effected (Table 4). The tension independent heat was reduced in all the experimental preparations.

Table 4

Tension Dependent Heat, Tension Independent Heat and Actomyosin ATPase
Activity (%C)

PREPARATION	P	T	PT2-3	PT4-5
TDH/P_{TW}	77	159	6	146
TIH/g	50	80	33	63
ATPase	70	174	90	124

DISCUSSION

Under normal conditions the cardiac output is adequate to meet the needs of the peripheral tissues and organs for oxygen. Congestive heart failure occurs when the cardiac output does not meet these metabolic needs. Very little is known about the molecular and cellular myocardial events which are involved in the transition from a normally functioning to a failing heart. From the data collected in the Framingham study it is clear that the risk of developing congestive heart failure is markedly increased in patients with hypertension and ECG or radiographic evidence of left ventricular hypertrophy (26). Myofibrils, isolated from the ventricular myocardium of patients who died in congestive cardiac failure with hearts hypertrophied secondary to hypertensive heart disease, had a 30% depression in ATPase activity (27). Sarcoplasmic reticulum, isolated from failing rabbit hearts, showed a decrease in the rate and amount calcium sequestered (28). These studies raised the question about the relationship of myocardial hypertrophy, contractile protein ATPase activity and excitation contraction coupling (EC) phenomena to congestive heart failure. This question was addressed by carrying out a detailed myothermal analysis on rabbit hearts hypertrophied secondary to pressure overload, thyrotoxicosis and various combinations of the two stresses. The myothermal measurements permit an in vivo assessment of contractile protein performance as well as EC phenomena.

In the P and T hearts there was substantial hypertrophy with no evidence of congestive heart failure. Tension dependent heat normalized for twitch tension (TDH/P_{TW}) and actin activated myosin ATPase were decreased in the P and increased in the T hearts. Thus the economy of the isometric twitch is greater than control in the P hearts and less in the T preparations. When the pressure overload and thyrotoxic stresses were combined the ATPase activity

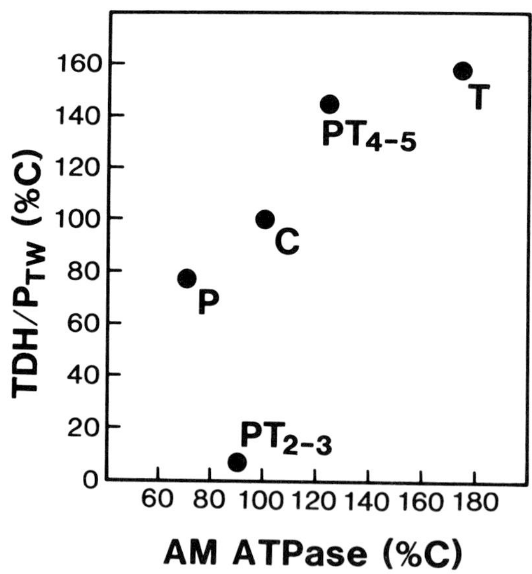

Figure 5. The relationship between actin activated myosin ATPase activity (AM ATPase) and the tension dependent heat normalized for twitch tension (TDH/-P_{TW}). The C, P and T groups are control, pressure overload and thyrotoxic hearts. The PT groups represent combined pressure overload and thyrotoxic stresses (see text for details).

was titratable between the two extremes. In the PT_2 group, where failure was present, there was a dissociation in the relationship between the ATPase activity and the TDH/P_{TW} (Fig. 5). In the PT_4 group where adaptation was successful (absence of congestive heart failure) the relationship between TDH/P_{TW} and ATPase activity was similar to that found in the controls and the other compensated hypertrophied hearts (Fig. 5). Since it is believed that tension dependent heat is a reflection of myosin cross-bridge cycling and ATP splitting, it is surprising not to find the expected association between the TDH/P_{TW} and the ATPase activity in the failing hearts. It suggests that under these conditions the values obtained with purified actomyosin do not reflect the interaction between actin and myosin in the intact highly organized myocyte.

It is informative to examine the tension dependent heat data in terms of an enzyme kinetic analysis of cross bridge cycling and tension development to clarify the observed changes in the economy of tension development and there relationship to the actin activated myosin ATPase activity (29). The basic cycle consists of two states, an "on" force developing state and an "off" non force developing state. In the "on" configuration force and work are produced when the cross-bridge head of the myosin molecule binds to the actin filament and rotates from the 90° to the 45° position. In the "off" state the actin and myosin are separated while a number of obligatory transformations occur which finally permits the actin and myosin to interact with each other. The following steps are involved in each of these states. The bound actomyosin (AM) is dissociated when ATP binds to it ($AM + ATP \rightarrow M^*ATP + A$). At this point in the "off" configuration the following obligatory transformation occurs: 1) $M^*ATP \rightarrow M^{**}ADPPi$ (This leaves the myosin in an energized but refractory state. $M^{**}ADPPi$ then undergoes a slow rate limiting transformation from the refractory to the non refractory state); 2) $M^{**}ADPPi \rightarrow M^{++}ADPPi$ ($M^{++}ADPPi$ is in a non refractory state and can combine with actin placing it in the "on" force generating configuration). In the "on" force developing state the following steps occur: 1) $A + M^{++}ADPPi \rightarrow AM^{++}ADPPi$ (cross-bridge head in the 90 position); 2) $AM^{++}ADPPi \rightarrow AMADPPi$ (cross-bridge head in the 45 force developing position non force generating position) and 3) $AMADPPi \rightarrow AM + ADP + Pi$ (the cycle is ready to start again). Tension dependent heat and force can be analyzed in terms of the cross-bridge cycling rate (f) and the "on" time. The force developed can be analyzed in terms of the average strength of the cross-bridge, the duration of the "on" force producing time and the rate of cross-bridge cycling. If it is assumed that the cross-bridge strength is the same for all preparations, then the values of the "on" time and cycling rate can be calculated from the tension dependent heat measurements and the isometric twitch force (30). The average "on" time for the P hearts is 154% of normal while the cycling rate (f) is 65% of normal. For the T hearts the "on" time and cycling rates are 47% and 156% of normal, respectively. The compensated double treated preparation (PT_{4-5}) falls on a line intermediate between the C and T hearts. In contrast the failing group (PT_{2-3}) has an "on" time and cycling rate which are 454% and 3% of normal, respectively. Thus in that preparation the cross-bridges are cycling very slowly and stay in the on force producing position for a prolonged period of time. Force is produced very economically in these hearts. This, by itself, should not be the cause of failure. However, the rate of cross-bridge cycling requires that sufficient time be available for the development of force. Accordingly, for an analysis of the adaptation or its absence the cross-bridge behavior must be considered in conjunction with EC coupling phenomena.

EC coupling phenomena can be evaluated in terms of tension independent heat (TIH) and time to peak tension (TPT). TIH is reduced in all experimental preparations. TPT is increased in the P and decreased in the T hearts. In the former where the cross-bridge cycling rate is reduced to 65% of normal and the "on" time is increased to 154% of normal, the increase in TPT is coordinated with these other changes to permit a longer period of time for force development. Even though the TIH in this preparation is reduced to 50% of normal the uptake of calcium is slowed sufficiently (TPT) to permit time for adequate force to be developed. Similarly in the T and PT_{4-5} preparations where the cross-bridge cyling rate is increased and the "on" time decreased, there is reduced TPT which allows the heart to develop force and relax quickly. In these hearts the TIH (Ca^{++} cycling) is sufficient for activation. In each of these cases there is a coordinated interaction between the contractile and EC coupling systems. In contrast in the PT_{2-3} animals where the cycling rate is markedly decreased and the "on" time substantially increased, TPT is reduced. This constellation represents a mismatch of the intracellular responses to the stresses applied with the contractile system slowing down and the EC coupling system accelerating. In addition the TIH is 30% of normal which, in conjunction with the decrease in TPT, provides an inadequate quantity of free Ca^{++} for activation. It is hypothesized that this mismatch is the cause of the congestive failure under these circumstances.

313

Extreme caution must be used in extrapolating from the data present here
to the situation found in human congestive heart failure. Congestive heart
failure in the PT_2 rabbit model may be uniquely related to the specific timing
of the sequential application of the two stresses. However, this particular
regimen of stresses illustrates that it is possible to have two organelle
systems (contractile and EC coupling) respond to the stresses differently.
This inappropriate differential response of the contractile and EC coupling
systems are antagonistic and therefore may be the cause of failure under these
circumstances. Another concern is that the studies were carried out on the
animals which survived the regimen of stresses. A significant number of
rabbits succumbed during the planned waiting period. It is important to know
whether they died in congestive heart failure with features similar to that
seen in the PT_{2-3} group. This is the direction of our future experiments.

SUMMARY

Myothermal, mechanical and biochemical studies were carried out on three
types of hypertrophied hearts. Pressure overload (P) was produced by reducing
the size of the pulmonary artery. Thyrotoxic (T) hypertrophied was produced
by daily injections of L-thyroxine. The third group of hypertrophied hearts
was produced by the sequential combination of the two stresses with the T
following the P stress by 2, 3, 4 and 5 weeks. Compensated hypertrophy was
present in the P, T and PT_{4-5} animals. Congestive heart failure occurred in
the PT_{2-3} group. Actin activated myosin ATPase activity was titratable
between the low values for the P hearts and the high values for the T hearts.
Tension dependent heat normalized for peak twitch tension (TDH/P_{TW}) was low in
the P hearts, and high in the T hearts with the PT_{4-5} falling between the
control and T preparations. These values correlated with the ATPase measurements. In contrast the TDH/P_{TW} was very low in the PT_{2-3} group and did not
correlate with the ATPase values. This data was analyzed in terms of a enzyme
kinetic actomyosin cross-bridge scheme and indicated that in the P hearts the
"on" force producing time was prolonged while the cyling rate was decreased
(154%N and 65%N). In the T preparations these values were 47% and 156% of
normal. The compensated double treated animals (PT_{4-5}) fell on a line between
the controls and the T group. The failing group had a marked prolongation of
the "on" time (454%N) and a major reduction in the cycling rate (3%N). In the
P hearts tension independent heat (TIH) was decreased and time to peak tension
(TPT) was increased. This change in EC coupling in conjunction with the
decrease in the contractile protein cross-bridge cycling rate and increase in

"on" time is coordinated so that there is more time for the slower muscle to develop force. In the compensated T and PT_{4-5} preparations, the cycling rate increases while the "on" time is shortened. In these hearts TIH and TPT are decreased. Thus there is a coordination between the contractile and EC coupling events. In the failing group (PT_{2-3}) the cycling rate is markedly slowed, the "on" time is increased and, surprisingly, the TPT is decreased. We hypothesize that this mismatch between the contractile protein cross-bridge behavior and the EC coupling performance is the cause of congestive heart failure in this group of animals.

BIBLIOGRAPHY

1. Frank, O. (1895): Zur Dynamik der Herzmuskels. Ztschr. F. Biol. 32:570
2. Starling, E.H., (1918): The Linacre Lecture on the Flow of the Heart, Given at Cambridge, 1914. Longmass, Green and Co, et al London.
3. Bowditch, H.P. (1871): Uber die Eigenthumlichkeiten der Reizbarkeit welche die Muskelfasern des Herzen Zeigen. Ber. Verhandl. Sachs. Akad. Wiss. 23:652-689.
4. Sarnoff, S.J. and Mitchell, J.H. (1962): The control of function of the heart. In: <u>Handbook of Physiology. Section 2. Circulation, Vol. 1.</u> edited by W.F. Hamilton and P. Dow, pp489-532. American Physiological Society, Washington D.C.
5. Kennedy, J.W., Twiss, R.D., Blackmon, J.R., and Dodge, H.T. (1968): Quantitative Angiography III Relationship of left ventricular pressure, volume and mass in aortic valve disease. Circulation 38:838-845.
6. Pfeffer, M.A., Pfeffer, J.M., and Frolich, E.D. (1976): Pumping ability of the hypertrophying left ventricle of the spontaneously hypertensive rat. Circ. Res. 38:423-429.
7. Sandler, H., and Dodge, H.T. (1963): Left ventricular tension and stress in man. Circ. Res. 13:91-104.
8. Alpert, N.R, and Mulieri, L.A. (1982): Myocardial adaptation to stress from the viewpoint of evolution and development. In: <u>Basic Biology of Muscles: A Comparative Approach.</u> Edited by B.M. Twarog, R.J.C. Levine and M.M. Dewey. Raven Press, New York pp. 173-188.
9. Hill, A.V. (1970): <u>First and last experiments in muscle mechanics.</u> Cambridge University Press, Cambridge, England.
10. Hartree, W. (1926): Heat production of tortoise muscle. J. Physiol. (Lond.), 61:255-260.
11. Woledge, R. (1968): The energetics of tortoise muscle. J. Physiol. (Lond.), 197:685-707.
12. Close, R. (1964): Dynamic properties of fast and slow skeletal muscles of the rat during development. J. Physiol. (Lond.), 173:74-75.
13. Close, R. (1969): Dynamic properties of fast and slow skeletal muscle of the rat after nerve cross union. J. Physiol. (Lond.), 204:331-346.
14. Schine, L. (1982): <u>The mechanical performance of the pressure overloaded, thyrotoxic and double treated hypertrophied hearts.</u> Masters Thesis, University of Vermont.
15. Barany, M. and Close, R. (1971): The transformation of fast and slow muscles of myosin in cross innervated rat muscles. J. Physiol. (Lond.), 213:455-474.
16. Gibbs, C. and Gibson, W.R. (1972): Energy production of rat soleus muscle. Am. J. Physiol. 223:864-871.
17. Hill, A.V. (1938): The heat of shortening and the dynamic constants of

muscle. Proc. Roy. Soc. Lond. (Biol.), 126:136-195.

18. Wendt, I.R. and Gibbs, C. (1973): Energy production of rat extensor digitorum longus muscle. Am. J. Physiol., 224:1081-1086.

19. Alpert, N.R., Hamrell, B.B., and Halpern, W. (1974): Mechanical and biochemical correlates of cardiac hypertrophy. Circ Res. 34/35(Suppl. II): 71-82.

20. Hamrell, B.B., and Alpert, N.R. (1977): The mechanical characteristics of hypertrophied rabbit cardiac muscle in the absence of congestive heart failure. Circ. Res., 40:20-25.

21. Banerjee, S.K. Flink, I.L., and Morkin, E. (1976): Enzymatic properties of native and N-Ethylmaleimide-modified cardiac myosin from normal and thyrotoxic rabbits. Circ. Res. 39: 319-326.

22. Mulieri, L.A., Luhr, G., Trefry, J. and Alpert, N.R. (1977): Metal film thermopiles for use with rabbit right ventricular papillary muscles. Am. J. Physiol. 233: 146-156.

23. Hamrell, B.B., Panaanen, R., Trono, J., and Alpert, N.R. (1975): A stable, sensitive, low-compliance force transducer. J. Appl. Physiol. 38:190-193.

24. Thomas, L.L. and Alpert, N.R. (1977): Functional integrity of the SH_1 site in myosin from hypertrophied myocardium. Biochim. Biophys. Acta 481:680-688.

25. Alpert, N.R. and Mulieri, L.A. (1982): Heat, mechanics and myosin ATPase in normal and hypertrophied heart muscle. Fed. Proc. 41: 192-198.

26. Kannel, W.B., Castelli, W.P. McNamara, P.M., McKee, P.A., and Feinleib, M. (1972): Role of blood pressure in the development of congestive heart failure. The Framingham Study. New England J. Med. 287: 781-787.

27. Alpert, N.R. and Gordon, M.S. (1962): Myofibrillar adenosine triphosphatase activity in congestive heart failure. Am. J. Physiol. 202:940-946.

28. Schwartz, A., Sordahl, L.A., Entman, M.L., Allen, J.C., Reddy, Y.S., Goldstein, M.A., Luchi, R.J. and Wyborny, L.E. (1976): Abnormal biochemistry in myocardial failure. In Congestive Heart Failure. Mechanisms, Evaluation and Treatment. Edited by Mason, D.T. Yorke Medical Books, Dun-Donnelley Publishing Corp., New York, 25-44.

29. Eisenberg, E. and Hill, T.L. (1978): A cross-bridge model of muscle contraction. Prog. Biophys. Molec. Biol. 33: 55-82.

30. Alpert, N.R., Mulieri, L.A. and Litten, R.Z. (1979): Functional significance of altered myosin adenosine triphosphatase activity in enlarged hearts. Am. J. Cardiol. 44: 947-953.

20

MITOCHONDRIAL OXIDATIVE PHOSPHORYLATION AND CALCIUM TRANSPORT IN CARDIAC
HYPERTROPHY DUE TO PRESSURE OVERLOAD IN PIGS*

G.N. PIERCE, B.S. TUANA, M.P. MOFFAT, P.K. SINGAL, V. PANAGIA and N.S. DHALLA

1. INTRODUCTION

By virtue of their ability to generate energy in the form of ATP,
mitochondria are known to play an important role in the maintenance of
cardiac function (1). In addition, heart mitochondria have a remarkable
capacity to accumulate a large quantity of calcium and are generally
considered to serve as calcium sink in the myocardium under a wide variety
of pathological conditions (2,3). In fact, an increase in Ca^{2+} uptake and
a depression in oxidative phosphorylation activity have been reported in
heart mitochondria isolated from animals with chronic potassium deficiency
(4) and early stages of bacterial cardiomyopathy (5). Similar observations
were also made with mitochondria isolated from Ca^{2+}-paradoxic hearts
obtained after a successive perfusion with Ca^{2+}-free medium and Ca^{2+}-containing
medium (6,7). Although mitochondria from different types of failing
hearts have been reported to show depressed Ca^{2+} uptake and energy production
(5, 8-10), the functional significance of these changes is not clear because
similar results were also obtained upon prolonged ingestion of alcohol
under which conditions cardiac contractile force was unaltered (11).

Some investigators have studied mitochondrial functions in hypertrophied
non-failing hearts but the results are conflicting. Cardiac hypertrophy
in rabbits due to pressure overload upon aortic stenosis was found to be
associated with a decrease in mitochondrial Ca^{2+}-uptake and an increase
in oxidative phosphorylation activity (10). On the other hand, an increase
in Ca^{2+}-uptake without any changes in mitochondrial oxidative phosphorylation
was observed in hypertrophied rabbit heart produced by inserting a
catheter into the left ventricle through the right carotid artery (5).
Furthermore, both energy production and Ca^{2+} uptake activities of

---

* This work was supported by a grant from the Medical Research Council of
Canada.

mitochondria were slightly depressed in non-failing enlarged hearts of the cardiomyopathic hamsters (9). Since cardiac hypertrophy has been described to be either physiological or pathological in nature (12) it appears that the conflicting reports on changes in mitochondrial functions may be due to differences in the stage of heart hypertrophy. In this study therefore we have examined mitochondrial changes at two stages of cardiac hypertrophy induced by pressure overload due to supravalvular banding of the aorta in pigs for 4 and 8 weeks. On the basis of alterations in the contractile properties of isolated cardiac muscle, we have previously suggested that heart hypertrophy in this experimental model was physiological and pathological in nature at 4 and 8 weeks of aortic banding, respectively (13).

2. MATERIALS AND METHODS

Left ventricle hypertrophy was induced in pigs by banding the supravalvular aorta for 4 and 8 weeks as described earlier (13). Sham operated animals without aortic banding were used as controls. All these animals were hemodynamically assessed and found to show no signs of heart failure (14). The animals were sacrificed by a stunning bullet blow on the forehead and the left ventricular tissue was used in this study. Mitochondria were isolated by the method of Sordahl and Schwartz (15). The techniques for the determination of mitochondrial Ca^{2+} binding, Ca^{2+} uptake, ATPase activities and oxidative phosphorylation activities were same as those employed previously (5). Mitochondrial Ca^{2+}-binding (25°C) was studied in the presence of 4 mM ATP and 50 μM Ca^{2+} whereas the medium for Ca^{2+} uptake (37°C) contained 5 mM inorganic phosphate and 5 mM sodium succinate. Mitochondrial oxidative phosphorylation activities were studied by using either 1.5 mM pyruvate and 0.3 mM malate or 1.5 mM succinate with 1 μM rotenone as a substrate. State 3 respiration was initiated by the addition of 200 nmol of ADP whereas state 4 respiration ensued when all the ADP was phosphorylated. The respiratory control index (RCI) was calculated as the ratio of oxygen uptake rates in state 3 and 4. The methods for determining subcellular contamination, gel electrophoresis patterns of proteins, and phospholipid composition was same as employed in our laboratory (5,16). Since values for the sham control for 4 and 8 weeks did not differ from each other, these results were grouped together. The data were analyzed statistically using the Student's t-test and a P value < 0.05 was taken to indicate a significant difference.

3. RESULTS

Mitochondria isolated from both control and hypertrophied hearts did not show any detectable Ca^{2+}-stimulated Mg^{2+} dependent ATPase activity indicating the absence of contamination by sarcoplasmic reticulum as well as myofibrils. When pyruvate-malate was used as a substrate, the respiratory and oxidative phosphorylation activities of the 4 and 8 week hypertrophied heart mitochondria were not different from the control values (Table 1). Likewise, no significant changes in the mitochondrial respiration and ADP:O ratio was evident in the hypertrophied heart when succinate was employed as a substrate except that RCI was significantly depressed in the 8 week hypertrophied hearts (Table 1).

TABLE 1. Mitochondrial oxidative phosphorylation in the presence of (A) pyruvate-malate or (B) succinate from sham control and hypertrophied pig left ventricle.

Animal Group	Oxygen Consumption (natoms O/mg protein/min)		RCI	ADP:O Ratio
	State 3	State 4		
(A) Pyruvate-malate as a substrate:				
Sham Control N = 12	165 ± 11	20 ± 1.6	8.5 ± 0.4	3.0 ± 0.1
4 week Hypertrophy N = 5	168 ± 4	18 ± 1.1	9.3 ± 0.4	2.8 ± 0.2
8 week Hypertrophy N = 5	163 ± 20	23 ± 2.7	7.1 ± 0.7	2.8 ± 0.5
(B) Succinate as a substrate:				
Sham Control N = 8	219 ± 11	66 ± 4.7	3.5 ± 0.2	2.2 ± 0.1
4 week Hypertrophy N = 5	220 ± 9	63 ± 5.5	3.6 ± 0.4	2.3 ± 0.1
8 week Hypertrophy N = 5	192 ± 29	76 ± 11	2.6 ± 0.3*	2.2 ± 0.2

* $P < 0.05$

The data in Table 2 indicate that the ATPase activity of mitochondria

TABLE 2. Mitochondrial ATPase activities in sham control and hypertrophied pig left ventricle.

Animal Group	ATPase activities (μmoles Pi/mg protein) at different times of incubation			
	1 min	2 min	5 min	10 min
Sham control N = 12	0.33 ± 0.03	0.50 ± 0.06	0.88 ± 0.12	1.50 ± 0.18
4 week Hypertrophy N = 9	0.38 ± 0.02	0.62 ± 0.05	1.10 ± 0.11	1.92 ± 0.22
8 week Hypertrophy N = 8	0.34 ± 0.02	0.60 ± 0.06	1.06 ± 0.12	1.75 ± 0.19

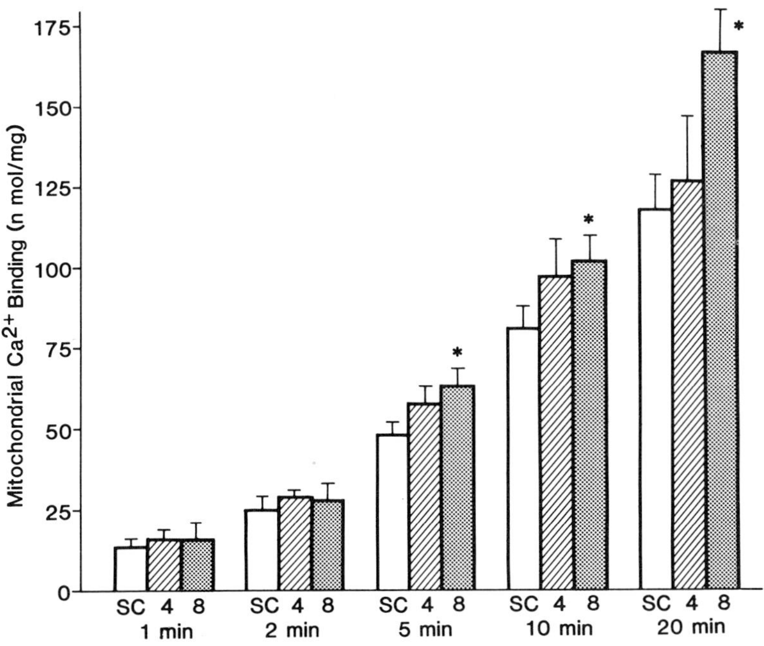

FIGURE 1. Mitochondrial Ca^{2+} binding of control (SC), 4 weeks (4) hypertrophied and 8 weeks (8) hypertrophied pig hearts at different times of incubation. Each value is a mean ± of 7 to 8 experiments. Data from 4 and 8 weeks control were pooled together. * - significant ($P < 0.05$).

from 4 or 8 week hypertrophied heart was not different from the control values. Although mitochondrial ATPase was markedly inhibited by 5 mM sodium azide, no difference in the degree of this inhibition was seen between the control and hypertrophied preparations.

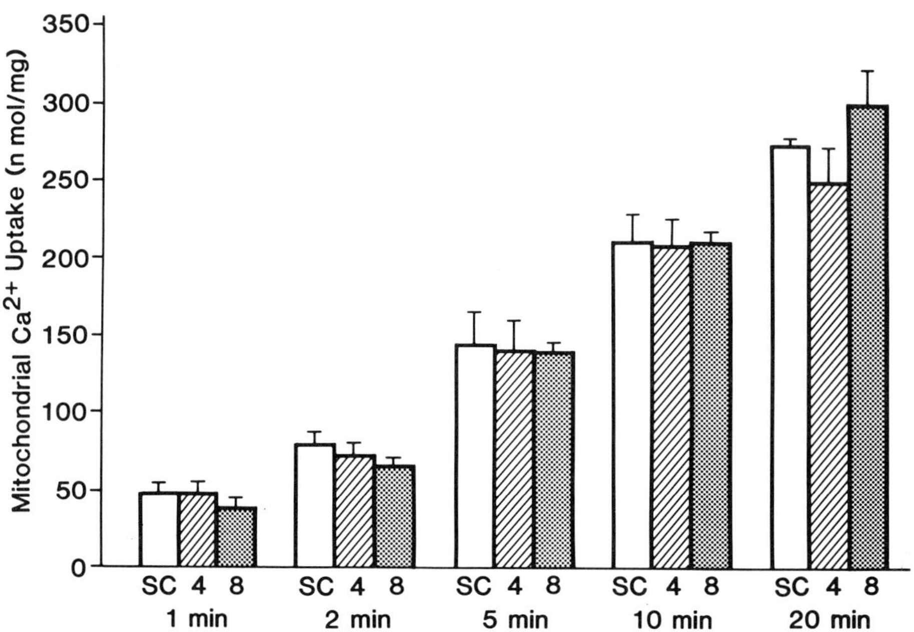

FIGURE 2. Mitochondrial Ca^{2+} uptake of control (SC), 4 weeks (4) hypertrophied and 8 weeks (8) hypertrophied pig hearts at different times of incubation. Each values is a mean ± S.E. of 7 to 8 experiments. Data from 4 and 8 weeks control were pooled together.

The time-course of Ca^{2+} binding activities of control and hypertrophied heart mitochondria was studied and the results are shown in Fig. 1. No difference between the control and 4 week hypertrophied preparations was evident but mitochondria for 8 week hypertrophied heart showed a significant increase in Ca^{2+}-binding at 5 to 20 min of incubation. On the other hand, mitochondrial Ca^{2+} uptake activities of control, 4 weeks hypertrophied and 8 week hypertrophied hearts were not significantly different each other (Fig. 2).

The phospholipid and protein composition of the mitochondria from control and experimental hearts was also examined. The data in Table 3 show

TABLE 3. Phospholipid composition of mitochondrial fractions isolated from sham control and hypertrophied pig left ventricle.

Phospholipid	Sham control	4 week Hyper.	8 week Hyper.
	nmol lipid Pi/mg protein		
Total Phospholipids	189.9 ± 21.2	269.0 ± 19.7*	280.5 ± 19.5*
Phosphatidylcholine	63.0 ± 7.1	99.5 ± 6.5*	97.0 ± 6.8*
Phosphatidylethanolamine	49.6 ± 5.9	82.1 ± 9.0*	81.2 ± 6.9*
Lysophosphatidylcholine	4.3 ± 0.9	4.1 ± 0.8	5.3 ± 1.2
Sphingomyelin	11.1 ± 2.2	11.4 ± 2.1	12.1 ± 1.8
Diphosphatidylglycerol	24.7 ± 6.5	32.3 ± 3.9	42.0 ± 4.8*
Phosphatidylserine	7.5 ± 1.8	10.8 ± 2.1	11.8 ± 1.1
Phosphatidylinositol	10.9 ± 2.5	11.5 ± 2.0	12.3 ± 1.1
Phosphatidic Acid	4.6 ± 1.3	2.5 ± 1.2	2.4 ± 1.2
Unknowns	13.8 ± 2.7	14.6 ± 3.7	16.1 ± 3.5

The data for 4 and 8 weeks sham controls were pooled. * Significantly (P < 0.05) different from sham control values.

that the total phospholipid contents in mitochondria from 4 and 8 weeks hypertrophied hearts were significantly increased in comparison to the control preparations. This increase was mainly due to an elevation of the phosphatidylcholine and phosphatidylethanolamine contents in the hypertrophied heart mitochondria. Although diphosphatidylglycerol contents were also increased in hypertrophied heart mitochondria, this increase was not significant in 4 weeks hypertrophied preparation. The protein gel profiles of the control, 4 weeks and 8 weeks hypertrophied heart mitochondria are shown in Fig. 3. No new protein peak was evident as well as none of the peaks were missing from the hypertrophied heart mitochondrial gel patterns; however, the magnitude of certain peaks in the hypertrophied preparations was quantitatively different from the control.

4. DISCUSSION

In this study we have demonstrated that mitochondria isolated from 4 and 8 weeks hypertrophied pig heart showed normal respiratory and oxidative phosphorylation activities when pyruvate-malate was used as a substrate. Similar results were also obtained by using succinate as a substrate except that the RCI values were significantly depressed in 8 weeks

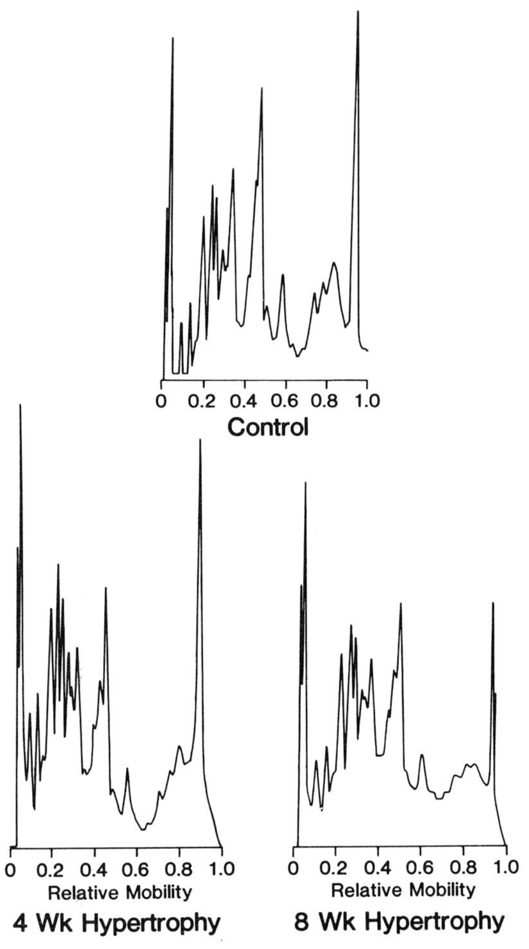

FIGURE 3. SDS-polyacrylamide gel electrophoretic pattern of mitochondria from control, 4 weeks hypertrophied and 8 weeks hypertrophied pig hearts. Each tracing is a typical for at least 4 experiments in each group.

hypertrophied hearts only. Thus it appears that the ability of mitochondria to produce energy did not change during the physiological hypertrophy at 4 weeks of aortic stenosis in pigs where the cardiac contractile
function has been reported to be normal or supernormal (13). On the other
hand, there seems to be some subtle defect in the process of energy
production by mitochondria in 8 weeks of aortic stenosis where the cardiac

contractile function was depressed and the hypertrophy at this stage was considered to be of pathological nature (13). It is highly unlikely that such a small change in mitochondrial RCI would cause a depression in the contractile function of isolated cardiac muscle from 8 weeks hypertrophied heart; however, the observed change may reflect the beginning of some biochemical defect in the mitochondrial membrane. In this regard it should be noted that the activity of mitochondrial ATPase, which is considered to be responsible for energy transduction, did not change during the development of cardiac hypertrophy in this experimental model.

Although there is a great deal of controversy concerning the involvement of mitochondria in the regulation of calcium during cardiac contraction and relaxation cycle under normal conditions (1-3), their role in diseased heart has not been evaluated adequately. We have shown that ATP-dependent Ca^{2+} binding with mitochondria from 4 weeks hypertrophied heart was unaltered whereas that from 8 weeks hypertrophied heart was significantly increased. Since Ca^{2+} uptake activity of mitochondria was not affected during 8 weeks of cardiac hypertrophy, it appears that increased mitochondrial Ca^{2+} binding may be due to some alterations in the mitochondrial membrane rather than due to any abnormality of the Ca^{2+}-transport system. In our earlier studies with this experimental model, we have observed that the rate of sarcoplasmic reticular Ca^{2+} uptake, but not Ca^{2+} binding, was increased at 4 weeks and decreased at 8 weeks of cardiac hypertrophy (17). Sarcolemmal changes favouring increased Ca^{2+}- influx at 4 weeks and decreased Ca^{2+} efflux at 8 weeks have also been observed during the development of cardiac hypertrophy in this animal model (18). These results suggest that there occur sequential alterations in different membrane systems of the heart during the development of cardiac hypertrophy; and in this experimental model changes in the sarcolemma and sarcoplasmic reticulum precede those seen in mitochondria. Since a depression in the sarcoplasmic reticular Ca^{2+} uptake activity as well as in sarcolemmal Ca^{2+} efflux mechanisms at 8 weeks of hypertrophy can be seen to raise the intracellular concentration of Ca^{2+} in the myocardium, it is possible that the observed increase in mitochondrial Ca^{2+} binding may occur as an adaptive change to protect the cell from the adverse effects of the intracellular Ca^{2+} overload (3). Such adaptative changes in mitochondria may be a consequence of alterations in the composition of these organelles. In this regard it should be noted that the contents of diphosphatidylglycerol, which is known to bind Ca^{2+},

were increased in mitochondria from 8 weeks hypertrophied heart and this
may explain the observed increase in mitochondrial Ca^{2+} binding activity
at this stage of hypertrophy. Although the contents of other phospholipids
such as phosphatidylcholine and phosphatidylethanolamine were increased
in mitochondria from both 4 and 8 weeks of cardiac hypertrophy, the
significance of these changes is not clear at present.

5. SUMMARY

The oxidative phosphorylation and Ca^{2+} transport activities of
mitochondria isolated from pig hypertrophied hearts were studied after
inducing pressure overload due to supravalvular aortic stenosis for 4 and
8 weeks. Sham control animals were used as control. No changes in
respiratory and oxidative phosphorylation activities were observed when
pyruvate-malate or succinate were used as substrates except that a significant decrease in mitochondrial RCI at 8 weeks cardiac hypertrophy was
evident in the presence of succinate only. Mitochondrial ATPase and Ca^{2+}
uptake activities were not altered at 4 and 8 weeks but mitochondrial
Ca^{2+} binding was increased at 8 weeks of aortic stenosis. Although
phosphatidylcholine and phosphatidylethanolamine contents in mitochondria
were increased during the development of cardiac hypertrophy, a significant
increase in diphosphatidylglycerol, which binds Ca^{2+}, was observed only at
8 weeks of cardiac hypertrophy. These results indicate that mitochondria
may play an adaptive role in regulating the intracellular concentration
of Ca^{2+} during the development of pathological hypertrophy.

REFERENCES

1. Dhalla NS, Ziegelhoffer A, Harrow JAC: Regulatory role of membrane
    systems in heart function. Can J Physiol Pharmacol (55): 1211-1234,
    1977.
2. Dhalla NS, Das PK, Sharma GP: Subcellular basis of cardiac contractile
    failure. J Mol Cell Cardiol (10): 363-385, 1978.
3. Dhalla NS, Pierce GN, Panagia V, Singal PK, Beamish RE: Calcium
    movements in relation to heart function. Basic Res Cardiol (77):
    117-139, 1982.
4. Ledwoch W, Greef K, Heinen E, Noack E: The influence of chronic
    potassium deficiency on energy production, calcium metabolism and
    phospholipid composition of isolated heart mitochondria. J Mol Cell
    Cardiol (11): 77-89, 1979.
5. Tomlinson CW, Lee SL, Dhalla NS: Abnormalities in heart membranes
    and myofibrils during bacterial infective cardiomyopathy in the
    rabbit. Circ Res (39): 82-92, 1976.
6. Lee SL, Dhalla NS: Subcellular calcium transport in failing hearts

due to calcium deficiency and overload. Am J Physiol (231): 1159-1165, 1976.

7.   Dhalla NS, Singh JN, McNamara DB, Bernatsky A, Singh A, Harrow JAC: Energy production and utilization in contractile failure due to intracellular calcium overload. Adv Exp Med Biol (161): 305-316, 1983.

8.   Morrison ES, Scott RF, Lee WM, Frick J, Kroms M, Cheney CP: Oxidative phosphorylation and aspects of calcium metabolism in myocardia of hypercholesterolaemic swine with moderate coronary atherosclerosis. Cardiovasc Res (11): 547-553, 1977.

9.   Lindenmayer GE, Harigaya S, Bajusz E, Schwartz A: Oxidative phosphorylation and calcium transport of mitochondria from cardiomyopathic hamster hearts. J Mol Cell Cardiol (1): 249-259, 1970.

10. Sordahl LA, McCollum WB, Wood WG, Schwartz A: Mitochondria and sarcoplasmic reticulum function in cardiac hypertrophy and failure. Am J Physiol (224): 497-502, 1973.

11. Bing RJ, Tillmanns H, Fauvel J-M, Seeler K, Mao JC: Effect of prolonged alcohol administration on calcium transport in heart muscle of the dog. Circ Res (35): 33-38, 1974.

12. Wikman-Coffelt J, Parmley WW, Mason DT: The cardiac hypertrophy process. Analyses of factors determining the pathological vs. physiological development. Circ Res (45): 697-707, 1979.

13. Singal PK, Dhillon KS, Panagia V, Dhalla NS: Cardiac muscle function during the development of hypertrophy in pigs due to pressure overload. In: Jacob R, Gulch RW, Kissling G (eds) Cardiac Adaptation in Hemodynamic Overload, Training and Stress. Dr. D. Steinkopff, Verlag, Darmstadt, 1983, pp. 189-196.

14. Sharma GP, Singal PK, Dhalla NS: Hemodynamic adaptation of the left ventricle during aortic stenosis in pigs. J Mol Cell Cardiol (12, Suppl 1): 151, 1980.

15. Sordahl LA, Schwartz A: Effects of dipyridamole on heart muscle mitochondria. Mol Pharmacol (3): 509-515, 1967.

16. Alto LE, Dhalla NS: Role of changes in microsomal calcium in the effects of reperfusion of Ca^{2+}-deprived rat hearts. Circ Res (48): 17-24, 1981.

17. Dhalla NS, Alto LE, Heyliger CE, Pierce GN, Panagia V, Singal PK: Sarcoplasmic reticular Ca^{2+}-pump adaptation in cardiac hypertrophy due to pressure overload in pigs. Europ Heart J: in press, 1983.

18. Panagia V, Michiel DF, Khatter JC, Dhalla KS, Singal PK, Dhalla NS: Sarcolemmal alterations in cardiac hypertrophy due to pressure overload in pigs. This volume.

21

ABNORMALITIES IN THE CALCIUM PUMP MECHANISM IN CARDIOMYOPATHY

JOHN H. MCNEILL

Long term diabetics have a higher incidence and greater mortality from cardiac disease. Cardiac disease in the diabetic can result from atherosclerosis but may also be due to a combination of microangiopathy, macroangiopathy, autonomic neuropathy and other factors which could produce structural, functional and biochemical alterations in the heart (1). Clinical evidence for the development of a diabetic cardiomyopathy associated with small vessel disease has been cited (2) and, in addition, cardiac functional abnormalities independent of vascular changes have been reported in an experimental model, the alloxan treated dog (3). The study of the cardiac changes produced by the diabetic state in both acute and long term diabetes has elicited a great deal of interest and several groups, including my own, have published extensively on the problem. The importance of studying cardiac changes produced in long term chronic diabetes has become apparent since the clinical changes cited above occur only after the patient has suffered from the disease for some years.

We began our investigations by using female Wistar rats in which diabetes was chemically induced by either alloxan (65 mg/kg) or streptozotocin (65 mg/kg) given intravenously (4). In later studies these doses were reduced to 40 mg/kg (alloxan) and 50-55 mg/kg of streptozotocin (STZ) since the latter doses caused a reproducible diabetic state and had a considerably lower mortality than those used in the early studies.

Table 1. Certain features of control and diabetic rats.

(a)

Time, days	Treatment	Serum Insulin mg/dL	Serum Glucose mg/dL
7	Control (9)	17.5±2.6	70.8±6.9
	Alloxan (9)	7.5±1.7*	200.8±35.5*
	STZ (7)	8.8±1.7*	200.7±34.8*
30	Control (9)	20.9±2.5	100.3±8.5
	Alloxan (7)	13.1±2.2*	382.2±92.9*
	STZ (10)	16.7±0.9	252.8±68.4*
100	Control (11)	11.2±0.7	151.3±13.0
	Alloxan (7)	5.1±1.1*	501.4±87.7*
	STZ (9)	5.2±1.0*	500.6±91.8*
180	Control (10)	19.4±1.3	137.0±21.9
	STZ (11)	9.4±1.5*	349.3±32.2*
240	Control (7)	18.1±2.4	132.6±15.1
	Alloxan (10)	8.6±1.9*	391.5±89.7*
360	Control (9))	18.1±2.0	119.6±8.9
	STZ (9)	10.9±1.6*	345.4±49.7*

(b)

Time, days	Treatment	Body Wt. (g)	Wet Heart Weight (g)	Heart Wt./ Body Wt. mg/g	Coronary Flow mL/min per gram[b]
7	Control (9)	210±4	0.94±0.03	4.48±0.11	4.1±0.2
	Alloxan (9)	201±3	0.87±0.03	4.35±0.16	4.4±0.3
	STZ (7)	201±4	0.87±0.02	4.32±0.10	4.3±0.1
30	Control (9)	236±3	1.03±0.03	4.38±0.16	3.7±0.2
	Alloxan (7)	214±10*	0.85±0.04*	4.04±0.19	3.1±0.1
	STZ (10)	222±5	0.88±0.02*	3.96±0.06	3.6±0.2
100	Control (11)	305±5	–	–	–
	Alloxan (7)	236±15*	–	–	–
	STZ (9)	231±10*	–	–	–
180	Control (10)	312±8	1.41±0.05	4.55±0.10	3.2±0.2
	STZ (11)	211±9*	1.10±0.05*	5.23±0.10*	3.1±0.9
240	Control (7)	324±8	1.41±0.06	4.36±0.16	3.2±0.1
	Alloxan (10)	239±7*	1.20±0.04*	5.00±0.21*	3.3±0.3
360	Control (9)	372±13	1.53±0.06	4.16±0.16	3.2±0.2
	STZ (9)	249±10*	1.30±0.04*	5.29±0.20*	3.1±0.2

NOTE: All the values are expressed as mean ± S.E. Numbers in parentheses are the number of rats used at that time point.
* Represents significant difference from control value at p < 0.05.
[a] Wet heart weight and coronary flow measurements were not made at this time point.
[b] Coronary flow measurements were made during the initial 5-min period of retrograde perfusion at 45 cm H_2O aortic perfusion pressure before the heart was switched to the working heart perfusion mode.

Hearts were removed from the animals at various time points, ranging from 7 days to one year, and perfused by the working heart technique (4). In addition the diabetic state was assessed in all animals by measuring serum insulin, serum glucose, body weight and heart weight. Representative data are illustrated in Table 1.

Treatment with either diabetogenic agent resulted in a decrease in serum insulin and an increase in serum glucose values as early as 7 days following injection of the drug. Diabetic animals did not maintain normal growth patterns and in 30 days (alloxan) or 100 days (STZ) were significantly lighter than their age-matched controls. Heart weights of diabetic animals were less than control at 30 days. Coronary flow values were similar in all groups of animals indicating that vascular changes were not implicated in the cardiac functional alterations that were subsequently observed.

Cardiac function, determined as (+) and (-) dP/dt and left ventricular developed pressure, was determined by altering the filling pressure (preload) from 5.0 to 22.5 cm H_2O. After 7 days of diabetes hearts from all groups performed normally but after 30 days hearts from the alloxan animals exhibited depressed function, particularly at higher filling pressures. In our initial study (4) hearts from STZ animals showed decreased function at 100 days. In a later study (6) the time point was more accurately determined to be 6 weeks after the onset of diabetes. A summary of the (-) dP/dt data at one filling pressure is shown in Figure 1. Note that function decreased at 30-100 days and remained lower than control up to the final time point of one year. Similar results were obtained when (+) dP/dt or left ventricular pressures were monitored.

Since the sarcoplasmic reticulum (SR) is known to be involved in both relaxation and contraction it was decided to examine the ability of SR obtained from both normal and diabetic animals to take up calcium in the presence of oxalate (7,8). Initial studies (7) revealed that SR obtained from 120 day, but not from 7 day, diabetic hearts showed a

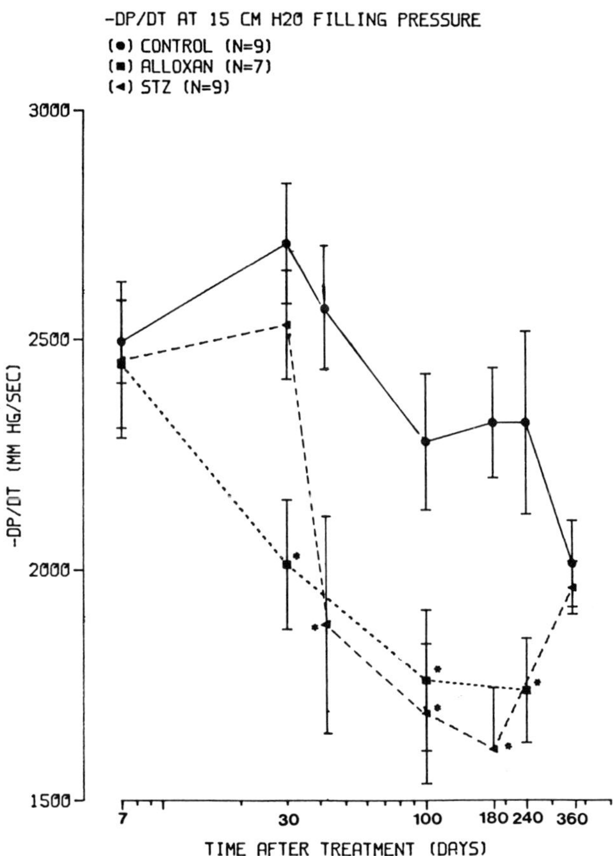

FIGURE 1. The effect of time on (-) dP/dt in control and diabetic rat hearts perfused on the working heart apparatus at 15 cm H_2O atrial filling pressure. Redrawn from data of Vadlamudi <u>et al</u> (4) and Tahiliani <u>et al</u> (6).

significant decrease in the rate of ATP-dependent tris oxalate facilitated Ca^{2+} transport over a range of Ca^{2+} concentrations (0.2-5.0 μM free Ca^{2+}) as shown in Figure 2. Ca^{2+}-ATPase activity in diabetic SR was similarly reduced. These changes corresponded with our previously reported decreases in cardiac function (4). Long chain acylcarnitine levels were increased in SR from 120 day diabetic animals and we were able to confirm that palmityl carnitine, the most

abundant long chain acyl carnitine could inhibit both Ca^{2+}-
ATPase and SR calcium uptake (Figure 3). We thus evolved the
working hypothesis that a buildup of long chain acylcarnitines in diabetic cardiac SR inhibited Ca^{2+}-ATPase and
Ca^{2+} uptake and thus interfered with both relaxation and
contraction in the diabetic myocardium.

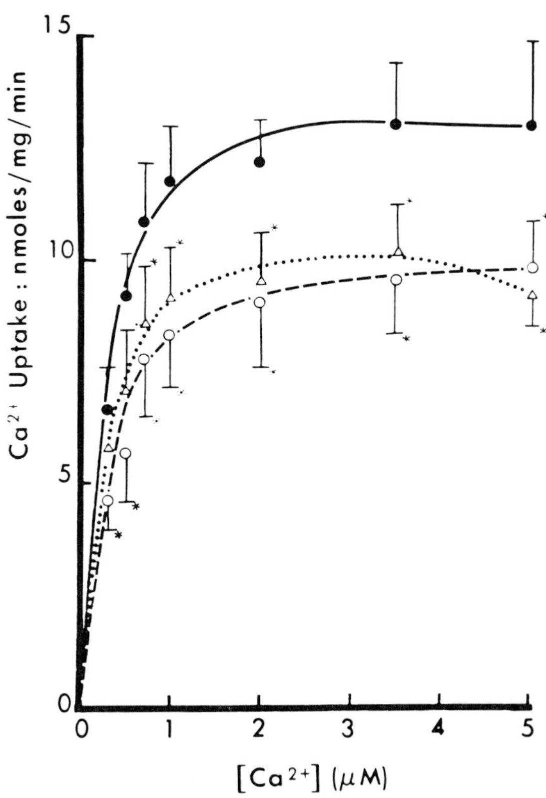

Figure 2. Effect of chronic diabetes (120 days) on cardiac
sarcoplasmic reticulum Ca^{2+}-uptake at various Ca^{2+}
concentrations. Ca^{2+} uptake, over a 5-min period, and
free Ca^{2+}-concentrations were determined in sarcoplasmic
reticulum preparations derived from control (●——●), streptozotocin-treated (○----○), or alloxan-treated rats
(△····△). The results shown are the mean $\pm$ SD of observations from seven controls, six streptozotocin-, and five
alloxan-treated rats. * indicates significantly different
than control $p < 0.05$. Redrawn from Lopaschuk et al (7).

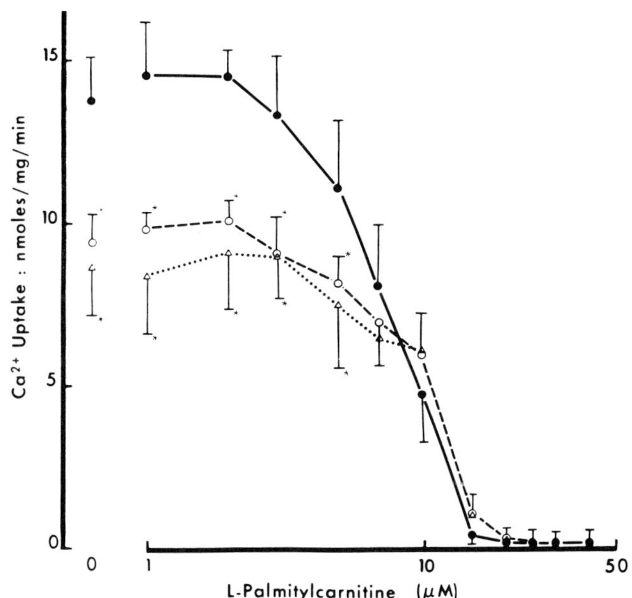

Figure 3. Effect of L-palmitylcarnitine on Ca^{2+}-uptake
in sarcoplasmic reticulum preparations from the chronically
diabetic rat (120 days). Ca^{2+}-uptake was measured in the
presence of 2 μM free Ca^{2+} in sarcoplasmic reticulum
preparations from control (●——●), streptozotocin-treated
(O----O), or alloxan-treated (△····△) rats. The results
shown are the mean ± SD of observations from six controls,
five streptozotocin-, and four alloxan-treated rats. * indicates significantly different than control $p < 0.05$. Redrawn
from Lopaschuk et al (7).

We next attempted to answer the question as to whether
or not treatment of the diabetic animals could prevent or
reverse the diabetes-induced cardiac changes. Two protocols
were drawn up in order to answer this question. In the prevention studies rats were made diabetic and treatment was
begun within 2-3 days following positive determination of
diabetes and continued over a 6-week period. In the reversal
study animals were made diabetic and left untreated for a 6
week period. At that time treatment was initiated and continued for a period of four weeks. In one limited study a
few animals that had been diabetic for 5 months were treated

for four weeks. At the end of the treatment schedule the animals were killed and cardiac and SR function was examined. Cardiac SR levels of long chain acylcarnitine and blood levels of glucose and plasma levels of insulin were also monitored. Glycosylated hemoglobin was used as an index of glucose control. Insulin (9 U/kg/day) was the first treatment examined. Insulin both prevented the cardiac changes when treatment was initiated immediately following the onset of diabetes and reversed the changes after a 6 weeks development period. The dose used restored body weight and heart weight to normal as well as blood glucose and plasma insulin levels. Glycosylated hemoglobin levels were normal in diabetic animals treated with insulin for the 6-week period and were restored towards normal in the six week diabetes-four week treatment study. SR uptake of calcium and levels of long chain acylcarnitines were normal in insulin treated animals. In the 5 month diabetes plus 4 week treatment study described above insulin partially, but not completely, restored cardiac function. Biochemical studies were not carried out on this set of animals.

Thus, as might have been expected, insulin was able to restore both biochemical and mechanical functional changes in the relatively short term diabetic rat heart. Complete restoration was not obtained in the 5 month diabetic animals. This may have been because the changes induced by diabetes had become irreversible by 5 months. Alternatively the four week treatment schedule may simply have been too short to totally reverse the changes. We are continuing to examine the latter possibility.

A number of studies (9-11) led us to speculate that carnitine administration to diabetic rats might lower the levels of long chain acylcarnitines. Carnitine was administered orally (3 g/kg/day) for a 6 week period in order to try to prevent the onset of the diabetes induced changes. Carnitine treatment did not affect the diabetes induced changes in blood glucose, plasma insulin or glycosylated hemoglobin values. It did, however, restore SR function and

SR levels of long chain acylcarnitines to normal (Table 2).
Unfortunately, carnitine had no positive effect on the

Table 2. Cardiac sarcoplasmic reticulum levels of carnitine
and long chain acylcarnitines from 6 week diabetic and
control carnitine treated rats.

Condition	Metabolites	Tissue levels (nmol carnitine/mg SR $\pm$ S.E.M.)
control (n, 8)	acid-soluble carnitine	7.01 ± 0.63
	fatty acylcarnitine	0.74 ± 0.09
control plus carnitine (n, 5)	acid-soluble carnitine	6.78 ± 0.56
	fatty acylcarnitine	0.85 ± 0.09
diabetic (n, 5)	acid soluble carnitine	7.33 ± 0.41
	fatty acylcarnitine	1.82 ± 0.40[1]
diabetic plus carnitine (n, 6)	acid soluble carnitine	7.67 ± 0.76
	fatty acylcarnitine	0.86 ± 0.14

[1] Significantly different from control ($p < 0.05$, analysis
of variance, followed by the Newman-Keuls test).

Hearts were isolated from control and diabetic rats 42 days
after the induction of diabetes with streptozocin (50 mg/kg
i.v.). Carnitine treated rats received D,L-carnitine (3
g/kg/day) orally throughout the study period, commencing 3
days after the induction of diabetes.

depression of cardiac function induced by diabetes. In fact,
hearts from diabetic animals treated with carnitine did not
respond to pressure changes as well as did non-treated diabetic hearts.

Our working hypothesis was that SR levels of long chain
acylcarnitines and SR function changes were intimately involved in the mechanical changes induced in the heart by diabetes. The carnitine experiment did not support the hypothesis
since SR function and long chain acylcarnitine levels were
restored to normal while contractile function remained
impaired. There does, however, still appear to be a relationship between the impairment of SR calcium uptake and the
level of long chain acylcarnitines in the SR.

One additional treatment was also tried. Diabetes is known to produce a mildly hypothyroid state (12). Hypothyroidism in turn is known to decrease myosin ATPase (13) and SR calcium transport (14). We thus considered it to be possible that the effect of diabetes on the heart could be a result of hypothyroidism. Dillman (15) has previously shown that triiodthyronine (30 μg/kg/day) can restore myosin ATPase to normal in STZ diabetic rats. This dose of thyroid hormone was used in our study and was administered for a 6 week period as described for the insulin and carnitine studies. Triiodothyronine treatment did not affect the diabetesinduced changes in body weight, heart weight, plasma glucose or plasma insulin found in diabetic rats. The dose used did restore the plasma triodothyronine levels of the diabetic animals to normal (Table 3). Cardiac function, SR function and SR long chain acylcarnitine levels were not affected by the thyroid hormone treatment. Thus, hypothyroidism does not account for the cardiac changes seen in diabetes (16).

Table 3. General features of T_3 treated and untreated control and diabetic rats.

(a)	Body Weight (g)	Plasma Glucose (mg%)	Glycosylated Hemoglobin (mol HFM/g globin)	Plasma Insulin (U/ml)
Control (8)	218±6	129±8	1.59±0.12	18.7±0.6
Control Treated (7)	211±4	119±8	1.33±0.09	19.1±0.7
Diabetic (7)	170±7*	403±25*	3.04±0.17*	5.6±0.4*
Diabetic Treated (6)	176±7*	339±29*	3.32±0.11*	7.1±0.6*

(b)	Heart Weight	Heart Weight/ Body Weight	T_3B Index (%)
Control (8)	0.60±0.005	2.73±0.03	53.3±2.7
Control Treated (7)	0.66±0.01	2.97±0.03	68.8±6.0*
Diabetic (7)	0.55±0.02	3.25±0.07*	45.9±0.8*
Diabetic Treated (6)	0.59±0.02	3.35±0.06*	54.7±4.1

(*p < 0.05)

In summary: While initial studies showed a correlation between disturbances in SR uptake of calcium and calcium function in diabetic rat hearts more recent findings have disassociated the two. It is possible to restore SR calcium uptake, using carnitine treatment, without restoring contractile function. Insulin is capable of restoring all of the diabetes-induced changes in the heart and was the only treatment tried that was successful. Since insulin control of diabetes in humans is not always totally successful in preventing the secondary complications of diabetes it is important to develop additional treatments to prevent, control and/or reverse such secondary complications. Experiments along these lines are currently underway in our laboratory.

ACKNOWLEDGMENTS

Work described was supported by grants from the MRC(C), B.C. Heart Fdn., Canadian Diabetes Association, B.C. Branch of the Canadian Diabetes Association and the B.C. Health Care Research Fund. The contributions of my colleagues R.V.S.V. Vadlamudi, A.G. Tahiliani, G.D. Lopaschuk and S. Katz are gratefully acknowledged.

REFERENCES

1. Ledet T, Neubauer B, Christensen NJ, Lundback K: Diabetic Cardiopathy. Diabetologia (16): 207-209, 1979.

2. Hamby RI, Zoneraich S, Sherman MD: Diabetic Cardiomyopathy. J Am Med Assoc (229): 1749-1754, 1974.

3. Regan TJ, Ettinger PO, Khan MI, Jesrani MU, Lyons MM, Oldewurtel HA, Weber M: Altered myocardial function and metabolism in chronic diabetes mellitus without ischemia in dogs. Circ Res (35): 222-237, 1974.

4. Vadlamudi RVSV, Rodgers RL, McNeill JH: The effect of chronic alloxan- and streptozotocin-induced diabetes on isolated rat heart performance. Can J Physiol Pharmacol (60): 902-911, 1982.

5. Vadlamudi RVSV, McNeill JH: Effect of experimental diabetes on rat cardiac cyclic AMP, phosphorylase and inotropy. Am J Physiol (244): H844-H851, 1983.

6. Tahiliani AG, Vadlamudi RVSV, McNeill JH: Prevention
    and reversal of altered myocardial function in diabetic
    rats by insulin treatment. Can J Physiol Pharmacol (61):
    516-523, 1983.

7. Lopaschuk GD, Katz S, McNeill JH: The effect of alloxan-
    and streptozotocin-induced diabetes on calcium transport
    in rat cardiac sarcoplasmic reticulum. The possible
    involvement of long chain acylcarnitines. Can J Physiol
    Pharmacol (61): 439-448, 1983.

8. Lopaschuk GD, Katz S, McNeill JH: Effect of oral
    carnitine treatment on cardiac sarcoplasmic reticulum
    function in streptozotocin-induced diabetic rats. Proc
    West Pharmacol Soc (26): 39-43, 1983.

9. Regitz V, Hadach RJ, Shug AL: Carnitine deficiency. A
    treatable cause of cardiomyopathy in children.
    Klinische Wochenschrift (60): 393-400, 1982.

10. Genuth SM, Hoppel CL: Plasma and urine carnitine in
    diabetic ketosis. Diabetes (28): 1083-1087, 1979.

11. Shug AL, Thomsen JH, Folts JD, Bittar N, Klein MI, Kohe
    JR and Huth PJ: Changes in tissue levels of carnitine
    and other metabolites during myocardial ischemia and
    anoxia. Arch Biochem Biophys (187): 25-33, 1978.

12. Pittman CS, Suda AK, Chambers JB, Ray GY: Impaired
    $3,5,3'$-triiodothyronine (T_3) production in diabetic
    patients. Metab. (28): 333-338, 1979.

13. Thyrum PT, Kritcher EM, Luchi RJ: Effect of L-thyroxine
    on the primary structure opf cardiac myosin. Biocnemica
    et Biophysica Acta (197): 335-336, 1970.

14. Suko, J: The calcium pump of cardiac sarcoplasmic
    reticulum. Functional alterations at different levels
    of thyroid state in rabbits. J Physiol (228): 563-582,
    1973.

15, Dillman WH: Influence of thyroid hormone on myosin
    ATPase activity and myosin isoenzyme distribution in the
    heart of diabetic rats. Metabolism (31): 199-204,
    1982.

16. Tahiliani AG, McNeill JH: Lack of effect of thyroid
    hormone on diabetic rat heart function and biochemistry.
    Can J Physiol Pharmacol (in press) 1984.

22

ROLE OF CALCIUM IN HEART FUNCTION AND METABOLISM

NIELS HAUGAARD AND MARILYN E. HESS

That calcium ions play a role in the regulation of cardiac contraction was realized by Sidney Ringer, who reported in 1883 that the presence of calcium ions in the extracellular fluid was necessary to maintain the beating of the isolated, perfused heart (1). The history of the gradual development of our knowledge of the specific function of calcium ions in coupling excitation with contraction has been outlined in excellent fashion by Olson (2) and by Naylor and Merrillees (3) in their chapters in the book "Calcium and the Heart," edited by Harris and Opie. More recently, Braunwald (4) and Herzig (5) have presented summaries of our present knowledge of the mechanisms by which calcium regulates cardiac contractility. Braunwald, in particular, emphasized the involvement of calcium ions in a variety of cardiovascular disorders and discussed the potential value of using slow-channel calcium blockers in treating circulatory diseases.

The current concepts of the regulation of cardiac contraction by calcium have been derived from extensive studies of heart morphology, chemistry of contractile proteins and electrophysiological properties of myocardial cells. After depolarization of the sarcolemmal membrane calcium ions enter the cell and there is considerable evidence that the influx of calcium causes release of additional calcium ions from the sarcoplasmic reticulum and possibly from the sarcolemmal membrane itself. Subsequently, the concentration of calcium in the myoplasm rises and calcium ions combine with a subunit of troponin. An interaction between the myosin bridges and actin then occurs in the presence of ATP, which allows movement of the actin toward the center of the sarcomere, resulting in shortening of the muscle. Relaxation is associated with a reversal of these processes. An integral part of the mechanism of lowering cytoplasmic calcium to promote relaxation is the extrusion of this ion by the action of a calcium-stimulated ATP-ase present on the sarcolemmal membrane, as well as reuptake of calcium by the sarcoplasmic reticulum. For bibliography and extensive discussions of calcium fluxes in the heart and the role of calcium ions in regulating cardiac contractility, see references 4 and 5 and the reviews by Dhalla and coworkers (6), and by Katz (7).

Most of the calcium present in heart cells is sequestered in mitochondria. These organelles have the ability to take up and release calcium, but the role of these processes in the regulation of the contractile activity of the myocardium is uncertain. Because the reactions involved are not fast enough at the low concentrations of free calcium present in the cytoplasm of cells in normal hearts, mitochondrial calcium fluxes are probably of little importance in the cycle of contraction and relaxation of the heart (8). Many excellent studies have been made of the factors that influence mitochondrial calcium uptake. These investigations have shown that calcium entry into mitochondria is supported by energy from the breakdown of ATP or by energy derived from respiration (8). Much less is understood about the mechanisms involved in the release of calcium from mitochondria. There is evidence that an increase in intracellular sodium ion concentration promotes mitochondrial release of calcium (9). Other studies have shown that phosphoenolpyruvate has an action, not shared by other glycolytic intermediates, in that it causes extrusion of calcium ions from mitochondria (10).

Future studies of mitochondrial uptake and release of calcium ions can be expected to define more precisely the significance of these processes in heart function. It is possible that intramitochondrial calcium may play a significant role in the regulation of energy production by mitochondria or that mitochondrial calcium uptake may be a factor in defending the myocardium against ischemia and other insults.

The importance of calcium ions for normal cardiac contraction is reflected by results from studies of the actions of a group of drugs generally referred to as slow-channel calcium blockers. These agents have unusual selectivity in inhibiting the transmembrane influx of calcium into myocardial cells. The prototype of this class of drugs, verapamil, was shown originally by Fleckenstein (11) to decrease isometric tension of the perfused heart without significantly affecting the resting potential or the velocity of the upstroke of the cardiac action potential (11). Depression of contractility produced by verapamil was dose-dependent and reversible. Studies performed in our laboratory showed that the negative inotropic effect of verapamil in rat hearts perfused continuously with the drug dissipates with time (12). These findings are presented in Figure 1.

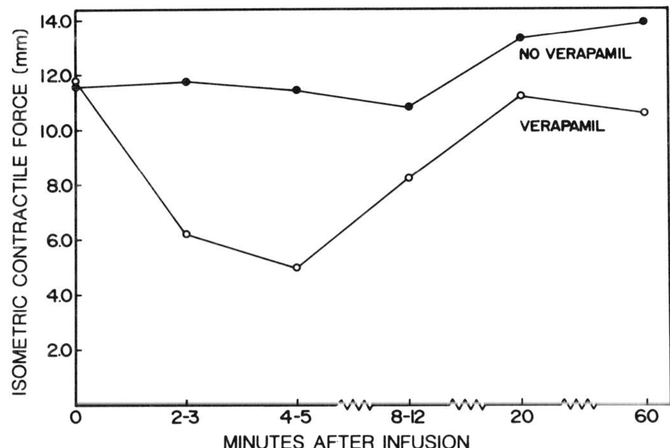

FIGURE 1. Effect of continuous perfusion of verapamil on isometric contractile force in the isolated rat heart. Concentration of verapamil in the perfusion fluid was 25 μg L^{-1}. The points on each curve are means of 5–9 experiments.

This phenomenon was seen with a concentration of verapamil that caused a 50% reduction of the force of contraction. Although the mechanism for the recovery of contractile force is not known, one obvious possibility is that verapamil, after a certain period of time, no longer exerts its effects on the sarcolemmal membrane to inhibit calcium influx. Another possibility is that intracellular calcium is mobilized and made available to the contractile proteins when the drug is administered continuously. It would be of interest to ascertain whether escape from the depressant effects of verapamil can also be demonstrated in intact animals given a constant, uninterrupted infusion of the drug.

Thus far, we have been discussing the involvement of calcium ions in regulating cardiac contractility. The influence of calcium on heart metabolism is also of major import. A prime example of drug-induced alterations in myocardial metabolism, dependent on a rise in intracellular calcium, is observed when the heart is stimulated by catecholamines. Associated with the positive inotropic effect of these drugs, there is a dramatic increase in glycogenolysis with a concomitant outpouring of lactate. While it is clear that cyclic AMP is a mediator of the glycogenolytic response, an elevation of cytoplasmic calcium is also essential for this metabolic effect to occur. Enzyme studies

have revealed that an important site of action of calcium in this process is phosphorylase
b kinase, rather than adenylate cyclase (13). It should be pointed out that calcium ions,
in addition, activate phosphodiesterase (14,15), thereby promoting the breakdown of
cyclic AMP and hastening the termination of catecholamine–induced glycogenolysis.
Intimately involved in the activation of both phosphorylase b kinase and
phosphodiesterase is the regulatory protein, calmodulin (15). These sites of action of
calcium are illustrated in Figure 2.

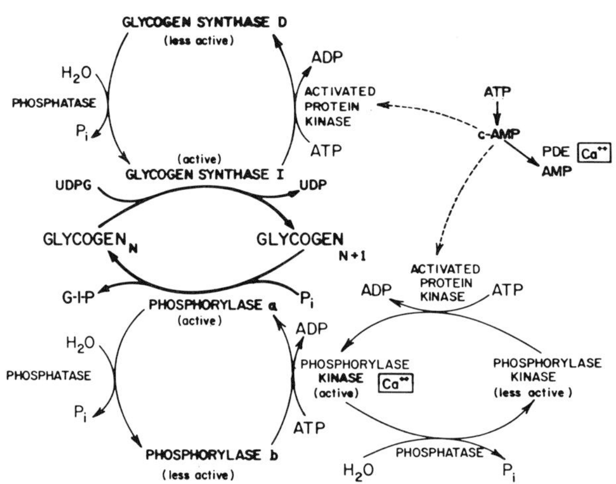

FIGURE 2. Sites of action of calcium ions in regulating the activities of glycogen
synthase and phosphorylase.

Another major site at which calcium influences myocardial metabolism is the
mitochondrion, where calcium ions act at the mitochondrial membrane to increase
pyruvate dehydrogenase activity. Denton and his coworkers (16) demonstrated that this
stimulatory effect of calcium was due to an activation of pyruvate dehydrogenase
phosphatase causing a transformation of PDH to its active dephosphorylated form. From
these studies, it is apparent that both glycogenolytic and oxidative reactions are
promoted by increases in the intracellular concentration of calcium.

In the intact heart, activation of oxidative reactions by a catecholamine have
been clearly shown. For example, Figure 3 depicts results of experiments with the
isolated rat heart perfused with pyruvate, showing that infusion of epinephrine doubled

the rate of pyruvate utilization (17). In light of the enzyme studies described earlier, this phenomenon is very likely a consequence of an increase in intracellular calcium produced by the catecholamine.

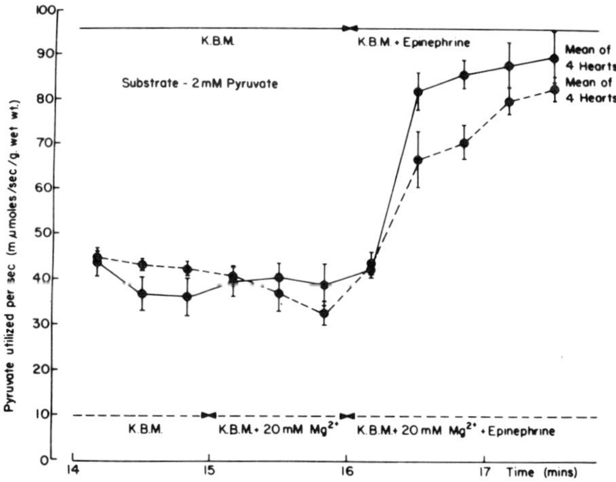

FIGURE 3. Effect of epinephrine infusion (5 μg min^{-1}) on the rate of pyruvate utilization by isolated perfused rat heart. Experiments with Krebs-Ringer bicarbonate solution (KRB) are indicated by solid line. Experiments with KRB containing 20 mM magnesium are indicated by broken line. (From Paddle and Haugaard, 1971).

The changes in heart function and metabolism just discussed have been concerned with the effects of moderate changes in intracellular calcium. However, it should be pointed out that when cytoplasmic calcium reaches excessively high concentrations, severe cellular damage occurs to the myocardium. Rona and coworkers (18) first observed the development of myocardial necrosis following administration of a large dose of isoproterenol to rats. Later, Fleckenstein and colleagues (19,20) showed that the myocardial lesions produced by the high dose of catecholamine could be prevented by simultaneous administration of a calcium antagonist. This group of investigators subsequently elucidated the mechanism of the catecholamine-induced necrosis, when they demonstrated that the damage to the myocardium was associated with a dramatic loss of intracellular high-energy phosphate compounds and a corresponding increase in inorganic phosphate. These changes in adenine nucleotides and creatine phosphate were prevented by the concomitant administration of calcium channel blockers (21). In addition to the protective effect of the organic calcium antagonists, certain cations, such as magnesium, can inhibit the transmembrane influx of calcium and catecholamine-induced necrosis.

The interaction between calcium and magnesium ions in the regulation of cardiac metabolism has been demonstrated in experiments from our laboratory. We showed that epinephrine-stimulated glycogenolysis in the isolated, perfused rat heart was abolished by raising the concentration of magnesium in the perfusion fluid from 1.3 to 20 mM, although contractility was minimally affected. Later, these experiments were extended by Levin and coworkers (22). Results of experiments by the latter investigators are illustrated in Figure 4.

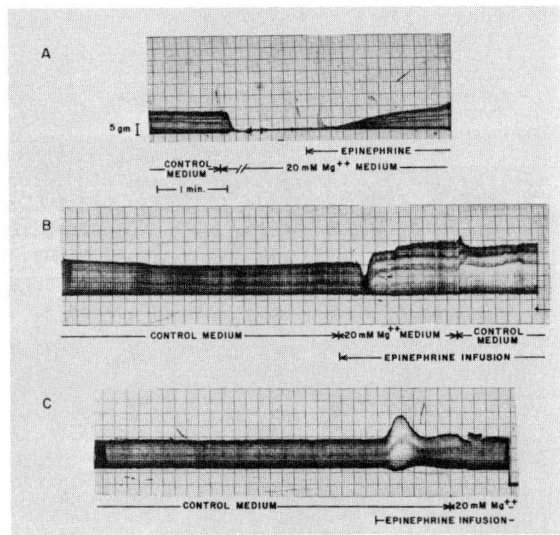

FIGURE 4. Effect of epinephrine infusion (5 µg min^{-1}) on isometric contractile force of the isolated perfused rat heart perfused with KRB solution or KRB with 20 mM magnesium. (From Levin et al., 1976).

In panel A, it is seen that, when the control perfusion fluid of the isolated rat heart was changed to one containing 20 mM magnesium, there was an abrupt and severe depression of contractility in the absence of epinephrine. When the catecholamine was subsequently infused in the presence of high magnesium, the force of contraction gradually increased. Results given in panel B, showed that the simultaneous infusion of epinephrine and perfusion with 20 mM Mg solution caused a large increase in force of contraction. When subsequently the perfusion fluid was changed to the control medium while continuing the epinephrine infusion, force of contraction was unaffected. The bottom panel illustrates the effect of raising the magnesium concentration in the perfusion fluid one minute after the beginning of an epinephrine infusion. Under these circumstances, there was also little change in contractility as a result of introducing the high magnesium. We interpret these inotropic effects of magnesium to mean that magnesium ions act at the sarcolemmal membrane to inhibit calcium influx during the normal cycle of cardiac contraction. This depressant action of magnesium can be overcome by catecholamines which increase calcium influx by activation of beta-receptors. The inability of excess magnesium to alter contractility significantly in the heart stimulated by a high dose of catecholamine, provides particularly strong support for the view that receptor-mediated calcium influx is much less sensitive to the antagonistic action of the magnesium ion than is potential-dependent calcium uptake. The low sensitivity of receptor-mediated calcium entry to inhibition by magnesium is similar to the phenomenon seen with slow channel calcium blockers. Braunwald (4) has pointed out that potential-dependent calcium entry is more readily blocked by these drugs than is calcium influx mediated by receptor stimulation.

In similar experiments, we measured the efflux of lactate from hearts perfused with control or high magnesium media in the presence and absence of epinephrine (22). The concentration of calcium in the perfusion fluid was varied over the range 1.3 to 3.9 mM. Results obtained from these experiments are illustrated in Figure 5.

In the absence of epinephrine, there was essentially no formation of lactate, regardless of the concentration of calcium or magnesium in the perfusion fluid. When epinephrine was administered to hearts perfused with the control medium containing 1.2 mM magnesium, lactate production was markedly increased. As the calcium concentration was raised in the perfusion fluid, lactate output was further elevated. Perfusion with a medium containing 20 mM magnesium almost abolished the output of lactate customarily seen following epinephrine administration. When the calcium concentration in the perfusion fluid was raised to 2.6 or 3.9 mM, lactate output again increased. At a calcium concentration of 3.9 mM, with the high magnesium medium, the rate of lactate efflux was the same as that in the control medium which contained only 1.3 mM calcium. Such data illustrate the interaction between extracellular calcium and magnesium in modulating glycogenolysis in the heart.

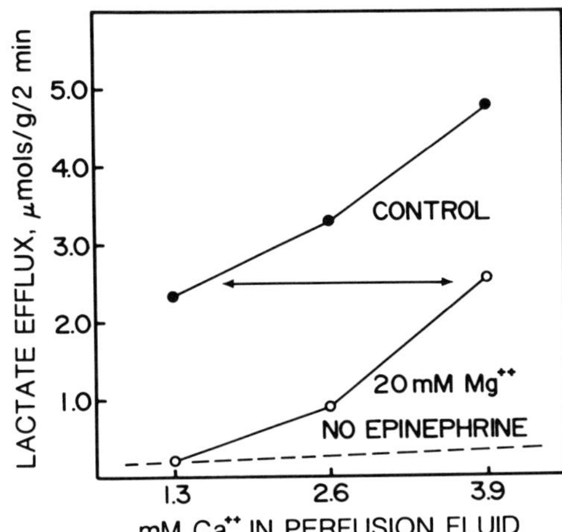

FIGURE 5. Lactate production by the isolated perfused rat heat in response to varying concentrations of calcium. The hatched line represents lactate formation in the absence of epinephrine. The line with solid circles indicates lactate efflux in response to a 2 min infusion of epinephrine (5 μg min^{-1}) in hearts perfused with KRB solution. The line with open circles indicates lactate efflux in similar experiments with hearts perfused with KRB solution containing 20 mM magnesium.

Results of experiments in which the concentration of magnesium was alternated between 1.2 and 20 mM during continuous infusion of epinephrine are illustrated in Figure 6.

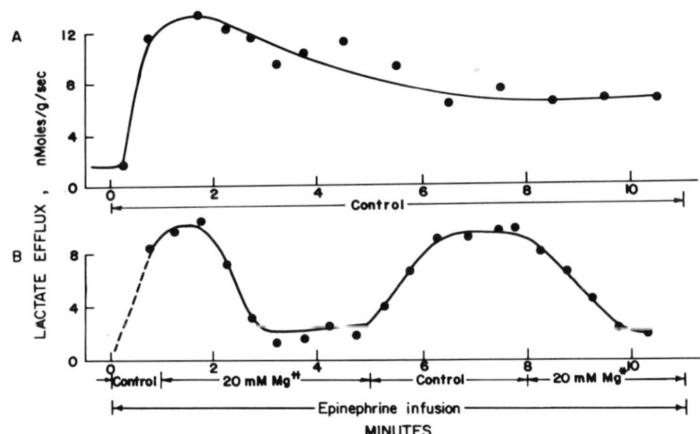

FIGURE 6. Lactate efflux by the isolated rat heart during constant infusion of epinephrine (5 µg/min) with varying the concentrations of magnesium in the perfusion fluid.

In panel A, epinephrine was given to a heart perfused with control Krebs-Ringer bicarbonate; lactate efflux was measured every 30 seconds and expressed as nmols/g/sec. Epinephrine infusion caused a rapid increase in the rate of lactate formation which reached a maximum at 2 minutes. This was followed by a slow decline leading to a plateau after about 6 minutes with a final rate of lactate production approximately 60% of the maximum. In panel B, we have illustrated experiments in which the perfusion medium was changed several times from control Krebs-Ringer bicarbonate to the same solution containing 20 mM magnesium. Within a very short time after altering the medium, the rate of lactate efflux changed from a high level in the control to almost immeasurable values when the high magnesium medium was introduced. It should be emphasized that these metabolic changes occurred with minimal alterations in the force of contraction.

Experiments designed to investigate the mechanism of action of magnesium ions in inhibiting the glycogenolytic effect of epinephrine revealed that changes in cyclic AMP and phosphorylase _a_ activity produced by the high magnesium concentration were small and could not explain the depressant effect of magnesium on catecholamine-stimulated cardiac metabolism. However, it was found that the high concentration of magnesium, as shown in the original experiments by Fleckenstein (21), effectively protected the heart against the undesirable decreases in high-energy phosphate compounds caused by excess cytosolic calcium ions following exposure to epinephrine. We concluded that the severe reduction in ATP and the increases in AMP and inorganic phosphate, seen after administration of epinephrine to hearts perfused with control medium, were the principal factors in releasing the constraints on glycogenolysis during administration of the catecholamine. At the high concentration of magnesium, the changes in intracellular levels of high-energy phosphate compounds following epinephrine were minimal and the rate of glycogenolysis was not greatly affected despite large increases in myocardial cyclic AMP and phosphorylase _a_ activity.

Investigations of effects of calcium on cardiac function and metabolism in animals with endocrinopathies or with other pathological conditions constitute an important area of research and will be discussed extensively in this symposium. For example, the increase in beta adrenergic receptors in the heart in experimental hyperthyroidism can be expected to lead to an enhanced calcium influx in response to a beta agonist. The symptomatic relief by beta adrenergic blocking agents of some of the cardiovascular complications seen in the hyperthyroid state may be explained on this basis.

Considerable excitement has been generated by the results of studies of myocardial metabolism in diabetes. It has been suggested that abnormalities of calcium fluxes are involved in mediating some of the alterations in heart metabolism in this disease. Miller and colleagues (23), Vadlamudi and McNeill (24), as well as ourselves (25), have shown that the stimulatory effect of catecholamines on phosphorylase activity in rat hearts is potentiated in diabetes. These observations could not be explained by an increased formation of cyclic AMP or an accentuated activation of cyclic-AMP-sensitive protein kinase. It was suggested by Miller and his associates (23), and Vadlamudi and McNeill (24) that in diabetes, alterations in the movement of calcium ions are involved in the accentuated response of phosphorylase to catecholamines. Ingebretsen and his group (26) observed that the action of cyclic AMP in activating glycogen phosphorylase is enhanced in hearts from diabetic rats, and suggested that in diabetic tissue, phosphorylase _b_ kinase is more sensitive to activation by calcium or that there is an increase in the availability of calcium for the activation of this enzyme in cardiac cells from diabetic animals. Results of recent experiments in our laboratory (25) on the action of isoproterenol on phosphorylase activity of isolated perfused hearts from normal and diabetic rats are illustrated in Figure 7. The normal and diabetic animals were placed on a diet of regular Purina Chow or a diet fortified by the addition of sucrose and raw corn starch.

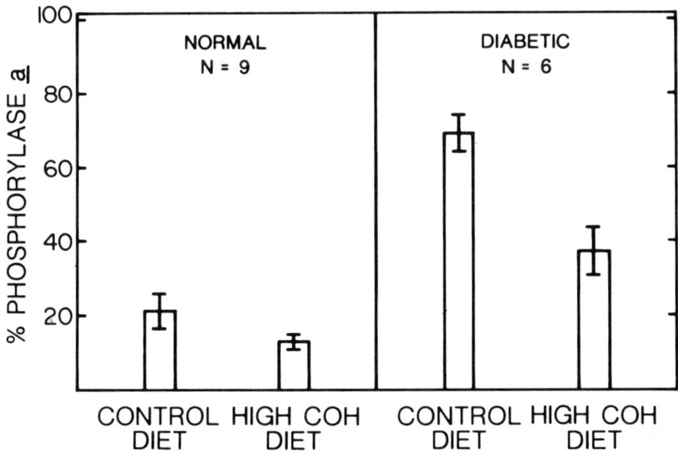

FIGURE 7. Phosphorylase $\underline{a}$ activity of perfused rat hearts after administration of isoproterenol (bolus of 0.01 µg in 0.2 ml).

Basal values of phosphorylase activity are not presented in the figure, but averaged between 5 to 8%. It is seen that in confirmation of the results from other laboratories, when a submaximal dose of catecholamine was administered, the activation of phosphorylase was much smaller in hearts from normal than from diabetic animals. In addition, we have shown that diet can influence catecholamine-induced activation of phosphorylase. Both in normal and diabetic animals, one week of exposure to a high carbohydrate diet caused a marked decrease in the sensitivity of phosphorylase to activation by a catecholamine. Whether changes in calcium homeostasis are involved in this phenomenon is open to further investigation, but the observations indicate that subtle differences in cardiac energy supply can markedly influence cardiac metabolism and the responses of the heart to catecholamines and possibly other drugs.

In concluding this discussion, I would like to focus attention to studies showing that enzymes involved in many metabolic pathways in the heart are located in membranes and in close apposition to each other. This is certainly true for the mitochondrial enzyme pyruvate dehydrogenase (16), but is also the case for the enzymes concerned with the synthesis and degradation of glycogen. For example, Entman and coworkers (27) isolated fragments of cardiac sarcoplasmic reticulum that contained glycogen and enzymes associated with glycogenolysis. Among the enzymes found in these particles were adenylate cyclase, cyclic AMP-dependent protein kinase, phosphorylase b kinase, phosphorylase and debrancher enzyme. Enzymes involved in the synthesis of glycogen in skeletal muscle also have been demonstrated to be closely associated with membranes (28). That enzymes located in cell membranes catalyze an entire metabolic sequence of reactions is evident from the finding that in skeletal muscle incorporation of glucose into glycogen occurs without penetration of free glucose into the cell (29).

The presence of enzymes in membranes that are readily accessible to the ionic milieu of extracellular fluid favor the hypothesis that important metabolic pathways are vulnerable to regulation by calcium and other ions in the extracellular environment. Based on this reasoning, it may well be appropriate to use the term "excitation-metabolism coupling" to describe alterations in cell metabolism produced by changes in extracellular ion concentrations.

REFERENCES

1. Ringer S.: A further contribution regarding the influence of direct constituents of the blood on the contractions of the heart. J Physiol (4):29-42, 1883.
2. Olson RE: Introduction. In: Harris P, Opie LH (eds) Calcium and the heart. Academic Press, London and New York, 1971, pp 1-23.
3. Naylor WG, Merrillees NCR: Cellular exchange of calcium. In: Harris P, Opie LH (eds) Calcium and the heart. Academic Press, London and New York, 1971, pp 24-65.
4. Braunwald E: Mechanism of action of calcium-channel-blocking agents. New Eng J. Med (307): 1618-1627, 1982.
5. Herzig, JW: The role of calcium ions in the regulaton of myocardial contractility. Triangle (22): 31-37, 1983.
6. Dhalla NS, Ziegelhoffer A, Harrow JAC: Regulatory role of membrane systems in heart function. Can J Physiol Pharmacol (55): 1211-1234, 1977.
7. Katz AM: Role of the contractile proteins and sarcoplasmic reticulum in the response of the heart to catecholamines: an historical review. Adv Cyclic Nucleotide Res (11): 303-343, 1979.
8. Carafoli E: The uptake and release of calcium by mitochondria. In: Lee CP, Schatz G, Dallner D (eds) Mitochondria and microsomes. Addison-Wesley Publishing Co, Inc, 1981, pp 357-374.

9. Crompton M, Cepano M, Carafoli E: The sodium-induced efflux of calcium from heart mitochondria. A possible mechanism of the regulaton of mitochondrial calcium. Eur J Biochem (69), 453-462, 1976.

10. Chudapongse P, Haugaard N: The effect of phosphoenol-pyruvate on calcium transport by mitochondria. Biochim Biophys Acta (307): 599-606, 1973.

11. Fleckenstein A: Experimentelle Pathologie der akuten und chronischen Hertzinsuffizienz. Verh dtsch Ges Krieslaufforsch (34): 15-34, 1968.

12. Shanfeld J, Hess ME, Levine NB: Effects of verapamil on myocardial contractility, cardiac adenosine 3',5'-monophosphate and heart phosphorylase. J. Pharmacol Exp Ther (193): 317-326, 1975.

13. Meyer WL, Fischer EH, Krebs EG: Activation of skeletal muscle phosphorylase $\underline{b}$ kinase by Ca^{2+}. Biochemistry (3): 1033-1039, 1964.

14. Cheung WY: Cyclic 3',5'-nucleotide phosphodiesterase: pronounced stimulation by snake venom. Biochem Biophys Res Commun (19): 478-482, 1967.

15. Cheung NY: Calmodulin plays a pivotal role in cellular regulation. Science (207): 19-27, 1980.

16. Denton RM, Randle PJ, Martin BR: Stimulation by calcium ions of pyruvate dehydrogenase phosphate phosphatase. Biochem J (128): 161-163, 1972.

17. Paddle BM, Haugaard N: Role of magnesium in effects of epinephrine on heart contraction and metabolism. Am J Physiol (221): 1178-1184, 1971.

18. Rona G, Chappel CI, Balazs J, Gaudry R: An infarct-like myocardial lesion and other toxic manifestations produced by isoproterenol in the rat. AMA Arch Path (67): 443-455, 1959.

19. Fleckenstein A: Myokardstoffwechsel und Necrose. In: Heilmeyer L, Holtmeier H-J (eds) VI Symposium der Deutsch Ges Für Fortschritte auf dem Gebiet der Inneren Medizin über "Hertz infarkt und Schock." Georg Thieme Verlag, Stuttgart, 1968, pp 94-109.

20. Fleckenstein A, Döring HJ, Leder O: The significance of high-energy phoshate exhaustion in the etiology of isoproterenol-induced cardiac necrosis and its prevention by iproveratril, compound D600 or prenylamine. In: Lamarch M, Royer R (eds) Symposium international on drugs and metabolism of myocardium and striated muscle. Nancy, 1969.

21. Fleckenstein A: Specific inhibitors and promoters of calcium action in the excitation-contraction coupling of heart muscle and their role in the prevention or production of myocardial lesions. In: Harris P, Opie LH (eds) Calcium and the heart. Academic Press, London and New York, 1971, pp 135-188.

22. Levin RM, Haugaard N, Hess ME: Opposing actions of calcium and magnesium ions on the metabolic effects of epinehrine in rat heart. Biochem Pharmacol (25): 1963-1969, 1976.

23. Miller TB Jr, Praderio M, Wolleben C, Bullman J: A hypersensitivity of glycogen phosphorylase activation in hearts of diabetic rats. J Biol Chem (256): 1798-1753, 1981.

24. Vadlamudi RVSV, McNeill JH: Effect of experimental diabetes on rat cardiac cAMP, phosphorylase and inotropy. Am J Physiol (244): H844-H851, 1983.

25. Haugaard N, Hess ME, Locke CL, Torbati A, Wildey G: Metabolic effects of acarbose administration in normal and diabetic rats. Biochem Pharmacol Submitted for publication.

26. Ingebretsen WR Jr, Peralta C, Monsher M, Wagner LK, Ingebretsen CG: Diabetes alters the myocardial cAMP-protein kinase cascade system. Am J Physiol (240): H375-H382, 1981.

27. Entman ML, Kanike K, Goldstein MA, Nelson TE, Bornet EP, Futch TW, Schwartz A: Association of glycogenolysis with cardiac sarcoplasmic reticulum. J Biol Chem (251): 3140-3146, 1976.

28. Bailey PJ, Dougherty HW, Mandel L, Reese AC, Landau BR: Distribution of enzymes of glycogen metabolism and calcium uptake in skeletal muscle. Arch Biochem Biophys (161): 592–600, 1974.
29. Haugaard ES, Haugaard N: The action of insulin on glycogen synthesis in rat diaphragm from intracellular and extracellular glucose. Biochim Biophys Acta (338): 309–316, 1974.

23

EXCITATION-CONTRACTION IN CARDIAC MUSCLE OF THE ADULT AND
SENESCENT RAT

EDWARD G. LAKATTA

The impact of adult aging on many aspects of myocardial
function in animals and man has recently been reviewed (1,2,3).
The present discussion will focus on excitation-contraction and
aging of the myocardium. I will try to integrate the findings of
recent and earlier studies in order to formulate alternative
hypotheses regarding the mechanisms of age-related alterations of
excitation-contraction coupling.

The myocardial excitation-contraction cycle begins with depolarization of the sarcolemma which causes a transient increase
in myoplasmic $[Ca^{2+}]$ which results in transient Ca^{2+} activation
of the myofilaments which causes a transient increase in force.

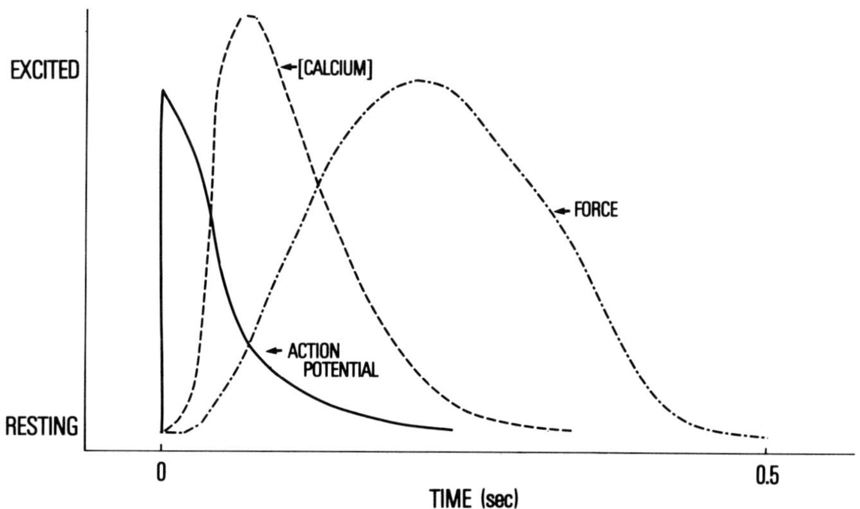

FIGURE 1. Schematic representation of the time course of the
transmembrane action potential, myoplasmic $[Ca^{2+}]$ transient as
reflected in aequorin luminescence in many studies, e.g. (4), and
contractile force upon excitation of the myocardial ventricular
cell.

The precise role of each transsarcolemmal ionic flux (e.g. via Na channel, slow channel, or Na-Ca exchange) in triggering the release of Ca^{2+} from intracellular or inner sarcolemmal storage sites, or in mediating transsarcolemmal Ca^{2+} influx in cardiac muscle is not precisely known and continues to be intensively studied. Although the relative contributions of intracellular Ca^{2+} stores and transsarcolemmal Ca^{2+} influx as the source of Ca^{2+} which activates the myofilaments remains to be definitively elucidated, it need be emphasized that the relative contribution of each to the transient increase in myoplasmic $[Ca^{2+}]$ need not be fixed but may vary with the level of "contractility" or "inotropic state" within a species and may vary among species.

Myocardial adult aging has been most often studied in the rat (1). Rat myocardium, however, has often been avoided in studies attempting to define the mechanisms of the coupling of excitation to contraction and is often labeled as being "different" from most other species. One apparent difference between cardiac muscle from rat and other species is that when bathed in given Ca^{2+} environment (stimulated at low rates at moderate temperatures), rat ventricular myocardial cells appear to gain more Ca^{2+} than those from other species. Recent evidence for this comes from comparison of scattered light intensity fluctuations, (SLIF), as a function of bathing fluid $[Ca^{2+}]$ in muscles from various species (5,6). SLIF measurements monitor microscopic cellular mechanical oscillations (7) which are driven by spontaneous cell Ca^{2+} oscillations (8,9) the frequency and magnitude of which seem to vary with the extent of cell Ca^{2+} loading (8). Since the Ca^{2+} oscillations that cause SLIF do not require depolarization of the sarcolemma (5-8), and since SLIF are abolished by caffeine and ryanodine in unstimulated muscle (7,8), it has been hypothesized (7) that SLIF are caused by Ca^{2+} oscillations resulting from spontaneous Ca^{2+} induced Ca^{2+} release from sarcoplasmic reticulum of the type previously described in isolated cardiac cells (10). Figure 2 compares the dependence of these cellular Ca^{2+} oscillations on extracellular $[Ca^{2+}]$, $([Ca^{2+}]_e)$, in isolated stretched rat and cat ventricular muscle stimulated at 2 min^{-1} at 29°C. Note that SLIF measured in the interstimulus interval at this slow rate of stimulation occur in

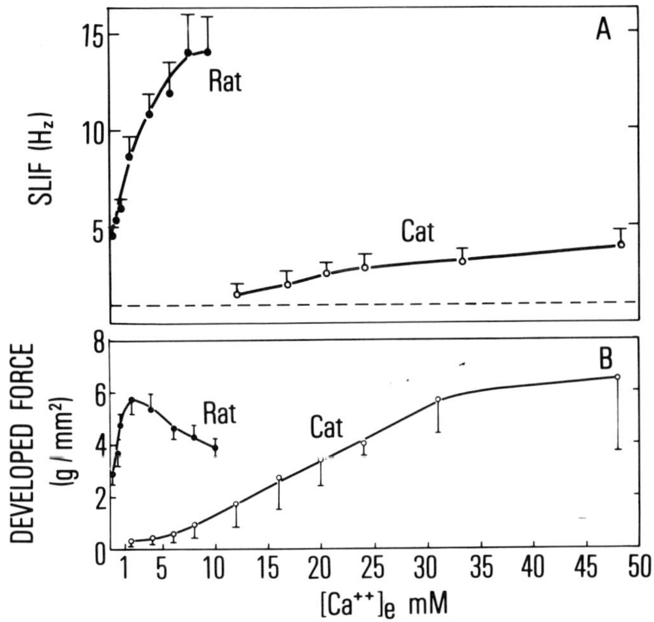

FIGURE 2. The effect of $[Ca^{2+}]_e$ on scattered light intensity fluctuations, (SLIF), in a rat and cat papillary muscle measured during the interstimulus interval during stimulation at 2 min^{-1} (A) and twitch force in response to the stimulus (B). Redrawn from Lakatta and Lappe (5).

rat myocardium at $[Ca^{2+}]_e$ as low as 0.25 mM but do not become detectable in cat muscle until $[Ca^{2+}]_e$ approaches 10 mM. Thus, at $[Ca^{2+}]_e$ usually employed in studies of excitation-contraction coupling (1-2 mM) it might be inferred the extent of cell Ca^{2+} loading in rat myocardium is high relative to the cat. This may account for the previous observations that the $[Ca^{2+}]_e$ dependence of force of contraction elicited by an externally applied depolarization, i.e. an action potential, under the conditions noted above, plateaus in rat myocardium at $[Ca^{2+}]_e$ of approximately 2.5-3 mM (11) as illustrated in Figure 2B. When $[Ca^{2+}]_e$ is increased further, more cell Ca^{2+} loading, manifest as a further increase in SLIF frequency, causes no change or a decline in the force of contraction. Excessive Ca^{2+} loading may account in part for the negative inotropic aspect of activation, NIAA (12).

At a given $[Ca^{2+}]_e$ cell Ca^{2+} loading in some species can be enhanced transiently by increasing the frequency of stimulation and this is reflected in a transient increase in SLIF measured post stimulation (5). Following a period of stimulation twitch force can exhibit persistent rest potentiation, or decay, depending on the level to which cell Ca^{2+} decays with time during the rest period. This can be monitored by SLIF measurements (Figure 3). In rat muscle, the rest potentiation and SLIF

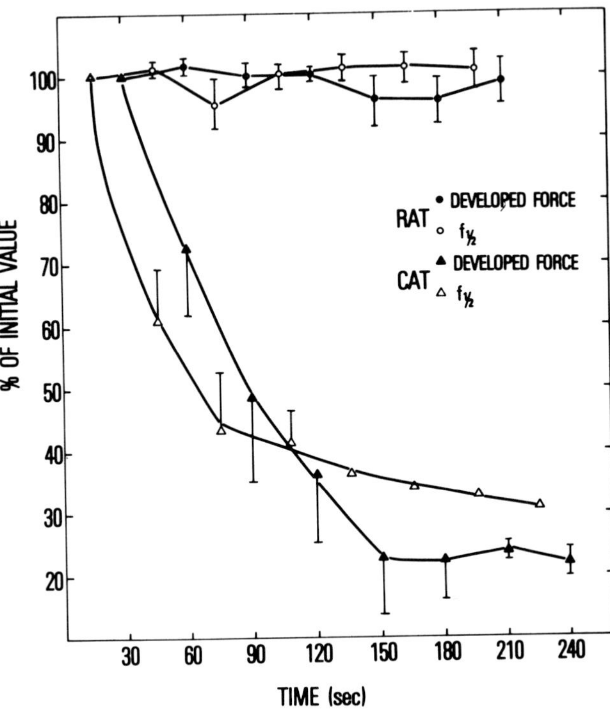

FIGURE 3. The decay of SLIF, $(f_{½})$, and twitch force in a tes beat at various times following stimulation in rat (n=4) and cat papillary muscles (n=4). All data have been normalized to th value measured in the initial time period; for twitch force this was 30 seconds after train of stimulation and for $f_{½}$ this was the average value measured from 5-29 seconds following the last stimulation in the train at 60 min^{-1} $[Ca^{2+}]_e$ was 4 mM and temperature was 29°C. Twitch force at 30 seconds was 9.5+3.0 g/mm^2 in cat and 12.1 +4.2 g/mm^2 in rat muscles. $F_{½}$ averaged over the period of 5-29 msec following the last stimulus in the train averaged 4 and 10 Hz in cat and rat muscles respectively. Redrawn from Lakatta and Lappe (5). It is noteworthy that in more recent studies in rat muscles, measurements made by time gating during the initial 30 second period following stimulation indicate that both $f_{½}$ and twitch force increase with time during this interval to achieve the steady levels noted above (13).

persist even in low $[Ca^{2+}]_e$ whereas in cat and rat muscle, a decline in cell Ca^{2+} loading results in rest decay of both SLIF and twitch force (5,13). These considerations and the results of other studies as well (14-17) indicate that the behavior of cardiac muscle depends on the extent of cell Ca^{2+} loading. This suggests that the same basic mechanisms that regulate excitation

-contraction coupling in other species might be present in the rat, albeit, set at a different level because of the difference in cell Ca^{2+} loading in a given experimental milieu.

An intimate relationship between the extent and duration of depolarization and the extent and duration of force during a contraction has been demonstrated to occur in many species (18). To examine in the rat the excitation-contraction mechanisms which have been studied extensively in other species, $[Ca^{2+}]_e$ must first be reduced in order to achieve a level of cell Ca^{2+} loading that is more comparable to that present in other species. When this is done some of the previous confusion regarding species differences in intrinsic mechanisms of excitation-contraction

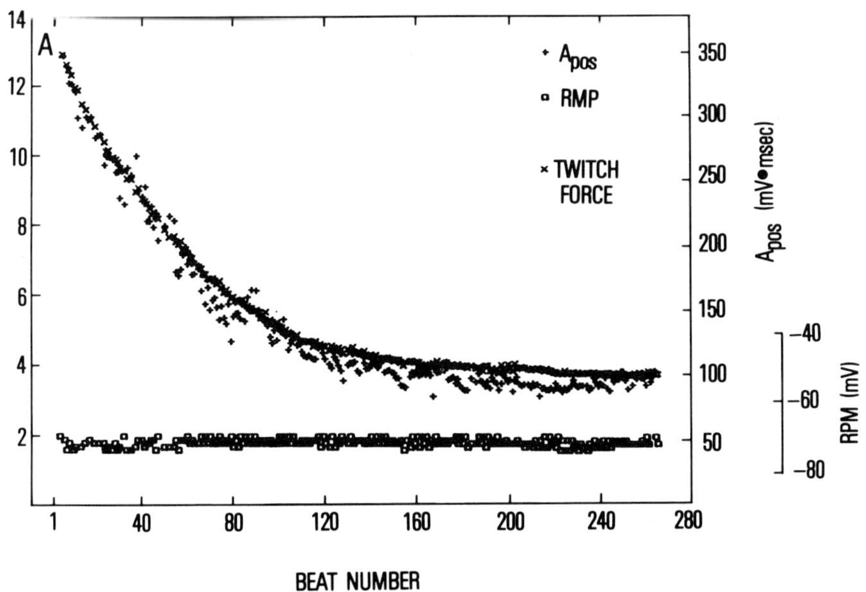

FIGURE 4. Transmembrane action potential area above zero, (A_{pos}), resting membrane potential, (RMP), and twitch force in a rat right ventricular papillary muscle in response to a reduction in $[Ca^{2+}]_e$ from 2.5 to 0.375 mM. Temperature was 29°C and the preparation was stimulated at 24 min^{-1}. Muscle cross-sectional area was 0.32 mm^2. From Wei et. al. (20).

mechanisms abates. For example, as illustrated in Figures 4 and 5 the relationship between changes in the extent and duration of

depolarization and changes in contractile force demonstrated in
other species (19) also can be demonstrated to occur in rat
myocardium (20,21).

In Figure 4 note that when $[Ca^{2+}]_e$ is lowered, i.e. over that
range where developed force declines from its maximal level, the
transient in the action potential area above zero is virtually
identical to transient in developed force.

In Figure 5, it is shown that the change in steady state action potential duration averaged from several cells among several
muscles in response to incremental β-adrenergic stimulation parallels the increment in contractile force in those muscles (20).

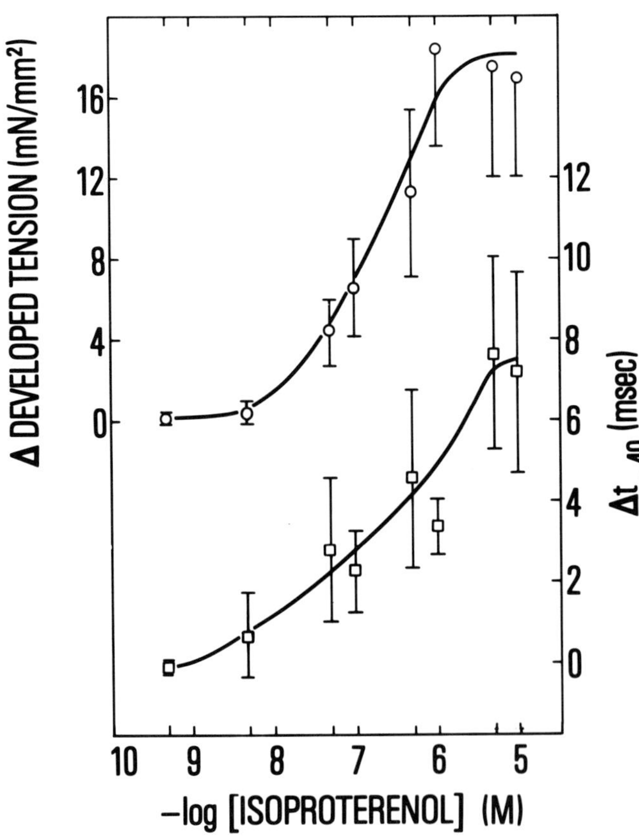

FIGURE 5. Average dose response (n=8) of the tension developed in the twitch and the transmembrane action potential depolarization time above −40 mV, (T_{40}), to isoproterenol in right ventricular
rat papillary muscles, stimulated at 24 min^{-1} at 29°C in $[Ca^{2+}]_e$ of 0.375 mM.
Cross-sectional area averaged 0.35+0.05 mm^2; before isoproterenol developed
tension, (DT), was 14.8+3.4 mN/mm^2 and T_{40} was 24.4+1.57 msec. The response
in DT was highly correlated to that in T_{40} (r = .86, regression analysis
of the means). From Wei et. al. (21).

From Figures 4 and 5, it might be argued that events that
occur during depolarization of the cell membrane modulate con-

traction in rat muscle as in other species, even though the total duration of the rat transmembrane potential relative to contraction is shorter than that in other species.

Transmembrane action potential, (TAP), measurements in low and high $[Ca^{2+}]_e$ have recently been measured in isolated isometrically contracting muscles from adult and senescent rats (20). The average TAP parameters measured at L_{max}, at 24 min^{-1} at 29°C in $[Ca^{2+}]_e$ of 0.375 and 2.5 mM are listed in Table 1. Note that while resting membrane potential, (RMP), was not affected by age, the extent and duration of depolarization, i.e. amplitude, (AMP), overshoot, (OS), area positive, (A_{pos}), and times to 75%, (T_{75}), and 90%, (T_{90}), repolarization, were greater in senescent than in adult muscle in both $[Ca^{2+}]_e$. Note also that an increase in

Table 1. The Effect of Age and $[Ca^{2+}]_e$ on TAP Parameters

| Parameter | $[Ca^{2+}]_e$ = 0.375 mM | | $[Ca^{2+}]_e$ = 2.5 mM | |
	6-8 mo	24-26 mo	6-8 mo	24-26 mo
N	(17)	(15)	(17)	(15)
RMP (mV)	−73.66+0.99	−70.51+0.91	−72.05+1.21	−70.53+0.81
Amp (mV)	81.50+2.08	84.93+1.86	89.75+1.45	96.57+1.86*
OS (mV)	9.12+1.50	13.83+1.68	18.61+1.63	26.99+1.63*
A_{pos} (mV.msec)	27.41+5.07	86.33+21.20**	87.26+12.47	219.50+30.90*
T_{75} (msec)	40.36+1.52	70.07+5.84*	31.43+1.52	62.23+5.45*
T_{90} (msec)	62.28+2.39	104.07+8.07**	67.39+4.21	128.71+10.55*

*P<0.001, **P<0.05 versus 6-8 mo

$[Ca^{2+}]_e$ caused a greater relative change in overshoot and the early part of TAP in the senescent versus adult muscles and that while on the average, T_{75} and T_{90} decreased with an increase in $[Ca^{2+}]_e$ in the younger adult muscles, T_{75} was unchanged and T_{90} increased in senescent muscles. Examples of the TAP in muscles from each age group are illustrated in Figure 6.

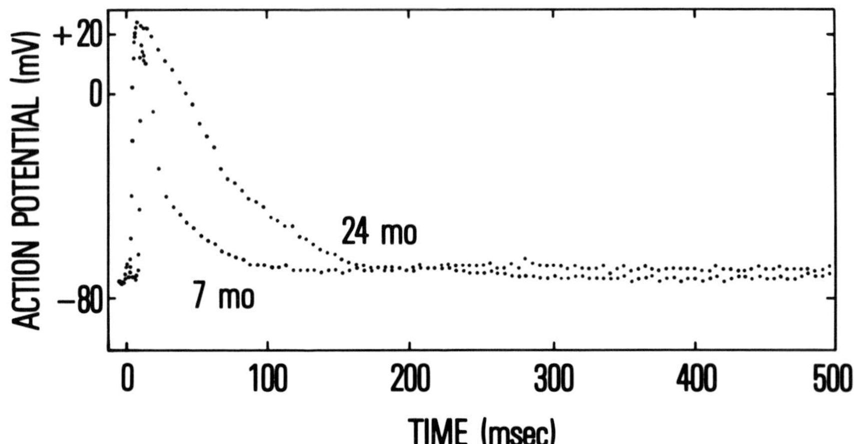

FIGURE 6. Computer (digital) resynthesizations of a typical action potential in isometrically contracting right ventricular muscles from adult (7 mo) and senescent (24 mo) rats. $[Ca^{2+}]_e$ was 2.5 mM and other conditions were as in Table 1. From Wei et. al. (20).

A typical contraction in muscles from each age group is illustrated in Figure 7.

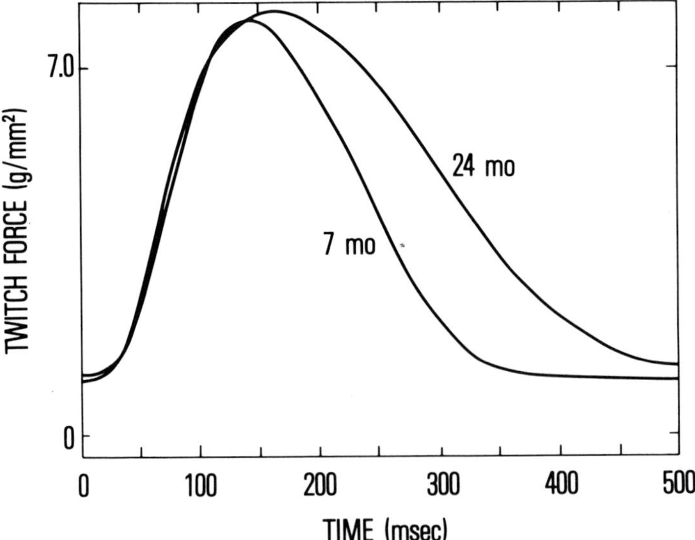

FIGURE 7. A typical isometric (auxotonic) contraction in 7 and 24 mo muscles measured simultaneously with TAP in Figure 6.

The isometric contraction force and duration parameters measured simultaneously with the action potential in both low and high $[Ca^{2+}]_e$ in the above experiments are listed in Table 2.

Table 2. The Effect of Age and $[Ca^{2+}]_e$ on Contractile Parameters

Parameter	$[Ca^{2+}]_e = 0.375$ mM		$[Ca^{2+}]_e = 2.5$ mM	
	6-8 mo	24-26 mo	6-8 mo	24-26 mo
N	(17)	(15)	(17)	(15)
RT (g/mm^2)	1.09+0.15	1.21+0.56	1.14+0.16	1.18+0.10
DT (g/mm^2)	2.14+0.28	2.71+0.47	5.72+0.69	7.14+1.01
dT/dt ($g/mm^2/sec$)	26.61+3.7	26.73+4.26	61.53+9.00	78.68+12.89
TPT (msec)	142.6+3.04	166.1+6.61*	148.5+3.37	164.5+2.19**
RT½ (msec)	92.7+3.68	115.9+6.54***	118.1+6.35	174.1+0.18*
CD (msec)	235.3+6.31	285.9+13.12*	266.6+9.37	339.1+11.1*

*P<.001, **P<.01, ***P<.05 versus 6-8 mo

While neither resting tension, (RT), peak developed tension, (DT), or its maximum derivative, (dT/dt), were altered with age in either $[Ca^{2+}]_e$, contraction duration indices, i.e. both time to peak tension, (TPT), and half relaxation time, (RT½), and their sum, (CD), were increased in senescent versus adult muscles in both $[Ca^{2+}]_e$. These results in right ventricular muscle are similar to those in left ventricular muscles in which both TPT and RT½, and time to peak stiffness and half relaxation of stiffness were observed to be prolonged (1,22). Note also in Table 2 that RT½ increased more in senescent than in adult muscles when $[Ca^{2+}]_e$ was increased.

When the change in contraction duration parameters and TAP repolarization parameters in response to an increase in $[Ca^{2+}]_e$ were compared in linear regression analysis, rather modest but significant correlations were observed. Figure 8 illustrates the relationship between the change in T_{75} and RT½. Note that the

less the shortening or the greater the prolongation of T_{75}, the
greater the prolongation in RT½. When comparisons were made

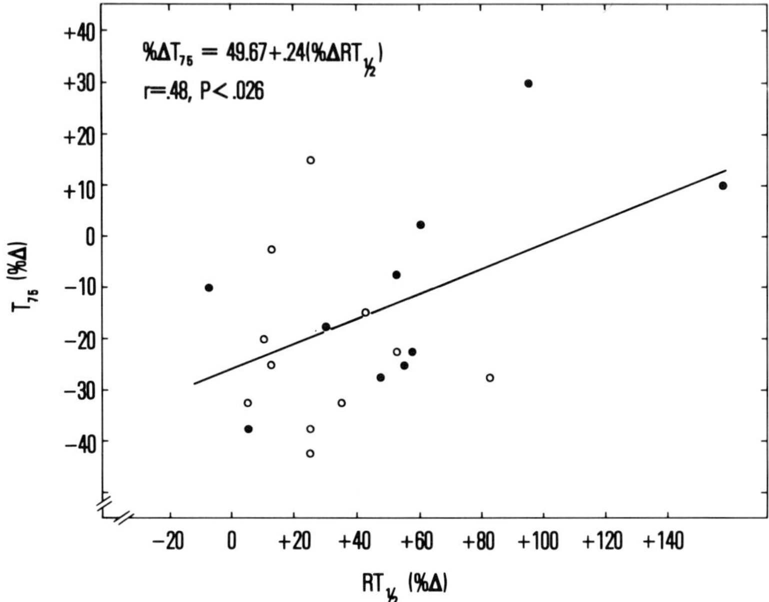

FIGURE 8. The relative change in steady state TAP time to 75%
repolarization, (T_{75}), versus that in steady state time for 50%
dissipation of peak twitch force, (RT½), in adult, 0, and senescent, ●, muscles when $[Ca^{2+}]_e$ was increased from 0.375 to 2.5 mM.
From Wei et. al. (20).

within each age group, only the senescent muscles exhibited significant correlations between TAP repolarization and contraction
duration indices (Table 3). Similarly only in the senescent muscles was the change in TAP duration with an increase in $[Ca^{2+}]_e$
correlated to the change in twitch force (Table 4). The prolonged excitation-contraction cycle in senescent hearts noted above
and that which also has been recently observed in high $[Ca^{2+}]_e$ in
an additional rat strain (23) and in guinea pig ventricular myocardium over a wide range of stimulation frequencies (24) when
senescent and maturational preparations were compared, may in
part at least account for the previous observations that senes-

cent muscles failed to demonstrate a contraction when the coupling interval between stimuli was progressively shortened to < 120 msec, while most adult muscle continued to do so (25).

Table 3. Correlation Coefficients, (r), and Significance, (p), for the Linear Regressions of the Relative Changes in TAP and Contraction Duration Indices in Response to an Increase in $[Ca^{2+}]_e$ from 0.375 to 2.5 mM

		Adult (6-8 mo)		Senescent (24-26 mo)		Adult + Senescent	
		r	p	r	p	r	p
T_{75}	versus						
	TPT	.24	.47*	.61	.04	.33	.12
	RT	.07	.82*	.65	.04	.48	.03
	CD	.06	.87*	.67	.03	.47	.03
T_{90}	versus						
	TPT	.43	.13*	.68	.02	.46	.02
	RT	.20	.40*	.74	.01	.67	.001
	CD	.30	.30*	.78.	.005	.67	.001

*Not significant

Table 4. Correlation Coefficients, (r), and Significance, (p), for the Linear Regression of the Relative Changes in T_{75} and T_{90} and DT and dT/dt in Response to an Increase in $[Ca^{2+}]_e$ from 0.375 to 2.5 mM

		Adult (6-8 mo)		Senescent (24-26 mo)		Adult + Senescent	
		r	p	r	p	r	p
T_{75}	versus						
	DT	.25	.41*	.73	.01	.57	.004
	dT/dt	.30	.34*	.72	.01	.60	.003
T_{90}	versus						
	DT	.44	.10*	.92	.0001	.81	.001
	dT/dt	.30	.26*	.90	.001	.76	.0001

*Not significant

The transient increase in myoplasmic $[Ca^{2+}]$ resulting from excitation has yet to be measured in adult and senescent muscles. However, the observations that peak twitch force is not altered during adult aging over a wide range of $[Ca^{2+}]_e$ (Figure 9A), coupled with the demonstration that the myofibrillar force pCA relation over the entire range of Ca^{2+} activation is not age-re-

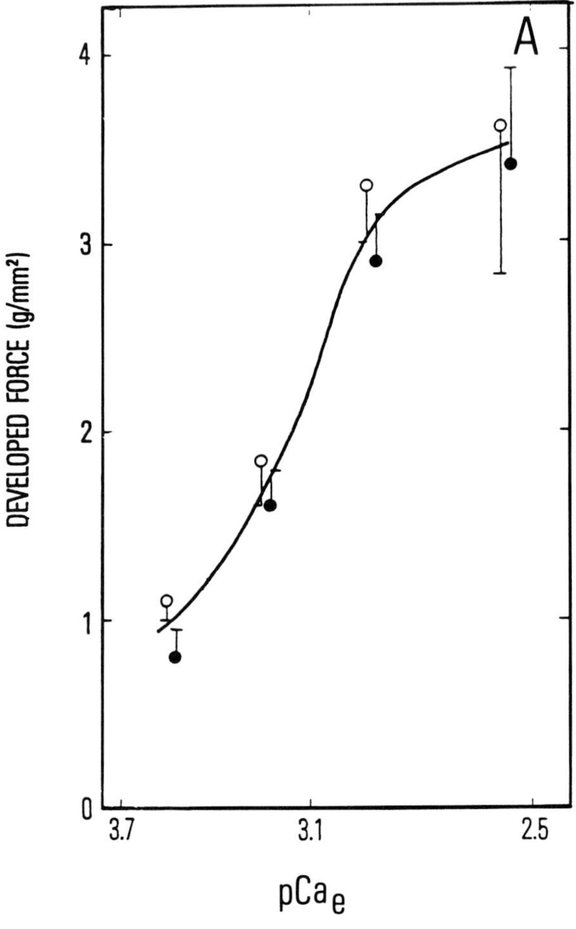

FIGURE 9A. Effect of age and perfusate $[Ca^{2+}]$ on isometric force development in trabeculae carneae isolated from adult (6-12 mo, ●) and senescent (25 mo, O) rat hearts. Muscles were stimulated via plate electrodes at a rate of 24 min^{-1} at 29 °C at the length at which force development was maximal. From Lakatta and Yin (1).

lated (Figure 9B and C) suggest that the peak myoplasmic $[Ca^{2+}]$ achieved following excitation is not age-related.

A diminution in Ca^{2+} accumulation rate has been observed in sarcoplasmic reticulum isolated from senescent versus adult (27) or maturational (28) myocardium (Figure 10). This would tend to prolong the $[Ca^{2+}]_e$ transient following excitation in senescent heart in a given contraction and could have a role in prolonging the twitch.

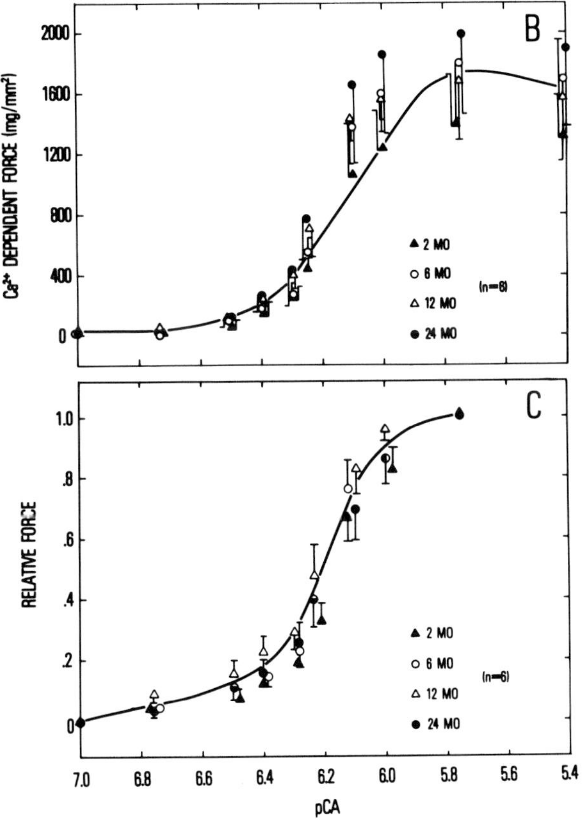

FIGURE 9B. The effect of pCa on force developed in Triton "skinned" papillary muscles from animals of varying age. Length was L_{max} and the Ca^{2+} independent force (pCa <7.0) has been subtracted.

FIGURE 9C. The data in Panel B have been normalized to the maximal value in each preparation in Panel A. From Bhatnagar et. al. (26).

In senescent heart compared to that in a younger adult a reduced Ca^{2+} sequestration rate might result in less total Ca^{2+} re-uptake by sarcoplasmic reticulum in a given beat, resulting in more Ca^{2+} loss from the cell across the sarcolemma via Na-Ca exchange or an ATP dependent pump prior to the next contraction. Indeed, the rate of Ca^{2+} transport in sarcolemmal vesicles prepared from senescent versus those from maturational hearts has been observed to be enhanced (28). Thus, while the considerations noted above suggest that the peak myoplasmic $[Ca^{2+}]$ following excitation might not be altered with adult age, in the senescent heart, the relative contribution from sarcoplasmic reticulum release may be less, and that from transsarcolemmal influx may be greater, as evidenced possibly by the greater TAP

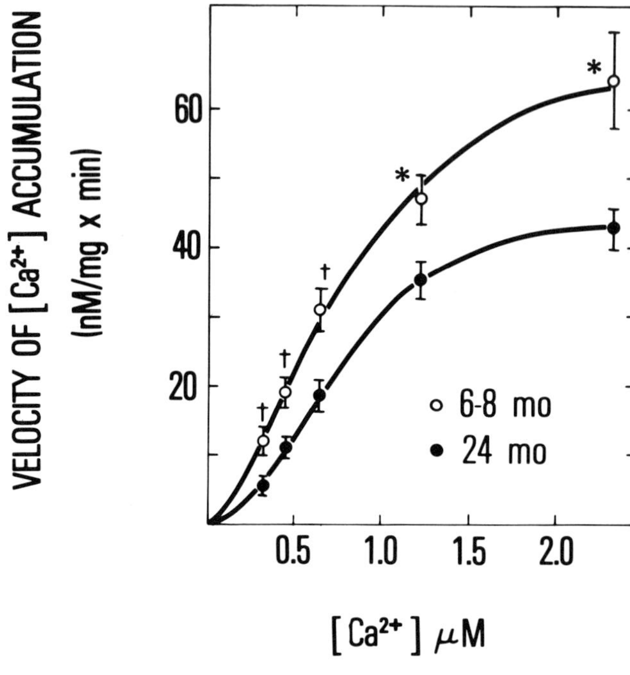

FIGURE 10. Effect of age on velocity of Ca^{2+} accumulation in microsomes isolated from adult (6 mo, 0) and senescent (24 mo, ●) hearts. All measurements were made at 25°C and are steady state rates measured over the initial 3-min reaction period in the presence of 1 mM oxalate. An age-related differential contamination of preparation by mitochondria was excluded by determining that succinate dehydrogenase activity in both mitochondria and microsomal preparations was not different in the 2 age groups. In addition, oligomycin and FCCP had no effect on Ca^{2+} accumulation under the experimental conditions used. Redrawn from Froehlich et. al. (27).

overshoot and duration in senescent muscles. A reduction in Ca^{2+} release by sarcoplasmic reticulum could permit a greater influx of Ca^{2+} with the depolarization that initiates the ensuing contraction since transsarcolemmal Na-Ca exchange or the slow Ca^{2+} channel resulting in Ca^{2+} influx would be subject to less Ca^{2+} inhibition (29). Thus, a diminished sarcoplasmic reticulum Ca^{2+} resequestration rate and uptake could not only account for prolonged relaxation but may prolong TAP by "allowing" more Ca^{2+} to flux into the cell via the slow inward current. (With sarcolemmal depolarization greater influx of Ca^{2+} via Na-Ca exchange would not be expected to prolong the TAP since this produces an outward current and would shorten the TAP (29)). This scheme provides an explanation for prolongation of both contraction and TAP in the senescent heart and the relationship observed between the two (Table 3). Stated in other words, a reduced rate of sarcoplasmic reticulum Ca^{2+} uptake and less sequestration during a given contractile cycle may result in less sarcoplasmic reticulum Ca^{2+} release in the subsequent contraction. While the peak myoplasmic $[Ca^{2+}]$ following excitation may not be age-related, a greater contribution could be made by transsarcolemmal influx in the senescent heart versus the adult heart and this might explain the relationship between TAP prolongation and increase twitch force in the senescent muscles (Table 4).

Alternatively, considering Ca^{2+} induced Ca^{2+} release as a mechanism to release Ca^{2+} from the sarcoplasmic reticulum, a greater slow inward current may be a more effective trigger for Ca^{2+} release from the sarcoplasmic reticulum and might elicit equal Ca^{2+} release in senescent and adult even with less Ca^{2+} preloading in senescent cell. Preliminary results suggest that Ca^{2+} release from sarcoplasmic reticulum in senescent cells requires a greater Ca^{2+} trigger than that in maturational cells (30). This particular scheme would require an _a priori_ increase in slow inward current or another Ca^{2+} trigger source in the senescent heart to account for the greater extent and duration of sarcolemmal depolarization and could also account for the observed relationship between the Ca^{2+} dependent changes in TAP and twitch force (Table 4). In this scheme prolonged sarcolemmal depolarization rather than a diminished sarcoplasmic reticulum Ca^{2+} sequestration rate, would be the primary mechanism to prolong the TAP and contraction duration parameters (Table 3, Figure 8).

The possible currents that may cause prolongation of TAP in the senescent heart and their likelihood of directly causing changes in the twitch are listed in Table 5. It might also be argued that K^{+} outward currents account for the prolonged TAP. This cannot per se account for either of the relationships observed in Figure 8 and Table 3 or Table 4. Measurements of the ionic currents that mediate the prolonged TAP in the senescent heart would help discriminate among these alternative hypotheses. Additionally, direct measurement of the peak and time course of the myoplasmic $[Ca^{2+}]$ transient elicited by excitation are required for more definitve modeling of how the specific age-related changes in excitation-contraction parameters interact to modify the cardiac contraction. The effect of physical conditioning

Table 5.

Possible Cause of Prolonged TAP in Senescent Ventricular Myocardium	Can Directly Explain TAP vs Twitch Duration Correlations in Senescent Muscles	Can Explain TAP vs Twitch Force Correlations in Senescent Muscles
1. $\downarrow$ Outward K Currents	–	–
2. Δ Na-Ca Exchange		
a. < Ca^{2+} Inward when E_m is more positive than E_R	–	–
b. > Ca^{2+} Outward when E_m is less positive than E_R	+	–
3. $\uparrow$ Slow Inward Current	+	+
4. $\uparrow$ T.I. Current	?	?
5. Combinations of above	+	+

on TAP may help differentiate among the hypotheses proposed,
since prolonged contraction in the senescent myocardium is
abolished following modest regular physical activity on a chronic
basis (22). Similarly, further elucidation of the mechanisms for
the diminished beta-adrenergic modulation of contactility in the
senescent heart (31-33) may also be enlightening in this regard.

I wish to thank Dr. Clive Orchard for a thoughtful reading of the
manuscript.

References

1. Lakatta EG, Yin FCP: Myocardial aging: functional alterations and related cellular mechanisms. Am J Physiol (242):
   H927-H941, 1982.
2. Lakatta EG: Heart and Circulation. In Finch CE, Schneider
   EL (eds) Handbook of the Biology of Aging. Van Nostrand
   Reinhold (2nd edition), 1984, in press.
3. Lakatta EG: Health, disease, and cardiovascular aging. Proc
   Natl Acad Sci, 1984, in press.
4. Allen DG, Kurihara S: Calcium transients in mammalian ventricular muscle. Eur Heart J (1): Suppl A, 15-15, 1981.
5. Lakatta EG, Lappe DL: Diastolic scattered light fluctuation,
   resting force, and twitch force in mammalian cardiac muscle.
   J Physiol (315): 369-394, 1981.
6. Kort AA, Lakatta EG: Light scattering identifies diastolic
   myoplasmic Ca^{2+} oscillations in diverse mammalian cardiac
   tissues. Circulation (64): IV-162, 1981.
7. Stern MD, Kort AA, Bhatnagar, GM, Lakatta EG: Scattered
   light intensity fluctuations in diastolic rat cardiac muscle
   caused by spontaneous Ca^{++}-dependent cellular mechanical oscillations. J Gen Physiol (82): 119-153, 1983.

8. Wier WG, Kort AA, Stern MD, Lakatta EG, Marban E: Cellular calcium fluctuations in mammalian heart: direct evidence from noise analysis of aequorin signals in Purkinje fibers. Proc Natl Acad Sci (80): 7367-7371, 1983.

9. Orchard CH, Eisner DA, Allen DG: Oscillations of intracellular Ca^{2+} in mammalian cardiac muscle. Nature (304): 735-738, 1983.

10. Fabiato A, Fabiato F: Contraction induced by a calcium-triggered release of calcium from the sarcoplasmic reticulum of single skinned cardiac cells. J Physiol (249) 469-495, 1975.

11. Lakattà EG: Excitation-contraction. In: Weisfeldt ML (ed) Aging, Volume 12, The Aging Heart: Its Function and Response to Stress. Raven Press, New York, 1980, pp 77-100.

12. Koch-Weser J, Blinks JR: The influence of the interval between beats on myocardial contractility. Pharmac Res (15): 601-652, 1963.

13. Kort AA, Lakatta EG: Rest potentiation in cardiac muscle is associated with cell Ca^{2+} oscillations. Circulation (68): III-166, 1983.

14. Forester GV, Mainwood GW: Interval dependent inotropic effects in the rat myocardium and the effect of calcium. Pflugers Arch (352): 289-296, 1974.

15. Leoty C: Membrane currents and activation of contraction in rat ventricular fibres. J Physiol (239): 237-249, 1974.

16. Meijler FL: Staircase, rest contractions, and potentiation in the isolated rat heart. Am J Physiol (202): 636-640, 1962.

17. Henderson AH, Brutsaert DL, Parmley WW, Sonnenblick EH: Myocardial mechanics in papillary muscles of the rat and cat. Am J Physiol (217): 1273-1279, 1969.

18. Morad M, Goldman Y: Excitation-contraction coupling in heart muscle: membrane control of development of tension. Prog Biophys Mol Biol (27): 257-313, 1973.

19. Reuter H: Exchange of calcium ions in the mammalian myocardium. Mechanisms and physiological significance. Circ Res (34): 599-605, 1974.

20. Wei JY, Spurgeon HA, Lakatta EG: Excitation-contraction in rat myocardium: alterations with adult aging. Am J Physiol, 1984, in press'.

21. Wei JY, Spurgeon HA, Lakatta EG: Electromechanical responsiveness of hyperthyroid cardiac muscle to β-adrenergic stimulation. Am J Physiol (243): E114-E122, 1982.

22. Spurgeon HA, Steinbach MF, Lakatta EG: Chronic exercise prevents characteristic age-related changes in rat cardiac contraction. Am J Physiol (244): H513-H518, 1983.

23. Capasso JM, Malhotra A, Remily RM, Scheuer J, Sonnenblich EH: Effect of age on mechanical and electrical performance of rat myocardium. Am J Physiol (245): H72-H81, 1983.

24. Rumberger E, Timmermann J: Age-changes of the force-frequency-relationship and the duration of action potential isolated papillary muscles of guinea pig. Eur J Appl Physiol (34): 277-284, 1976.

25. Lakatta EG, Gerstenblith G, Angell CS: Prolonged contraction duration in aged myocardium. J Clin Invest (55): 61-68, 1975.

26. Bhatnagar GM, Walford GD, Beard ES, Humphries SH, Lakatta EG:

ATPase activity and force production in myofibrils and twitch characteristics in intact muscle from neonatal, adult and senescent rat myocardium. J Mol Cell Cardiol, 1984, in press.

27. Froehlich JP, Lakatta EG, Beard E, Spurgeon HA, Weisfeldt ML, Gerstenblith G: Studies of sarcoplasmic reticulum function and contraction duration in young adult and aged rat myocardium. J Mol Cell Cardiol (10): 427-438, 1978.
28. Narayanan N: Differential alterations in ATP-supported calcium transport activities of sarcoplasmic reticulum and sarcolemma of aging myocardium. Biochim Biophys Acta (678): 442-459, 1981.
29. Mullins LJ: Ion Transport in Heart. Raven Press, New York, 1981, p 614.
30. Fabiato A: Calcium release in skinned cardiac cells: variations with species, tissues, and development. Fed Proc (41): 2238-2244, 1982.
31. Lakatta EG, Gerstenblith G, Angell CS, Shock NW, Weisfeldt ML: Diminished inotropic response of age myocardium to catecholamines. Circ Res (36): 262-269, 1975.
32. Guarnieri T, Filburn CR, Zitnik G, Roth GS, Lakatta EG: Contractile and biochemical correlates of β-adrenergic stimulation of the aged heart. Am J Physiol (239): H501-H508, 1980.
33. Filburn CR and Lakatta EG: Age altered β-adrenergic modulation of cardiac cell function. In: Johnson J Jr (ed) Aging and Cell Structure, Volume 2. Plenum Press, New York, 1984, in press.